Children with Handicaps

SECOND EDITION

Children
with
Handicaps

A Medical Primer

by

Mark L. Batshaw, M.D.
Associate Professor
The Johns Hopkins University
 School of Medicine, and
Developmental Pediatrician
The Kennedy Institute for Handicapped Children
Baltimore

and

Yvonne M. Perret, M.S.W.
Social Worker
Walter P. Carter Center
Baltimore

drawings by Elaine Kasmer

· P A U L · H ·
BROOKES
PUBLISHING CO.

Baltimore • London

Paul H. Brookes Publishing Co.
Post Office Box 10624
Baltimore, Maryland 21285-0624

First printing, August, 1986.
Second printing, May, 1987.
Third printing, December, 1988

Typeset by Brushwood Graphics Studio, Baltimore, Maryland.
Manufactured in the United States of America by
The Maple Press Co., York, Pennsylvania.

Library of Congress Cataloging-in-Publication Data

Batshaw, Mark L., 1945–
    Children with handicaps.
    Includes bibliographies and index.
    1. Handicapped children—Care and treatment.   2. Developmentally
disabled children—Care and treatment.   3. Child development deviations.   I. Perret, Yvonne M., 1946—   .   II. Title.
[DNLM: 1. Birth Injuries.   2. Child Development Disorders.   3. Handicapped.   4. Rehabilitation—in infancy & childhood. WS 368 B334c]
RJ138.B37   1986   618.92   86-4233
ISBN 0-933716-64-8

Contents

CONTENTS / ix

Automatic Movement Reactions
Walking and Movement
Disabilities Associated with Cerebral Palsy
Treatment
Case Histories of Children with Cerebral Palsy
Prognosis
Summary

Chapter 22 **Epilepsy**..325
What Is a Seizure?
Types of Seizures
Diagnosis of Epilepsy
Treatment of Epilepsy
What to Do in the Event of a Seizure
Case Histories of Children with Epilepsy
Prognosis
Summary

Chapter 23 **Caring and Coping: The Family of a Child with
Handicaps**..351
The Life Cycle of the Family
Effects on Parents
Effects on the Child with a Disability
Effects on Siblings
Effects on Grandparents
Society and Community Reactions
Role of the Professional
Case Study
Summary

Chapter 24 **Some Ethical Dilemmas**............................365
Genetic Screening
Prenatal Diagnosis, Therapeutic Abortion, and Fetal
    Therapy
Withholding Treatment
Experimental Treatment of and Research on Children with
    Handicaps
Sterilization
Institutionalization
Education for Children with Handicaps
Summary

Chapter 25 **Public Benefits, Legal Services, and Estate Planning**.......381
by John J. Capowski
Public Benefits
Advocacy and Legal Assistance
Estate Planning
Summary

Preface

The first edition of *Children with Handicaps: A Medical Primer* was published in 1981. While writing that book, we felt it would be most helpful to those who work with these children—special educators, physical therapists, occupational therapists, speech and language pathologists, child life specialists, and social workers. What we learned was that these professionals did read the book, but so did many others. We were pleased to find that many parents found the book beneficial to them, and that it answered many questions they had about caring for their child and the possible causes for their child's disability. In addition, other professionals such as developmental disability lawyers and other health care workers used the book.

In this second edition, the purpose of the book remains unchanged—to answer the question, "Why this child?" As is true of the first edition, this version discusses what happened before, during, or after birth to cause a child to have a developmental disability. In all the chapters, we have tried to address a number of new issues as well as to respond to suggestions made by our readers. Because of the rapid change in information in this field, all the chapters have been rewritten, updated, and expanded.

Thus, in the first part of the book, the reader becomes acquainted with heredity. New sections provide updates on the fragile-X syndrome and the diagnostic techniques used to detect abnormalities before birth. The chapter on prenatal diagnosis now also covers a more recent diagnostic approach called chorionic villus biopsy. Chapters on fetal development and the birth process and neonatal and early childhood development bring the first part of the book to a close. The special problems faced by premature and small for gestational age infants are also discussed.

The next portion of the book contains an examination of the various organ systems in the body—how they work and what can go wrong. These include the digestive tract, the nervous system, bones, muscles, vision, and hearing. Nutritional requirements and the special feeding problems of children with handicaps receive particular attention. Also covered in this section are inborn errors of metabolism and a new chapter on dental care of children with handicaps.

Comprehensive descriptions of mental retardation; visual impairments; hearing, speech, and language problems; autism; attention deficit disorder and hyperactivity; learning disabilities; cerebral palsy; and epilepsy comprise the next section of the book. Case studies are included to illustrate these conditions.

The last portion of the book concentrates on the emotional and financial aspects of life with a child who has a disability, and raises some of the ethical dilemmas faced by professionals and parents in caring for such a child. A new chapter covers public benefits, legal services, and estate planning for children with handicaps. Finally, appendices include a glossary of medical terms; a description of various syndromes; a list of resources for children with handicaps, their families, and professionals; and instruction on life-saving techniques.

Many individuals from The Kennedy Institute for Handicapped Children and The Johns Hopkins University School of Medicine reviewed the manuscript and gave us advice. We would like to thank them. They are: Marilee Allen, Seth Canion, Lauren Cohen, John Freeman, Brad Friedrich, Robin Gallico, Jackie Krick, Judy Levy, Jay Moore, Fred Palmer, Michael Repka, Harry Shaw, Harvey Singer, George Thomas, Vernon Tolo, Patricia Vining, Renee Wachtel, and Lana Warren. We would also like to thank Bill Diehl of The Kennedy Institute for the photographs he provided for several illustrations. And, finally, we want to express our appreciation to Susan Cascio for her patience, diligence, and untiring work in helping us bring this manuscript to fruition.

For the Reader

Throughout this book, the terms that are defined in the glossary (Appendix A) are indicated in **bold type** the first time that they appear.

The reference lists at the end of each chapter contain more references than those actually cited in the text. We felt that these additional references might be useful for anyone interested in doing further reading on a particular topic.

The case histories that are included in this book are based on actual or synthesized cases. The names used in these cases are fictitious.

To the families of children with handicaps

Children
with
Handicaps

Chapter 1

Understanding
Your Chromosomes

Upon completion of this chapter, the reader will:
—know the components of the cell and their functions
—be familiar with the various stages of mitosis and meiosis
—understand the differences between mitosis and meiosis
—be able to explain nondisjunction, translocation, and deletion

A child is born, and the preceding 9 months have witnessed a marvelous process. So complex and numerous are the steps involved from the fertilization of an egg to the birth of an infant that the chances for errors in that process would seem limitless. The surprise, then, is not that so many children are born with birth defects, but that so few are. Tracing the path of human development, beginning with the fertilized egg, quickly points out the opportunities that exist for mistakes to occur.

As an introduction to the discussion in the chapters that follow, this chapter describes the human cell, explains what chromosomes are, reviews the processes of **mitosis** and **meiosis**, and provides some illustrations of the errors that can occur in these processes. As you progress through this book, bear in mind that the purpose here is to focus on the abnormalities that can occur in human development; most infants are never troubled by these handicapping conditions.

THE CELL

The cell is divided into two compartments: a central, enclosed core, the nucleus, and an outer, gelatinous area, the cytoplasm (Figure 1.1). The nucleus contains the chromosomes, structures that consist of the genetic code for our physical and biochemical traits. The cell can divide into daughter cells containing this same genetic information. The cytoplasm, under the direction of the nucleus, turns out products that release energy, get rid of wastes, and are needed for the growth of the organism. The nucleus, then, provides the blueprint for an individual's eventual development, and the cytoplasm provides the products needed to complete the task.

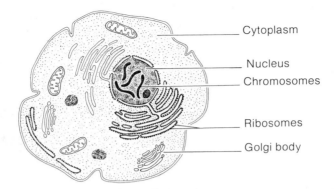

Figure 1.1.   An idealized cell. The chromosomes direct the creation of a product on the ribosome. The product is then packaged in the Golgi body and released from the cell.

CHROMOSOMES

Each organism has a fixed number of chromosomes. In humans, 46 chromosomes direct the cell's activities. Except for the **germ cells** (the egg and sperm), every cell contains 23 pairs of complementary chromosomes. In each pair, one chromosome comes from the mother, and one comes from the father, thus accounting for the total number of 46 chromosomes in each cell. This number is called the *diploid* number. The germ cells each contain 23 chromosomes, or half the diploid number; this number is termed the *haploid* number.

Except for the **sex chromosomes** (X and Y), the chromosomes in each pair resemble each other. The X and Y chromosomes look quite different from each other. The X chromosome is about twice as large as the Y and has a different shape (see Figure 1.3 on page 5). It is these chromosomes that determine the sex of the fetus. The remaining 22 pairs of chromosomes, called **autosomes**, define the other features of the individual.

Most types of cells divide, but not all cells divide at the same rate. Skin cells, for instance, divide rapidly and resurface the area of an abrasion in just a few days. On the other hand, the nerve cells in an adult brain do not appear to divide at all. It takes a sperm cell but a few hours to divide, while division of an egg takes years. The ability of cells to continue to divide is a major factor in the continued proper functioning of the organism. For example, the inability of nerve cells in adults to reproduce limits recovery after a stroke or other brain injury.

CELL DIVISION

The formation of a human being takes about 266 days. It is accomplished primarily through two kinds of cell division: mitosis and meiosis. There are two major differences between these kinds of cell division. In mitosis, or nonreductive division, two daughter cells are created from one parent cell, and each of the offspring cells contains 46 chromosomes. Meiosis, or reductive division, on the other hand, involves the formation of four daughter cells from one parent cell. (In the case of the egg, three of these daughter cells eventually disintegrate; only one daughter cell survives as a mature egg). Each of the offspring cells in meiosis contains 23 chromosomes. Although mitosis occurs in all cells, meiosis takes place only in the germ cells.

Mitosis

Mitosis occurs in four steps: *prophase, metaphase, anaphase,* and *telophase* (Figure 1.2). Most cells undergo mitosis throughout their lives. Between the periods of mitosis is a resting phase called *interphase*. During this phase the cell grows, and the chromosomes resemble a ball of loose yarn. During *prophase*, the cell division begins. The chromosomes thicken and shorten and begin to look like separate strands. In the next stage, *metaphase,* the chromosomes become double-stranded; each strand of the chromosome is a **chromatid**, and each chromatid contains the same genetic information as the chromosome. It is during this stage that one chromosome can be easily differentiated from another.

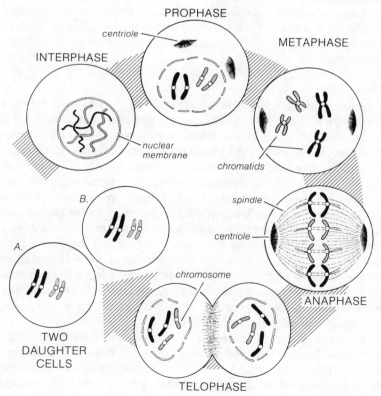

Figure 1.2.   Mitosis. This process produces two daughter cells, each containing a diploid number (46) of chromosomes.

If division is arrested at metaphase, the chromosomes appear under the microscope as large X-shaped bodies that can be counted and divided into groups according to size, shape, and **banding pattern**, a process called **karyotyping**. As an illustration, Figure 1.3 shows the karyotype of a child who has Down syndrome. Some of the child's white blood cells were obtained, and a chemical was added to start the cell division. Days later, another chemical was inserted to arrest the division in metaphase. The cell nucleus was then photographed under a microscope, and a print was made. The chromosomes were cut out, matched in pairs, and put into seven groups, A–G, according to size, shape, and banding pattern. In this case, the G group had an extra #21 chromosome as well as an X and a Y chromosome, the karyotype of a male who has Down syndrome.

In the next stage, *anaphase*, the chromatids line up in the center of the cell and become attached to tiny spindles. These spindles pull the chromatids toward the **centrioles**, or poles, in the two daughter cells (see Figure 1.2). Following mitosis, each daughter cell winds up with 46 chromosomes. If, for some reason, a pair of chromatids did not split during anaphase, one daughter cell would contain 47 chromosomes and one would have 45. If no split occurred in any of the pairs of chromatids, one daughter cell would have 92, and the other would have none. Often, when cells divide unequally, or undergo **nondisjunction**, they do not survive.

During *telophase,* the division is completed, and the two daughter cells separate from each other.

Meiosis

Since meiosis is a much more complicated process than mitosis, it is more often associated with abnormalities. Unlike mitosis, meiosis involves two cell divisions instead of one; each division has stages of prophase, metaphase, anaphase, and telophase. As already mentioned, chromosomes come in pairs. Thus, there are two #1 chromosomes, two #2 chromosomes, and so on. In prophase of the first meiotic division, the chromosomes thicken and shorten just as they do in mitosis. The same is true for the stage of metaphase, where each chromosome doubles and becomes two chromatids. It is in anaphase where a major difference between mitosis and meiosis exists. In mitosis, one of each of the doubled chromatids moves toward one daughter cell, and the other moves toward the second daughter cell. In anaphase of the first meiotic division, on the other hand, both chromatids of one #1 chromosome move toward one daughter cell, and both chromatids of the other #1 chromosome move toward the other daughter cell (Figure 1.4). At the end of the first meiotic division, each of the two daughter cells contains 23 double-stranded chromatids instead of 46 single-stranded chromosomes as in mitosis.

In the second meiotic division, the 23 double-stranded chromatids line up in the center of each daughter cell and undergo a mitotic division; that is, the doubled chromatids separate. Thus, the two daughter cells that formed after the first meiotic division split into two more cells; each of these cells contains 23 chromosomes. The end result is four daughter cells that have 23 chromosomes each. As stated earlier, meiosis occurs only in the germ cells. During fertilization, the 23 chromosomes from

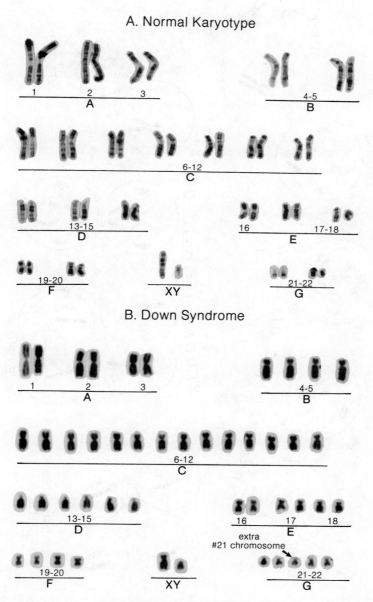

Figure 1.3. Illustrations of two chromosome patterns: A) a normal male, and B) a boy with Down syndrome. Note that the Down syndrome child has 47 chromosomes; the extra one is a #21. (Courtesy of Dr. George Thomas, Kennedy Institute for Handicapped Children, Baltimore.)

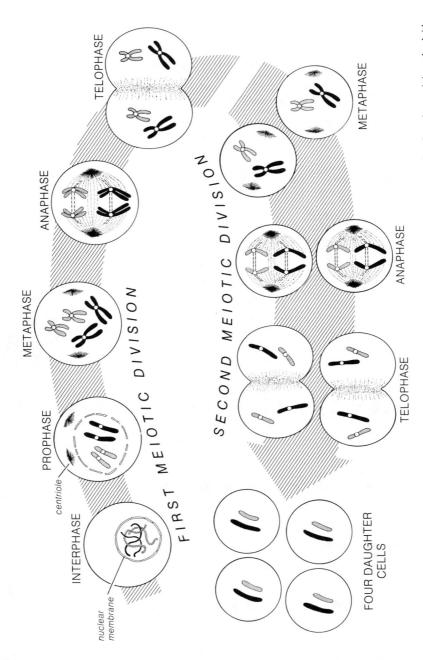

INTERPHASE

PROPHASE

METAPHASE

ANAPHASE

TELOPHASE

nuclear membrane

centriole

FIRST MEIOTIC DIVISION

SECOND MEIOTIC DIVISION

METAPHASE

ANAPHASE

TELOPHASE

FOUR DAUGHTER CELLS

Figure 1.4. Meiosis. This reductive division occurs only in the ovaries and the testes. Four daughter cells are produced, each containing a haploid number (23) of chromosomes.

each of the two germ cells, the sperm and the egg, combine. The resulting embryo emerges with the *diploid* number (46) of chromosomes.

WHAT CAN GO WRONG?

A number of events that subsequently affect a child's development can occur during cell division. One of these, *nondisjunction,* happens more often during meiosis than during mitosis. Nondisjunction can cause Down syndrome, as occurred in the case illustrated in Figure 1.3. (Another cause of Down syndrome, **translocation**, is discussed later in this chapter.) When nondisjunction occurs during the first meiotic division, both #21 chromosomes end up in one cell. Instead of both cells having 23 chromosomes, one cell has 24 chromosomes and the other has 22. This imbalance takes place far more often in the formation of an egg than in the formation of a sperm. The loss of a #21 chromosome makes it difficult for the egg containing 22 chromosomes to survive. However, the egg with 24 chromosomes can survive and, if a sperm containing 23 chromosomes then fertilizes it, the result is a child with 47 chromosomes who has Down syndrome, or trisomy 21—three #21 chromosomes (Smith & Wilson, 1973). Approximately 70% of individuals with Down syndrome acquire it as a result of nondisjunction of the egg and 20% from nondisjunction of the sperm (Manning & Goodman, 1981). The remaining 10% of the cases come from translocation.

The one disorder associated with survival despite the loss of a complete chromosome is **Turner's syndrome**. In this case, nondisjunction affects the X chromosome rather than one of the autosomes. The child is born with 45 instead of 46 chromosomes; she has a single X chromosome, but no second X or Y chromosome. All children with Turner's syndrome are female because the Y chromosome, responsible for the development of male sexual organs, is absent. These children are very short, have webbed necks, and have nonfunctional ovaries. Unlike children with Down syndrome, most of these children have normal intelligence. However, they do tend to have visual-perceptual problems that lead to learning disabilities.

The reason why a child with an X chromosome **deletion** can survive, whereas the deletion of an autosome would be fatal, is probably because females have two X chromosomes while males have only one. In effect, the male's chromosomal structure is similar to that of a female with Turner's syndrome except that the male has a Y chromosome and the Turner's syndrome female does not. At present, the Y chromosome is known to be responsible only for directing the development of male sexual organs.

Besides nondisjunction, other abnormalities in cell division can also lead to birth defects. Two examples are deletion and translocation. During mitosis and meiosis, the chromosomes are close together for extended periods of time. They may touch, stick to each other for a while, and then separate. When they separate, a segment of a chromosome may be pulled off and lost (deletion) or may attach itself to another chromosome (translocation). The **cri-du-chat** ("cat cry") **syndrome** is an example of a disorder resulting from a deletion. In this syndrome, a portion of a #5 chromosome is lost (Figure 1.5). The child looks unusual and has a high-pitched cry. These children also have severe retardation and resemble each other, just as children with Down syndrome share similar physical characteristics.

Translocation involves the transfer of a portion of one chromosome to a completely different chromosome (Figure 1.6). For example, a part of the #21 chromosome might attach itself to the #14 chromosome. If this occurs during meiosis, one cell will then have 23 chromosomes with one #21 and one #14/21 translocated chromosome. Fertilization of the egg or sperm containing the #14/21 translocated chromosome will result in a child with 46 chromosomes, including two #21 chromosomes and one #14/21 chromosome. This child, too, will have Down syndrome because of the partial trisomy 21 caused by the translocation.

With all these potential problems in cell division, one wonders why more children are not born with chromosomal abnormalities. The answer is that most fetuses with chromosomal abnormalities do not survive. Over 50% of the fetuses that are miscarried prior to 12 weeks gestation are found to have chromosomal abnormalities (Figure 1.7). As the fetus continues to develop, the frequency of both chromosomal abnormalities and spontaneous abortion, or miscarriage, decreases.

While the closeness of the chromosomes during meiosis may result in disorders, it also allows for the mutual transfer of some genetic information. This transfer, or

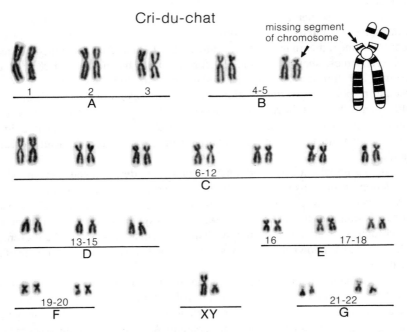

Figure 1.5. Karyotype of a child with severe retardation who has cri-du-chat ("cat cry") syndrome. This is an example of the effect of a partial chromosomal deletion. A complete deletion is usually fatal. (Courtesy of Dr. George Thomas, Kennedy Institute for Handicapped Children, Baltimore.)

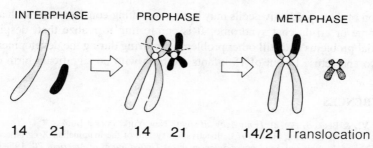

Figure 1.6. Translocation. During prophase of meiosis in a parent, there may be a transfer of a portion of one chromosome to another. In this figure, the long arm of #21 is translocated to chromosome #14, and the residual fragments are lost. The resulting translocated chromosome #14/21 places the parent at risk for having additional children with Down syndrome.

crossing over, is what enables us to be similar to but not exactly like our **siblings**. The only sibling relationship in which crossing over does not occur is in identical twins where division of the twins occurs after fertilization of the egg.

SUMMARY

Each human cell contains a full complement of genetic information entwined in 46 chromosomes. This genetic code not only determines our physical appearance and biochemical makeup, but it also is the legacy we pass on to our children. The unequal

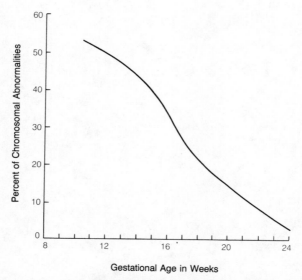

Figure 1.7. Incidence of chromosomal abnormalities among fetuses spontaneously aborted during the first two trimesters of pregnancy. (From Creasy, M.R., Crolla, J.A., & Alberman, E.D. [1976]. *Human Genetics, 31,* Figure 3, p. 188; reprinted by permission.)

division of the reproductive cells may have devastating consequences such as Down syndrome or cri-du-chat syndrome. It is comforting to realize that, despite these potential problems and still other problems occurring during the development of the embryo and fetus, 14 out of 15 infants are born with no significant birth defects.

REFERENCES

Apgar, V., & Beck, J. (1972). *Is my baby all right?* New York: Pocket Books.

Brown, S.W., & Chandra, H.S. (1973). Inactivation system of the mammalian X chromosome. *Proceedings of the National Academy of Sciences of the United States of America, 70,* 195–199.

Creasy, M.R., Crolla, J.A., & Alberman, E.D. (1976). A cytogenetic study of human spontaneous abortions using banding techniques. *Human Genetics, 31,* 177–196.

Emery, A.E.H. (1983). *Elements of medical genetics* (6th ed.). New York: Churchill Livingstone.

Erickson, J.D., & Bjerkedal, T.O. (1981). Down syndrome associated with father's age in Norway. *Journal of Medical Genetics, 18,* 22–28.

Fraser, F.C., & Nora, J.J. (1975). *Genetics of man.* Philadelphia: Lea & Febiger.

Gore, R. (1976). The awesome worlds within a cell. *National Geographic, 150,* 354–395.

Hook, E.B., & Porter, I.H. (1977). *Population cytogenetics.* New York: Academic Press.

Levitan, M., & Montagu, A. (1977). *Textbook of human genetics* (2nd ed.). New York: Oxford University Press.

Manning, C.H., & Goodman, H.D. (1981). Parental origin of chromosomes in Down's syndrome. *Human Genetics, 59,* 101–103.

Palmer, C.G., & Reichmann, A. (1976). Chromosomal and clinical findings in 110 females with Turner syndrome. *Human Genetics, 35,* 35–49.

Smith, C. (1974). Concordance in twins: Methods and interpretation. *American Journal of Human Genetics, 26,* 454–466.

Smith, D.W., & Wilson, A.C. (1973). *The child with Down's syndrome.* Philadelphia: W. B. Saunders.

Chapter 2

Heredity
A Toss of the Dice

Upon completion of this chapter, the reader will:

—know the differences and similarities between autosomal recessive, autosomal dominant, and sex-linked disorders

—be able to describe some of the major chromosomal abnormalities

—understand the ways in which environment and heredity contribute to the development of certain disorders

—be aware of the part genes play in some hereditary disorders

---

Whether or not we have brown or blue eyes is determined by genes carried on our parents' chromosomes. On the other hand, our height and weight are affected both by these genes and by our environment before and after birth. In a similar manner, genes and their interaction with environmental factors may lead to certain birth defects. **Phenylketonuria** and Tay-Sachs disease, for example, result from single-gene mutations within a chromosome, whereas **phocomelia** (shortened limb syndrome) may be induced by ingestion of the **teratogenic** drug thalidomide. And although **spina bifida** and cleft palate are products of the interaction of environment and heredity, the absence of a finger may happen spontaneously. This chapter describes the ways in which genetically determined birth defects are passed on from one generation to another.

GENETIC PRINCIPLES OF MENDEL

Gregor Mendel (1822–1884), an Austrian monk who enjoyed gardening, pioneered our understanding of genetics. He was the first to recognize the existence of genetic traits, that is, characteristics in organisms that show variability. While cultivating pea plants, he noted two different appearing types of plants—yellow and green plants. When he bred two plants with different appearances or traits, that is, yellow × green, the **hybrid** offspring all were green rather than mixed in color. Mendel, therefore, thought of the green trait as being dominant. He named the other trait (the yellow color), which did not appear in the hybrid offspring but sometimes appeared in subsequent generations, recessive. Later, it was determined that many birth defects are also inherited as autosomal recessive disorders. As mentioned in the introduction to this chapter, genes are what determine these various traits in human beings.

Genes

Each chromosome consists of thousands of genes; genes are responsible for the production of specific products, for example, a hormone, an enzyme, or blood type. The chromosome contains **deoxyribonucleic acid (DNA)** and looks like a double **helix**, a ladder like structure composed of "steps" of four **nucleotides**: cytosine (C), adenine (A), thymine (T), and guanine (G) (Figure 2.1). Pairs of nucleotides link to form each step: adenine links with thymine, and cytosine with guanine. The sides of the ladder are composed of sugar and phosphate molecules.

When a certain product is needed, the particular gene directing that production unzips so that a series of half steps are exposed. For example, if the complete step read AT, GC, GC, TA, AT, the half step would be AGGTA (see Figure 2.1). This half ladder then transcribes or rewrites the complementary message onto a single-stranded nucleic acid, called *messenger* **ribonucleic acid** (mRNA). A new nucleotide, uracil, is substituted for thymine so that the complementary message then reads UCCAU. This strand of mRNA then detaches from the DNA, and the double-stranded DNA zips back together. Next, the mRNA moves out of the nucleus into the cytoplasm. There it attaches to a **ribosome** (see Figure 1.1), a unit similar in function to a videocassette recorder. The ribosome reads out or translates this RNA strand in triplet groups—for example, GCU, CUA, UAG. Each triplet codes for a specific amino acid. As these triplets are read out, another type of RNA, called *transfer* RNA (tRNA), carries the requested amino acid to the ribosome. Other triplets code for the termination of production when all of the correct amino acids are in place, at which time they form a whole protein.

Once the protein is complete, this end product is either used by the cytoplasm or secreted. When the protein is secreted, it is transferred to the Golgi bodies (see Figure 1.1). These bodies package the protein in a form that can be released through the cell membrane and carried throughout the body.

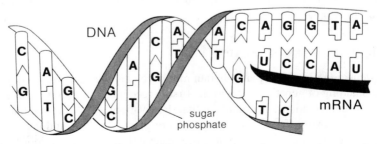

Figure 2.1.   Four nucleotides form the genetic code: G = guanine, C = cytosine, A = adenine, T = thymine. On the mRNA molecule, U (uracil) substitutes for thymine. The DNA unzips to transcribe its message to the mRNA.

Abnormalities in this process may result from a defective gene that can cause genetically inherited disease. An illustration of this is the production of hemoglobin, the pigment in blood. In people who have sickle cell anemia, one nucleotide is substituted for another, thymine for adenine, at one point in the gene that directs the production of hemoglobin. The triplet code is then misread, and the resulting hemoglobin is defective. This error causes the disorder of sickle cell anemia.

Such a substitution is called a **mutation**. A mutation can occur by chance or as the result of external factors such as radiation, viruses, or drugs. If the substitution occurs in the germ cells, that is, in the sperm or egg, the mutation becomes part of the person's genetic code and is passed on from one generation to another.

Geneticists generally believe that everyone carries at least four mutations, which they can pass on to their offspring. Some of these mutations are helpful and are part of the process of natural evolution. Others are harmful and predispose one to various diseases, including diabetes and cancer. Some have no observable effect and do not pose a serious threat to the well-being of our children.

Autosomal Recessive Disorders

Tay-Sachs disease is an example of an **autosomal recessive trait**. It is a progressive nervous system disease caused by the absence of an enzyme, hexosaminidase A, that normally converts a toxic nerve cell product into a nontoxic substance. In Tay-Sachs disease, this toxic product is not broken down, and it consequently builds up in the brain, leading to neurological damage and death.

The origin of the mutation leading to Tay-Sachs disease has been traced to Jewish families living in eastern Poland in the early 1800s. Prior to this time, Tay-Sachs disease did not exist. The original mutation occurred by chance. However, once the abnormality appeared, it was passed on from one generation to another.

Children with Tay-Sachs disease initially develop normally. At about 6 months of age, the child begins to deteriorate. He or she can no longer sit or babble and soon becomes blind and has severe **mental retardation**. Death usually occurs by 5 years of age.

Since all children with Tay-Sachs disease die, it may seem puzzling that the disease continues to be passed on from one generation to another. The reason is that Tay-Sachs disease is caused by a recessive gene. The following illustration explains this concept.

Two forms of the gene for hexosaminidase A are known. These alternate forms of the gene, called **alleles**, are the normal gene, symbolized by an "H," and the rare, disease-carrying allele, symbolized by "h" (see Figure 2.2). After fertilization, the embryo will have two genes that possibly could carry the Tay-Sachs disorder, one passed on from the father and one from the mother. The following combinations could occur; hh, hH, Hh, HH. Since this is a recessive disorder, two abnormal or "h" genes are needed to produce a diseased child. So, for the combinations just mentioned, hh would be a child with Tay-Sachs disease, hH or Hh would be a normal appearing child who is a carrier of Tay-Sachs disease, and HH would be a healthy noncarrier.

Autosomal Recessive Disorders

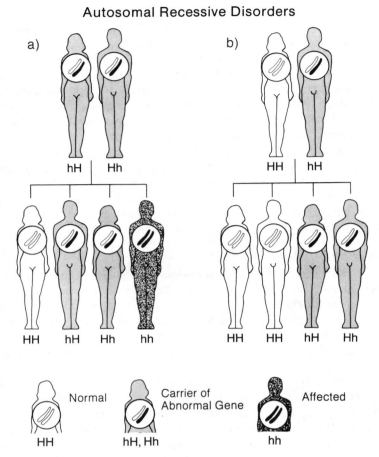

Figure 2.2.   Inheritance of autosomal recessive disorders: a) Two carriers mate, resulting, on average, in 25% normal children, 50% carriers, and 25% affected children. b) A carrier and a normal person mate, resulting in 50% normal children and 50% carriers. No children are affected.

Therefore, it is the carriers of the abnormal gene who pass on the disease from one generation to the next. If two carriers were to mate (hH × Hh), the following combinations could occur by chance: ¼HH, ¼hH, ¼Hh, and ¼hh (see Figure 2.2a). According to the law of probability, one-fourth of the children would be normal (HH), one-half would be carriers (hH or Hh), and one-fourth would have Tay-Sachs disease (hh). If a carrier mated with a noncarrier (hH × HH), half of the children would be carriers (hH, Hh), and half would be normal noncarriers (HH). None of these children would have Tay-Sachs disease (Figure 2.2b).

Remember that the 25% risk of having an affected child when two carriers mate is a *statistical* risk. This does not mean that if a family has one affected child, the next three will be normal. Each new pregnancy carries the same 25% risk; the parents could have three affected children in a row or 10 normal ones.

It is important to reemphasize, however, that recessive disorders can occur only if two carriers mate. A carrier mating with a noncarrier will always produce nonaffected children. Since it is unlikely for a carrier of one disease to meet another carrier of the same unusual disease by chance, these types of disorders are quite rare, ranging from 1 in 2,000 to 1 in 200,000 (Smith, 1982). However, when intermarriage occurs, the incidence of these disorders increases markedly because the cousin of a carrier is much more likely to be a carrier than is someone in the general population. This probably underlies the biblical proscription about marrying one's immediate relatives (Adams & Neel, 1967) (Figure 2.3).

Besides understanding the incidence of autosomal recessive disorders, it is important to keep in mind some other characteristics of these disorders. First, the mutation causing an autosomal recessive disorder often results in an enzyme deficiency of some kind. These enzyme deficiencies generally lead to biochemical abnormalities involving either the insufficiency of a needed product or the buildup of toxic materials (see Chapter 8); mental retardation or early death may result. Second, these disorders affect males and females equally. And third, a history of the disease in past generations rarely exists, unless blood relatives have mated (consanguinity).

Autosomal Dominant Disorders

Autosomal dominant disorders differ markedly from autosomal recessive disorders in mechanism, incidence, and clinical characteristics. The most significant difference is that an individual has the disease when he or she has a single abnormal gene. Therefore, a person with the **genotype**, Aa, is affected. This makes the incidence of autosomal dominant diseases greater than that of autosomal recessive disorders.

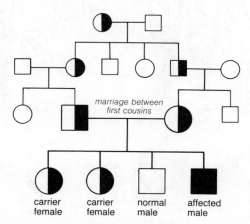

Figure 2.3. A family tree illustrating the effect of consanguinity (in this case, a marriage between first cousins) on the risk of inheriting an autosomal recessive disorder. If one parent is a carrier, the chance of the other parent being a carrier is usually less than 1 in 300. However, when first cousins marry, the chance rises to 1 in 4. The risk, then, of having an affected child increases almost 100-fold.

To better understand this, consider the disorder of **achondroplasia**, a form of short-limbed dwarfism. Suppose "A" represents a normal gene, and "a" indicates the abnormal gene for achondroplasia. If a person with achondroplasia, Aa, mates with a normal individual, AA, half of the children, statistically speaking, will have the disorder (Aa), and half will be normal (AA): Aa × AA ⟶ ½Aa + ½AA (Figure 2.4a). The normal children will not have the trait at all and, therefore, cannot pass it on to their children. If two affected parents (Aa × Aa) mate, a double dose of the disorder is likely to hit some of the children. This double dose is usually fatal. Thus, half of the affected parents' children, statistically speaking, would have achondroplasia (Aa), one-fourth would be normal (AA), and one-fourth would have a severe form of dwarfism (aa) that leads to early death (Figure 2.4b).

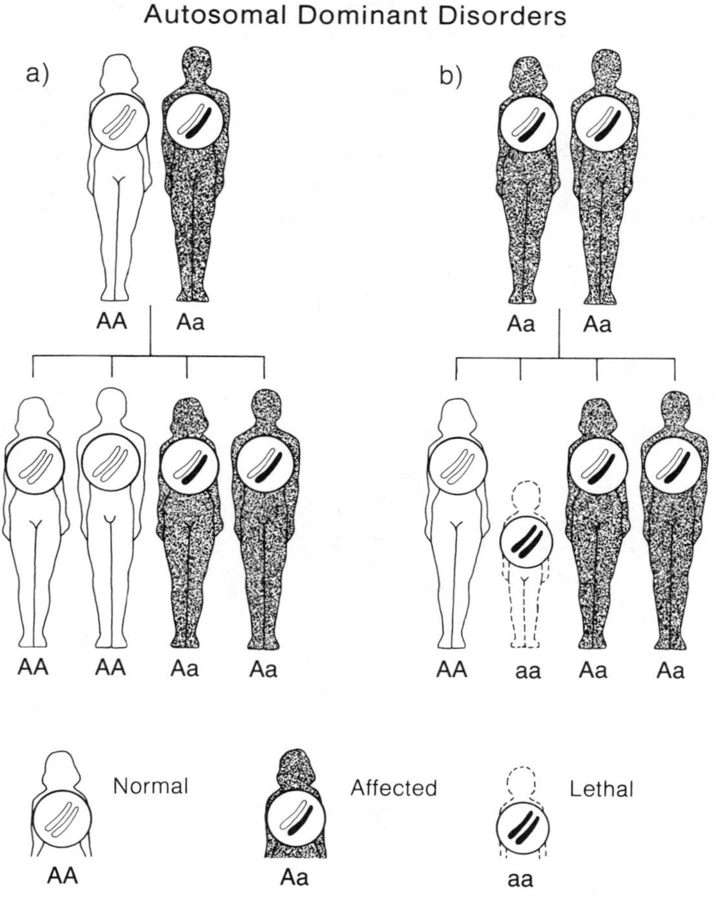

Autosomal Dominant Disorders

Figure 2.4.   Inheritance of autosomal dominant disorders: a) An affected person marries a normal person. Statistically, 50% of the children will be affected and 50% will be normal. b) If two affected people marry, 25% of the children will be normal, 50% will be affected, and 25% will have an often fatal double dose of the abnormal gene.

As with autosomal recessive disorders, males and females are equally affected. Unlike autosomal recessive disorders, these disorders usually involve structural (physical) rather than enzymatic abnormalities. Also, mental retardation is less common in individuals having these diseases. A family history of the disease, in which a sibling or parent is affected, is usual. However, some individuals who have the disorder will represent new mutations and will have no family history of the abnormality. Unlike autosomal recessive disorders, intermarriage is not a factor.

X-Linked Disorders

The two previous forms of heredity described by Mendel involved genes located on the 22 pairs of autosomes, or nonsex, chromosomes. The third form of genetic abnormality is called *sex-linked* or **X-linked recessive** because it involves genes located on the X, or female, sex chromosome. For this type of disorder, females are carriers, and males are affected. Muscular dystrophy, hemophilia, and color blindness are examples of sex-linked disorders. Recently, researchers have identified another sex-linked disorder, called fragile-X syndrome, that causes mental retardation. A brief discussion of some of these X-linked disorders follows.

Boys with Duchenne-type muscular dystrophy usually develop normally until 6–9 years of age. Then, muscle weakness becomes evident, progresses, and forces the child to be wheelchair-bound by adolescence. Since the disease affects all muscles, eventually the heart muscle and the diaphragmatic muscles needed for circulation and breathing are impaired. Muscular dystrophy is often fatal because of these complications.

Hemophilia is an equally devastating disease in which one of the blood-clotting factors is missing. As a result, a minor injury or accident can lead to uncontrolled bleeding. Injecting a concentrate of the missing clotting factor is needed to stop the bleeding. Therefore, children afflicted with hemophilia are frequently hospitalized and have a number of chronic disabilities.

Besides causing physical disabilities, X-linked disorders also contribute to intellectual impairment. Approximately 25% of the intellectual deficits in males are attributed to X-linked syndromes as well as about 10% of the learning disabilities in females (Uchida, Freeman, Jamro, et al., 1983). In the fragile-X syndrome, there is something visibly wrong with the X chromosome; an area at the end of the X chromosome is subject to breaking. It is called "a fragile site." In families that carry the fragile-X, a large number of the males have mental retardation. Affected boys have an unusual, elongated face, large ears, and a prominent jaw. They also develop enlarged testicles. Mental retardation generally falls in the moderate range. Under certain conditions, this syndrome can be diagnosed prenatally by looking for the fragile-X chromosome in fetal cells obtained by amniocentesis (see Chapter 3) (Jenkins, Brown, Brooks, et al., 1984). Attempts at using supplements of **folic acid** to improve the symptoms of this condition have had variable results (Brown, Jenkins, Friedman, et al., 1984).

Fortunately, not all sex-linked disorders are associated with mental retardation or are life threatening. For example, color blindness is also inherited in this way. The characteristic shared by these disorders is the way they are passed from one generation to another, from unaffected mother to affected son.

Since women have two X chromosomes, the carrier mother has one chromosome that bears the mutation (X^a) and one normal (X) chromosome. She is clinically normal but can pass the abnormality on to her children. The male child has one X chromosome and one Y chromosome; he is either normal (XY) or affected (X^aY). Suppose a woman who carries the gene for muscular dystrophy (X^aX) mates with a normal male (XY). Half of their sons (statistically speaking) would have muscular dystrophy (X^aY), and half would be normal (XY). Also, half of their daughters would be carriers for muscular dystrophy (X^aX), and half would be normal (XX) (Figure 2.5a). A family tree would usually reveal that maternal uncles and maternal grandfathers as well as male siblings have the disease.

If a woman who is a carrier of hemophilia mates with a hemophiliac (an extremely rare occurrence except in intermarriage), half of their children (statistically speaking) would have this disorder. Half of their sons would have hemophilia (X^aY), and half would be normal (XY). Half of their daughters would also have the disease (X^aX^a), and half would be carriers of hemophilia (X^aX) (Figure 2.5b). This is one way in which a female child could manifest a sex-linked disorder. Another way that a female can show signs of a sex-linked trait is if she is a carrier and inactivates her normal X chromosome. This is uncommon, occurring in less than 10% of women carriers of X-linked traits. However, because of this possibility, in a large family with the fragile-X syndrome, some women may also have retardation, but to a lesser degree than the men (Uchida, Freeman, Jamro, et al., 1983).

Thus, sex-linked disorders primarily manifest themselves in males but are passed on from carrier females. Consanguinity is not a factor.

Over 2,000 diseases are now known to be transmitted as Mendelian traits (McKusick, 1983). Approximately 1% of the population suffers from a Mendelian disorder (Table 2.1). Fortunately, some of these disorders can now be treated (see Chapter 8), and others can be diagnosed prenatally (see Chapter 3).

CHROMOSOMAL MALFORMATIONS

Although a single-gene mutation causes Mendelian diseases, other disorders involve the loss or addition of an entire chromosome, including many genes. These syndromes may affect either autosomes or sex chromosomes.

Autosomal chromosomal abnormalities usually lead to mental retardation and are characterized by a number of unusual physical findings. For example, in Down syndrome, the head is small and the eyes are slanted. Affected children have broad, flat noses and large tongues. **Congenital** heart defects and gastrointestinal malformations are common. Other trisomy or extra chromosome syndromes (involving chromosomes #13 or #18) produce even more severe abnormalities; children with these syndromes rarely live beyond infancy.

In the general population, the incidence of chromosomal aberrations of autosomes is about 4/1,000 live births, or 0.4%. However, in children with mental

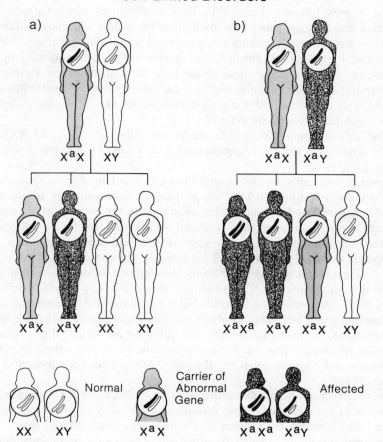

Sex-Linked Disorders

Figure 2.5. Inheritance of sex-linked disorders: a) A carrier woman marries a normal man. Of the male children, statistically speaking, 50% will be affected and 50% will be normal. Of the female children, 50% will be carriers and 50% will be normal. b) A carrier woman marries an affected man. Of the male children, 50% will be normal and 50% will be affected. Of the female children, 50% will be affected and 50% will be carriers.

Table 2.1.   Incidence of Mendelian disorders per 1,000 live births

Type of disorder	Number
Autosomal dominant	7.0
Autosomal recessive	2.5
X-linked	0.4
Total	9.9

Source: Ash et al. (1977).

retardation and multiple malformations, the incidence rises to between 8% and 14% (Nielsen, Hansen, Sillesen, et al., 1981). Thus, many parents of children with severe retardation and multiple congenital malformations have a chromosome analysis (karyotype) done to help in making a diagnosis and in providing genetic counseling.

Characteristically, the physical and intellectual problems caused by sex-chromosome abnormalities are less severe than those of autosomal chromosome syndromes. These syndromes also tend to occur more frequently than the autosomal ones. As with autosomal chromosome disorders, the sex-chromosome disorders usually result from nondisjunction.

The most common sex-chromosome abnormalities are 45 X, 47 XXY, and 47 XYY syndromes. The most frequent is 45 X, or Turner's syndrome, described in Chapter 1.

Another common sex-chromosome abnormality is Klinefelter's syndrome (47 XXY) (Caldwell & Smith, 1972). As in Turner's syndrome, the sexual organs develop abnormally in this disorder. The child is male, but because testosterone (the male sex hormone) is inadequately produced, he neither develops secondary sexual characteristics nor forms sperm. He appears as a tall, slender man with breast development and small genitalia. His IQ is generally close to normal. Thus, the extra X chromosome seems to interfere with the development of normal "maleness."

On the other hand, the XYY syndrome seems to have a very different effect (Hook, 1973). These men tend to be tall, have normal sexual development, but have lower intelligence. When a number of tall, male prisoners were found to have an extra Y chromosome, the media had a field day, calling it the "criminal chromosome." There was speculation that this extra chromosome predisposed these men to aggressiveness and criminal behavior. However, this has not been proven to be so (Pitcher, 1982).

Other sex-chromosome abnormalities exist: 47 XXX, 48 XXXY, 48 XXYY, and 49 XXXYY syndromes. Those disorders having all X chromosomes result in females. The presence of a single Y chromosome, even with a number of X chromosomes, results in a male. Abnormal physical, sexual, and mental development characterizes all of these syndromes. Compared to Turner's, Klinefelter's, and XYY syndromes (with a combined incidence of 1/300), these other disorders are extremely rare (Smith, 1982).

Finally, one chromosomal aberration, **mosaicism**, may involve either autosomal or sex chromosomes. Nondisjunction in the egg or sperm before or during fertilization causes the previously described syndromes. If nondisjunction happens after fertilization, mosaicism results. Suppose nondisjunction takes place shortly after fertilization when four cells are dividing to form eight cells in the **morula**. If one of the four cells divides unevenly, this would lead to 47 chromosomes in one daughter cell, 45 in another, and 46 in the remaining six cells (Figure 2.6). The cell containing 45 chromosomes will die. If the 47-chromosome cell contains a third #21 chromosome, all subsequent daughter cells of this cell will also have 47 chromosomes (trisomy 21). The end result will be a child who will have about 67% normal cells and 33% trisomic cells. The child will look like he or she has Down syndrome. However,

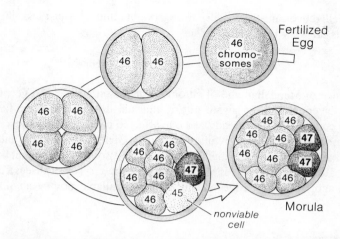

Figure 2.6. Mosaicism. Here nondisjunction occurs after fertilization. This results in a few cells with an additional or missing chromosome; the rest are normal. The cells with 45 chromosomes generally die, while those with 46 or 47 chromosomes survive and multiply. The child is a mosaic with some normal and some abnormal cells. If the abnormal cell contains an extra #21 chromosome, the child will look as though he or she has Down syndrome but will be less severely affected.

the physical abnormalities are less obvious, and the mental retardation is less severe (Fishler, Koch, & Donnell, 1976). Mosaicism is rare and accounts for fewer than 4% of all children with Down syndrome.

HEREDITARY-ENVIRONMENTAL INTERACTIONS

Some traits result not solely from Mendelian or chromosomal effects but rather from the interaction of heredity and environment. Weight and intelligence are traits inherited in this manner. Furthermore, in disorders such as cancer and hypertension, heredity and environment both play a role. Examples of birth defects that result from the interaction of heredity and environment include spina bifida, cleft palate (Fraser, 1970), and pyloric stenosis (Smith, 1971).

Several factors contribute to the total effect; no one factor is sufficient to produce the particular abnormality. Consider the predominantly male disorder of pyloric stenosis, a malformation of the stomach muscle that leads to a block in the passage of food from the stomach to the small intestine. For this abnormality to occur, it is thought that an intrauterine viral infection, male gender, and genetic factors must all be present. A viral infection alone, for example, will not produce the defect. Thus, although pyloric stenosis is uncommon in the general population (3/1,000 births), it carries a recurrence risk of 1/20 in a family with a previously affected child (Carter & Evans, 1969).

Similarly, bright parents have a greater chance of having bright children, and obese parents more often have obese children. However, since a number of factors are interacting, including the environment inside and outside the uterus, two people of average intelligence can still produce a very bright child. It is just less likely than if both parents are very bright themselves.

SUMMARY

The incidence of Mendelian and of chromosomal disorders is rare. Yet, it remains important for couples to be aware of any unusual disorders in their families. In addition, a couple who has already had one affected child needs to know about any increased risk of recurrence in future children. Genetic counseling and prenatal diagnosis may therefore be obtained. Many of these disorders still cannot be detected prenatally. However, progress in the detection of these types of disease continues. Ten years ago, the knowledge and techniques available now were not thought possible.

REFERENCES

Adams, M.S., & Neel, J.V. (1967). Children of incest. *Pediatrics, 40,* 55–62.

Ash, P., Vennart, J., & Carter, C.O. (1977). The incidence of hereditary disease in man. *Lancet, 1,* 849–851.

Bender, B., Fry, E., Pennington, B., et al. (1983). Speech and language development in 41 children with sex chromosome anomalies. *Pediatrics, 71,* 262–267.

Brown, W.T., Jenkins, E.C., Friedman, E., et al. (1984). Folic acid therapy in the fragile X syndrome. *American Journal of Medical Genetics, 17,* 289–297.

Caldwell, P.D., & Smith, D.W. (1972). The XXY (Klinefelter's) syndrome in childhood: Detection and treatment. *Journal of Pediatrics, 80,* 250–258.

Carter, C.O., & Evans, K.A. (1969). Inheritance of congenital pyloric stenosis. *Journal of Medical Genetics, 6,* 233–254.

Fishler K., Koch, R., & Donnell, G.N. (1976). Comparison of mental development in individuals with mosaic and trisomy 21 Down's syndrome. *Pediatrics, 58,* 744–748.

Fraser, F.C. (1970). The genetics of cleft lip and cleft palate. *American Journal of Human Genetics, 22,* 336–352.

Hagerman, R.J., & McBogg, P.M. (Eds.). (1983). *The fragile X syndrome.* Dillon, CO: Spectra Publishing Co.

Hook, E.B. (1973). Behavioral implications of the human XYY genotype. *Science, 179,* 139–150.

Jenkins, E.C., Brown, W.T., Brooks, J., et al. (1984). Experience with prenatal fragile X detection. *American Journal of Medical Genetics, 17,* 215–239.

Kaback, M.M. (1973). Heterozygote screening: A social challenge. (Editorial.) *New England Journal of Medicine, 289,* 1090–1091.

Ledbetter, D.H., Riccardi, V.M., Airhart, S.D., et al. (1981). Deletions of chromosome 15 as a cause of the Prader-Willi syndrome. *New England Journal of Medicine, 304,* 325–329.

McKusick, V.A. (1983). *Mendelian inheritance in man: Catalogs of autosomal dominant, autosomal recessive, and X-linked phenotypes* (6th ed.). Baltimore: Johns Hopkins University Press.

Milunsky, A. (1977). *Know your genes.* New York: Avon Books.

Nielsen, J., Hansen, K.B., Sillesen, I., et al. (1981). Chromosome abnormality in newborn children. Physical aspects. *Human Genetics, 59,* 194–200.

Pitcher, D.R. (1982). Chromosomes and violence. *Practitioner, 226,* 497–501.

Ratcliff, S.G. (1982). Speech and learning disorders in children with sex chromosome abnormalities. *Developmental Medicine and Child Neurology, 24,* 80–84.

Ratcliff, S.G., Bancroft, J., Axworthy, D., et al. (1982). Klinefelter's syndrome in adolescence. *Archives of Disease in Childhood, 57,* 6–12.

Shapiro, L.R., Wilmot, P.L., Brenholz, P., et al. (1982). Prenatal diagnosis of fragile X chromosome. *Lancet, 1,* 99–100.

Smith, C. (1971). Recurrence risks for multifactorial inheritance. *American Journal of Human Genetics,* *23,* 578–588.

Smith, D., with assistance of Jones, K.L. (1982). *Recognizable patterns of human malformation: Genetic, embryologic, and clinical aspects* (3rd ed.). Philadelphia: W.B. Saunders Co.

Stewart, D.A., Netley, C.T., & Park, E. (1982). Summary of clinical findings of children with 47,XXY, 47,XYY, and 47,XXX karyotypes. *Birth Defects, 18,* 1–5.

Thompson, J.S., & Thompson, M.W. (1980). *Genetics in medicine* (3rd ed.). Philadelphia: W.B. Saunders Co.

Turner, G., Daniel, A., & Frost, M. (1980). X-linked mental retardation, macro-orchidism, and the Xq27 fragile site. *Journal of Pediatrics, 96,* 837–841.

Uchida, I.A., Freeman, V.C., Jamro, H., et al. (1983). Additional evidence for fragile-X activity in heterozygous carriers. *American Journal of Human Genetics, 35,* 861–868.

Chapter 3

Birth Defects, Prenatal Diagnosis, and Fetal Therapy

Upon completion of this chapter, the reader will:
—know the risks and benefits of amniocentesis
—be familiar with the prenatal diagnostic procedures of chorionic villus biopsy and restriction enzyme analysis
—be aware of certain screening tests used to diagnose diseases prenatally
—understand the principles of fetoscopy and sonography, two other major prenatal diagnostic tools
—be informed about those instances in which fetal therapy is possible

Anne, in the fourth month of her second pregnancy, is undergoing amniocentesis. Her first child was born with spina bifida. By using the prenatal diagnostic technique of amniocentesis, her physician should be able to determine if the child Anne is now carrying has the same condition. Approximately 3 weeks later, Anne learns that this child, a boy, does not have spina bifida or any of the many diagnosable chromosomal abnormalities. Many of her fears are allayed.

Amniocentesis, along with fetoscopy, sonography, and some blood screening tests, are the major prenatal diagnostic tools used to identify a serious medical problem in a fetus. This chapter examines these various techniques and discusses the risks and benefits associated with them. Two new diagnostic methods, **chorionic** villus biopsy and restriction enzyme analysis, are also considered. The chapter concludes with the mention of a few instances where prenatal therapy is possible.

AMNIOCENTESIS

The use of amniocentesis for prenatal diagnosis has increased dramatically over the past 15 years. Yet only about 5% of women who are at risk for having a child with a diagnosable defect are now being evaluated by this procedure (Simpson, Dallaire, Miller, et al., 1976).

Over 250 genetic disorders are diagnosable by analyzing **amniotic fluid** and fetal cells. The most common of these is Down syndrome. As a woman ages, the risk of nondisjunction (discussed in Chapter 1) and resultant trisomy 21 (or Down syndrome) increases (Figure 3.1). In women 45 years old, the incidence is about 1 in 32 compared to 1 in 2,000 for women between 20 and 25 years old. In women 35 years old, the risk is 1 in 400, making Down syndrome a significant enough possibility to warrant amniocentesis (Hook & Fabia, 1978). This is why approximately 60% of all amniocenteses are performed on women 35 years of age or older.

For women younger than 35 who have already had one child with trisomy 21, the recurrence risk increases to 1 in 100 (Carter & Evans, 1961). For these women, amniocentesis is suggested in future pregnancies and accounts for an additional 20% of all amniocenteses performed in the United States. Some cases of Down syndrome, about 3%, are caused by #14/21 translocations (see Chapter 1) rather than by trisomy 21 (Wright, Day, Muller, et al., 1967). In the case of a translocation, one parent is normally a carrier, and the recurrence risk may be as high as 1 in 10, warranting amniocentesis for future pregnancies.

Besides its use in checking for Down syndrome or other chromosomal abnormalities, amniocentesis can be used to diagnose spina bifida (a malformation in which there is an opening in the spine) and some inherited inborn errors of metabolism. To diagnose spina bifida in a mother who has had a previously affected child, the

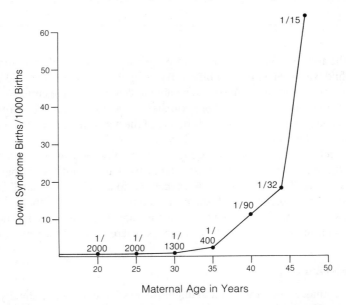

Figure 3.1. Incidence of trisomy 21 in mothers of various ages. The risk increases markedly after 35 years of age (Hook & Fabia, 1978).

concentration of a specific compound, alpha-fetoprotein (AFP), is measured in the amniotic fluid. What seems to happen is this: AFP is plentiful in the spinal fluid. With an open spine, the AFP leaks into the amniotic fluid and then can be measured. Since the risk of recurrence in a mother who already has a child with spina bifida is about 1 in 30, amniocentesis is offered to all such women (Laurence, 1969).

When testing for inborn errors of metabolism, such as Tay-Sachs disease, the fetal cells are studied for the presence of a defective enzyme. In the case of Tay-Sachs, the enzyme is hexosaminidase A. If the enzyme level is very low or is missing, the fetus is diagnosed as having the disease. Because many of these diseases are fatal, the parents may then elect to terminate the pregnancy.

In addition to looking for these abnormalities, one can also determine the sex of the fetus through amniocentesis. Gender determination is requested when parents are concerned about the possibility of having a child with a serious sex-linked disease that does not have a specific prenatal diagnostic test (Golbus, Loughman, Epstein, et al., 1979). These parents may choose to abort all males to avoid the risk of such a disorder recurring. Unfortunately, if they choose to do this, they will also abort, statistically speaking, an equal number of healthy males. Because no specific diagnostic tests for these disorders are available, many of these couples feel this is the only avenue open to them if they wish to have their own children but are unable to accept the risk of having another affected child.

The Procedure

The procedure of amniocentesis is fairly simple. It is usually performed between 14 and 17 weeks gestation, in the second trimester, when about 8 ounces of amniotic fluid surround the fetus. Amniocentesis involves inserting a needle below the mother's **umbilicus** and withdrawing about 1 ounce of this fluid.

Ultrasound monitoring is done at the same time. This provides a picture of the placenta and fetus using sound waves rather than X rays. The rationale is that this monitoring enables the obstetrician to do the procedure without puncturing a fetal part.

Once the amniotic fluid containing the fetal cells is removed, the cells are separated and put into a culture medium (Figure 3.2). To diagnose spina bifida, the fluid is tested for levels of AFP, and the results are available in a few days. To diagnose biochemical or chromosomal disorders, the amniotic cells are grown in a culture medium for about 2 weeks. After a sufficient number of cells have grown, either a karyotype is assembled to determine the gender and to analyze the chromosomes, or a specific enzyme analysis is performed.

Problems, Risks, and Benefits

Amniocentesis is done as an outpatient procedure, and few difficulties have been recorded. A study by the National Institute of Child Health and Human Development (NICHD National Registry, 1976) concluded that amniocentesis does not lead to a statistically significant increase in risk for the mother or the fetus. Yet, the literature has reported individual instances of the following complications: miscarriages within 12 hours of the procedure; infants born prematurely or with a needle hole in a part of

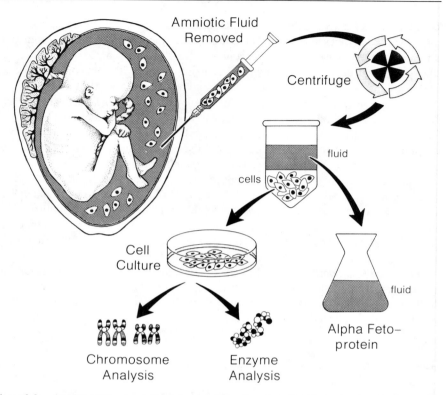

Figure 3.2.   Amniocentesis. Approximately one ounce of amniotic fluid is removed at 14 to 17 weeks gestation. It is spun in a centrifuge to separate the fluid from the fetal cells. The fluid is used immediately to test for spina bifida. The cells are grown for 2 weeks, and then a chromosome or enzyme analysis can be performed. Results are usually available about 3 weeks later.

the body; chronic leakage of amniotic fluid that increased the chances for an orthopedic abnormality in the fetus, and infections in the mother following the test (Brown, 1984). These problems point to the presence of some finite risk with this test.

As already mentioned, although these risks are small, only a fraction of the women who have a greater chance of having children with diagnosable diseases take advantage of amniocentesis. At least five factors might account for this low utilization. First, amniocentesis is expensive; in 1984, the cost averaged $500. Second, a large number of women are unaware of the availability of this procedure. Third, few diagnostic laboratories can perform the task. Fourth, prospective parents have an unjustifiable fear of the risk of amniocentesis to the mother and the fetus. Lastly, for religious reasons, many parents will not consider amniocentesis because they would never decide to abort an affected child.

Performed correctly, amniocentesis is an extremely useful procedure that can allay many fears and provide prospective parents with much-needed information (Simpson, Dallaire, Miller, et al., 1976).

CHORIONIC VILLUS BIOPSY

A new method that may eventually replace amniocentesis as the most common form of prenatal diagnosis is chorionic villus biopsy. This procedure is performed in the first trimester (8–10 weeks gestation) when the mother has just started to look pregnant and before she feels any movement from the fetus. The main advantage is that a decision to terminate a pregnancy is emotionally easier and medically safer for women at this stage of pregnancy. Also, the uncertainty of whether or not the fetus is affected lasts for a much shorter period of time. So far, this technique has been used successfully to measure the activity of specific enzymes, to detect certain chromosomal abnormalities, and to determine the sex of the fetus.

This diagnostic procedure is illustrated in Figure 3.3. An instrument is inserted through the vagina into the uterus, guided by ultrasound, and some chorionic tissue is removed by suction. This tissue is the fetal component of the developing placenta. The tissue is then examined under a microscope. Because fetal cells exist in the chorion in relatively large numbers, they can then be analyzed directly, without waiting 2–3 weeks for them to grow, as is done in amniocentesis (Jackson, 1985; Rodeck & Morsman, 1983; Rodeck, Nicolaides, Morsman, et al., 1983). An answer

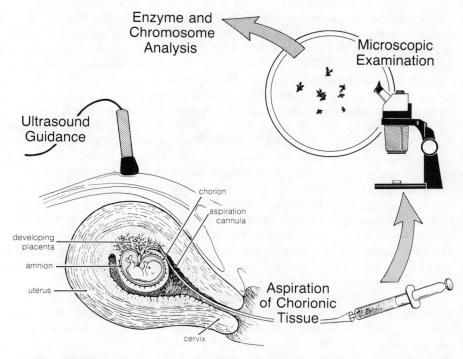

Figure 3.3. Chorionic villus biopsy. A hollow instrument is inserted through the vagina into the uterus, guided by ultrasound. A small amount of chorionic tissue is suctioned. The tissue is then examined under a microscope, and its chromosomes and enzymes are analyzed.

may then be available at about 10 weeks gestation instead of 17–20 weeks in the case of amniocentesis. Thus, this technique appears to be a good solution for many women who are concerned about the possibility of having a child with abnormalities but who feel that amniocentesis is available too late in pregnancy.

Unfortunately, right now, chorionic villus biopsy is not readily available, and the risk of infection as well as the incidence of bleeding and miscarriage are higher with this procedure than with amniocentesis. The rate of miscarriage is less than 2.5/1,000 following amniocentesis while, after chorionic villus biopsy, this rate is approximately 10/1,000 (Daker, 1983). Also, the technique is so new that the literature has few reports on its use. However, if the risks are reduced, it will become a great boon to prenatal diagnosis, as it is less expensive and more emotionally acceptable than amniocentesis.

RESTRICTION ENZYME ANALYSIS

Another recent advance in prenatal diagnosis is the use of a procedure called restriction enzyme analysis, or gene splicing. Using this technique, geneticists are now able to diagnose a number of diseases that previously had no prenatal diagnostic test.

This procedure is based on the ability of certain enzymes to break or cut DNA at certain points in the nucleotide sequence (see Chapter 2). The result is pieces of DNA of specific, set lengths. If the DNA has undergone a mutation, and the nucleotide sequence is changed, the enzyme may miss a cut and the length of the piece is different from normal. This kind of change occurs in sickle cell anemia, an autosomal recessive disorder that affects blacks and leads to severe anemia. The defect in the red blood cell results from a substitution of one nucleotide for another, which causes the formation of an abnormal hemoglobin, the pigment in the blood. Children who have this disorder are severely ill and may die in childhood. Until recently, prenatal diagnosis depended on drawing blood from the fetus and examining it. This technique carried a high risk to the fetus. Now, amniocentesis or chorionic villus biopsy is used to collect fetal cells. The DNA from these cells is then split using the appropriate restriction enzymes (Figure 3.4). Next, the size of these fragments of DNA is measured and compared with patterns in cells from normal individuals, from carriers of sickle cell anemia, and from those with the disorder. A normal fetus has two normal fragments, one derived from the mother and one from the father. If one abnormal fragment (1.35 Kb) and one normal fragment (1.15 Kb) are found, the fetus is a carrier of the disorder. Finally, if both fragments are abnormally long, the fetus has sickle cell anemia (Kan, Chang, & Dozy, 1982).

Another disorder that can now be diagnosed using this method is phenylketonuria (PKU). In this disorder, the defective enzyme, phenylalanine hydroxylase, does not exist in amniotic fluid cells or those in the chorion. However, using restriction enzyme analysis, scientists can look for genes that are close to or linked with the defective gene. If these genes show up in the fetal cells obtained through amniocentesis or chorionic villus biopsy, one can make the diagnosis that the fetus has phenylketonuria.

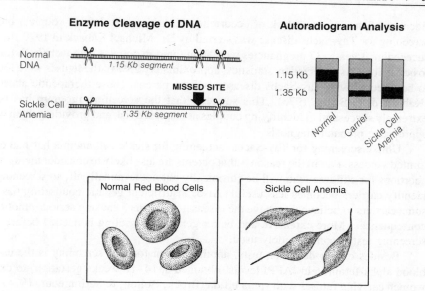

Figure 3.4.   Restriction enzyme analysis in sickle cell anemia. An enzyme breaks the DNA at certain points. When a mutation has occurred, the enzyme may miss a cut at a particular site, and the resulting fragment of DNA will be different than normal (for example, 1.35 Kb instead of the normal 1.15 Kb). Using autoradiogram analysis, one can determine whether the fetus is normal (with two fragments measuring 1.15 Kb), is a carrier (with one 1.35 Kb fragment and one 1.15 Kb fragment), or is affected (two 1.35 Kb fragments).

Besides its use for sickle cell anemia and PKU, this technique has recently been used to diagnose **cystic fibrosis**.

CARRIER DETECTION AND BLOOD SCREENING TESTS

Methods complementary to amniocentesis and chorionic villus biopsy now include carrier detection and blood screening tests. Carrier detection is used to diagnose two autosomal recessive disorders, Tay-Sachs disease and sickle cell anemia. In the past, these techniques could only be effective after a family already had at least one affected child. Now, a blood test can identify carriers of these diseases before they have a child with the disorder. If a couple is screened and both are found to be carriers—meaning they have a 25% risk of having an affected child—the woman can undergo amniocentesis or chorionic villus biopsy and choose to terminate her pregnancy if she is found to be carrying an affected child. This can enable a **heterozygote**, or carrier, couple to have a series of normal children without ever bearing an affected child.

One of the reasons Tay-Sachs screening has been successful is because it can be limited to a relatively small number of persons, the Ashkenazic Jewish population. The chance of a Jewish couple bearing a child affected with Tay-Sachs disease is about 1/2,500. Among non-Jewish couples, the incidence is about 1/360,000.

Because of the increased risk of occurrence in Ashkenazic Jewish couples, blood screening for Tay-Sachs disease was started by Dr. Michael Kaback in 1970. In the succeeding 3 years, 37 pregnancies were monitored in couples who were both found to be carriers. As expected by statistics, approximately 25% of the fetuses were found to be affected with Tay-Sachs disease, and the parents chose therapeutic abortion (Kaback & O'Brien, 1973). This suggests that the screening program has been extremely successful in identifying couples at increased risk and providing them with appropriate prenatal diagnosis.

Unlike screening for Tay-Sachs, screening for sickle cell anemia has had only limited success. Part of the reason is that parents are less likely to consider therapeutic abortions for children who will be chronically but not terminally ill, so screening to identify carriers becomes less useful. Also, insufficient genetic counseling has led some carriers to believe they have the disease, sometimes causing serious emotional consequences. More extensive and better genetic counseling is needed before this screening test becomes widely used.

Besides carrier detection tests, another recent form of screening is the use of blood alpha-fetoprotein (AFP) levels, obtained at 14–18 weeks gestation, to detect women carrying fetuses with spina bifida (Brock, Bolton, & Scrimgeour, 1974) and Down syndrome (Cuckle & Wald, 1984). About 12% of pregnant women with high blood levels of AFP have been found to be carrying spina bifida children. A smaller number of women with very low AFP levels have been identified as carrying Down syndrome babies. If a woman has either a very high or very low AFP level, she is offered amniocentesis to make a definitive diagnosis. The amniotic fluid should contain high levels of AFP in cases of spina bifida and low levels in those of Down syndrome. However, for every 10 women identified by this blood screening test, only 1 will actually be carrying an affected fetus. Combining this test with ultrasound, during which the fetal spine is observed, improves the precision of detecting spina bifida. Yet, even with this approach, many women will undergo prenatal diagnosis unnecessarily.

OTHER METHODS OF DIAGNOSIS

Although amniocentesis is the most common form of prenatal diagnosis, other methods are also available, including fetoscopy and sonography.

Fetoscopy

In this procedure, a small tube is inserted through the mother's abdominal wall into the amniotic cavity. Using a **fibro-optic** light source, the physician can see parts of the fetus—for example, a foot or hand (Figure 3.5). This information can be important for a family who has had a child with multiple congenital malformations. The finding of one of these abnormalities, such as an extra toe, would indicate that the child has the complete syndrome (Benzie, 1977).

Besides enabling the physician to see a part of the fetus, the fetoscope also contains a syringe needle at its end so that the doctor can locate a placental blood

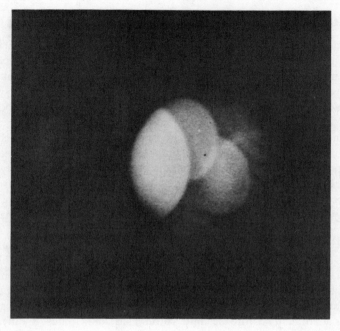

Figure 3.5. Fetal toes as seen through a fetoscope at 17 weeks gestation. (From Mahoney, M.J., & Hobbins, J.C. [1979]. Fetoscopy and fetal blood sampling. In A. Milunsky [Ed.], *Genetic disorders and the fetus: Diagnosis, prevention, and treatment*. New York: Plenum Publishing Corp.; reprinted by permission.)

vessel and withdraw blood. This aids in the fetal diagnosis of certain inherited blood diseases (Patrick, Perry, & Kinch, 1974). However, fetal blood sampling carries a significant risk of miscarriage. Thus, instead of using this technique, restriction enzyme analysis is now used to detect sickle cell anemia, thalassemia, and other inherited blood diseases.

Sonography

In sonography, or ultrasound, which carries no known risks, sound waves rather than X rays are used to outline the fetus (Bobrow, Blackwell, Unrau, et al., 1971). The sound waves bounce off structures with different densities. This allows, for example, visualization of the fetal spine and, as already stated, aids in the diagnosis of spina bifida. It is also used to determine head size. For families who have had a **microcephalic** child, this is especially important. Subsequent pregnancies can be monitored to see if the head size is increasing at the proper rate throughout the pregnancy. In addition, a physician can compare the gestational age of the fetus with its size to make sure it is growing normally. Finally, fetal sex can be determined with good accuracy by looking at the genital area in the late second trimester (Birnholz, 1983).

FETAL THERAPY

The ultimate goal of prenatal diagnosis is to identify affected fetuses and treat them before birth so that severe disabilities are prevented. So far, this approach has only been tried in a few instances. Two of these involve inborn errors of metabolism that are responsive to vitamin therapy (see Chapter 8). In one of these syndromes, **methylmalonic aciduria**, supplements of vitamin B_{12} correct this metabolic abnormality in some affected infants. In the second, **propionic acidemia**, another B vitamin, biotin, can lead to a similar improvement. One case of each of these disorders has been reported in the literature after successful *in utero* therapy (Roth, Yang, Allen, et al., 1982). In both cases, the mother, who had previously delivered an affected child, was found to be carrying a second child with the same disorder. The mothers received supplements of the vitamins, and the children continued to receive this therapy after they were born. Both children have done well. Unfortunately, most inborn errors of metabolism are not vitamin responsive.

A second example of *in utero* treatment involves **hydrocephalus**. Hydrocephalus is a condition in which an enlargement of the head is caused by a blockage of the normal flow of fluid from the head into the spine (see Chapter 12). Some cases of hydrocephalus exist during fetal development and can be diagnosed using ultrasound when a markedly increased head size is found. Recently, an attempt was made to correct this abnormality before the child's birth (Harrison, Golbus, & Filly, 1981). A shunt was implanted into the **ventricle** in the fetus's head to release the increased pressure and to prevent further enlargement of the head. The baby was then delivered at term by cesarean section. To date, too few operations have been done to determine if this approach improves the quality of life for these children.

SUMMARY

Currently, the various forms of prenatal diagnosis can identify well over 250 inherited disorders. The number increases each year. Real progress will come not only as more disorders are diagnosed but as measures are found to treat disorders before birth. Although prenatal diagnosis leads some parents to choose to abort an affected fetus, it also helps others to have more children. Without prenatal diagnosis, some parents would be unwilling to risk the recurrence of a severe defect in another child. It is also important to reemphasize that while prenatal diagnosis can tell a prospective parent about a specific abnormality, it cannot ensure anyone a normal child. Unfortunately, many causes of developmental disabilities are still not diagnosable prenatally.

REFERENCES

Allen, L.C., Doran, T.A., Miskin, M., et al. (1982). Ultrasound and amniotic fluid alpha-fetoprotein in prenatal diagnosis of spina bifida. *Obstetrics and Gynecology, 60,* 169–173.

Ampola, M.G., Mahoney, M.J., Nakamura, E., et al. (1974). *In utero* treatment of methylmalonic acidemia (MMA-EMIA) with vitamin B_{12}. *Pediatric Research, 8,* 387.

Benzie, R.J. (1977). Fetoscopy. *Birth Defects: Original Article Series, 13,* 181–189.

Birnholz, J.C. (1983). Determination of fetal sex. *New England Journal of Medicine, 309,* 942–944.

Bobrow, M., Blackwell, N., Unrau, A.E., et al. (1971). Absence of any observed effect of ultrasonic irradiation on human chromosomes. *Journal of Obstetrics and Gynaecology of the British Commonwealth, 78,* 730–736.

Brock, D.J., Bolton, A.E., & Scrimgeour, J.B. (1974). Prenatal diagnosis of spina bifida and anencephaly through maternal plasma-alpha-fetoprotein measurement. *Lancet, 1,* 767–769.

Brock, D.J.H., & Sutcliffe, R.G. (1972). Alpha-fetoprotein in the antenatal diagnosis of anencephaly and spina bifida. *Lancet, 2,* 197–199.

Brown, B.S. (1984). How safe is diagnostic ultrasonography? *Candian Medical Association Journal, 131,* 307–311.

Carter, C.O., & Evans, K.A. (1961). Risk of parents who have had one child with Down's syndrome (mongolism) having another child similarly affected. *Lancet, 2,* 785–788.

Cuckle, H. S., & Wald, M. J. (1984). Maternal serum alpha-fetoprotein measurement: A screening test for Down's syndrome. *Lancet, 1,* 926–929.

Daker, M. (1983). Chorionic tissue biopsy in the first trimester of pregnancy. *British Journal of Obstetrics and Gynecology, 90,* 193–195.

Golbus, M.S. (1982). The current scope of antenatal diagnosis. *Hospital Practice, 17,* 179–186.

Golbus, M.S., Loughman, W.D., Epstein, C.J., et al. (1979). Prenatal genetic diagnosis in 3000 amniocenteses. *New England Journal of Medicine, 300,* 157–163.

Harrison, M.R., Golbus, M.S., & Filly, R.A. (1981). Management of the fetus with a correctable congenital defect. *Journal of the American Medical Association, 246,* 774–777.

Hill, L.M., Breckle, R., & Gehrking, W.C. (1983). The prenatal detection of congenital malformations by ultrasonography. *Mayo Clinic Proceedings, 58,* 805–826.

Hook, E.B., & Fabia, J.J. (1978). Frequency of Down syndrome in live births by single-year maternal age interval: Results of a Massachusetts study. *Teratology, 17,* 223–228.

Hook, E.B., Schreinemachers, D.M., & Cross, P.K. (1981). Massachusetts Department of Public Health. Use of prenatal cytogenetic diagnosis in New York State. *New England Journal of Medicine, 305,* 1410–1413.

Jackson, L.G. (1985). First-trimester diagnosis of fetal genetic disorders. *Hospital Practice, 20,* 39–48.

Kaback, M.M., & O'Brien, J.S. (1973). Tay-Sachs: Prototype for prevention of genetic disease. *Hospital Practice, 8,* 107–123.

Kan, Y.W., Chang, J.C., & Dozy, A.M. (1982). Prenatal diagnosis by DNA analysis. *Birth Defects, 18,* 275–283.

Langman, J. (1981). *Medical embryology* (4th ed.). Baltimore: Williams & Wilkins Co..

Laurence, K.M. (1969). The recurrence risk in spina bifida cystica and anencephaly. *Developmental Medicine and Child Neurology, Suppl. 20,* 23–30.

Macri, J.N., & Weiss, R.R. (1982). Prenatal serum and alpha-fetoprotein screening for neural tube defects. *Obstetrics and Gynecology, 59,* 633–639.

Manning, C.H., & Goodman, H.O. (1981). Parental origin of chromosome in Down's syndrome. *Human Genetics, 59,* 101–103.

Milunsky, A. (1979). *Genetic disorders and the fetus: Diagnosis, prevention, and treatment.* New York: Plenum Press.

Milunsky, A. (1980). Prenatal detection of neural tube defects. VI. Experience with 20,000 pregnancies. *Journal of the American Medical Association, 244,* 2731–2735.

NICHD National Registry for Amniocentesis Study Group. (1976). Mid-trimester amniocentesis for prenatal diagnosis: Safety and accuracy. *Journal of the American Medical Association, 236,* 1471–1476.

Patrick, J.E., Perry, T.B., & Kinch, R.A. (1974). Fetoscopy and fetal blood sampling: A percutaneous approach. *American Journal of Obstetrics and Gynecology, 119,* 539–542.

Perret, Y.M. (1985). A woman's view of amniocentesis. *Great Expectations, 14,* 14–16.

Persson, P.H., Kullander, S., Gennser, G., et al. (1983). Screening for fetal malformations using ultrasound and measurements of alpha-fetoprotein in maternal serum. *British Medical Journal, 286,* 747–749.

Petres, R.E., & Redwine, F.O. (1982). Ultrasound in the intrauterine diagnosis and treatment of fetal abnormalities. *Clinical Obstetrics and Gynecology, 25,* 753–771.

Roberts, N.S., Dunn, L.K., Weiner, S., et al. (1983). Midtrimester amniocentesis. Indications, technique, risks, and potential for prenatal diagnosis. *Journal of Reproductive Medicine, 28,* 167–188.

Rodeck, C.H. (1982). Fetal blood sampling. *Birth defects, 18,* 255–261.

Rodeck, C.H., & Morsman, J.M. (1983). First-trimester chorion biopsy. *British Medical Bulletin, 39,* 338–342.

Rodeck, C.H., Nicolaides, K.H., Morsman, J.M., et al. (1983). A single-operator technique for first-trimester chorion biopsy. *Lancet, 2,* 1340–1341.

Roth, K.S., Yang, W., Allen, L., et al. (1982). Prenatal administration of biotin in biotin responsive multiple carboxylase deficiency. *Pediatric Research, 16,* 126–129.

Sanders, S.P., Chin, A.J., Parness, I.A., et al. (1985). Prenatal diagnosis of congenital heart defects in thoracoabdominally conjoined twins. *New England Journal of Medicine, 313,* 370–374.

Schwartz, D.B., Zweibel, W.J., Donovan, D., et al. (1983). Fetoscopic visualization in second trimester pregnancies. *American Journal of Obstetrics and Gynecology, 145,* 51–55.

Siggers, D.C. (1978). *Prenatal diagnosis of genetic disease.* Boston: Blackwell Scientific.

Simpson, N.E., Dallaire, L., Miller, J.R., et al. (1976). Prenatal diagnosis of genetic disease in Canada: Report of a collaborative study. *Canadian Medical Association Journal, 115,* 739–748.

Super, M., & Summers, E.M. (1982). Hazards of amniocentesis. *Lancet, 2,* 1459.

Verjaal, M., Leschot, N.J., & Treffers, P.E. (1981). Risk of amniocentesis and laboratory findings in a series of 1500 prenatal diagnoses. *Prenatal Diagnosis, 1,* 173–181.

Volodkevich, H., & Huether, C.A. (1981). Causes of low utilization of amniocentesis by women of advanced maternal age. *Social Biology, 28,* 176–187.

Wright, S.W., Day, R.W., Muller, H., et al. (1967). The frequency of trisomy and translocation in Down's syndrome. *Journal of Pediatrics, 70,* 420–424.

Chapter 4

Growth before Birth

Upon completion of this chapter, the reader will:
—understand the fertilization and implantation process
—be aware of the various stages of prenatal development
—be able to discuss the effects of maternal nutrition on fetal development
—know the various causes of malformations, including the different major teratogens
—be able to identify some of the causes of deformities
—be acquainted with some of the methods available to prevent birth defects

Many factors, both environmental and genetic, influence the formation of a human being from fertilization to birth. The environment in which the fetus grows is greatly affected by maternal health and nutrition. Radiation, drugs, and infections are a few of the factors that can contribute to the development of malformations. Genetically transmitted disorders can have equally devastating results. This chapter outlines prenatal development and describes how these various factors can lead to the birth of a child with developmental disabilities.

FERTILIZATION

An infant girl is born with 2 million oocytes, or immature ova. Over her lifetime, only about 500 of these will mature into fully developed eggs; by 45–55 years of age, all the remaining oocytes will have disappeared.

During a woman's reproductive years, one mature ovum typically ripens each month, is pushed from the ovary, and drops into the fallopian tube (Figure 4.1). Fertilization occurs about one-third of the way down the fallopian tube. If fertilization does not occur, the **menses** wash away the egg and the lining of the uterine wall. The cycle repeats itself unless conception takes place.

Unlike females, who are born with all the reproductive cells they will ever possess, males continue to produce sperm throughout their lives. With ejaculation during intercourse, hundreds of millions of sperm swim through the vagina to the cervix. Most of them die enroute. Midway through the woman's menstrual cycle, the

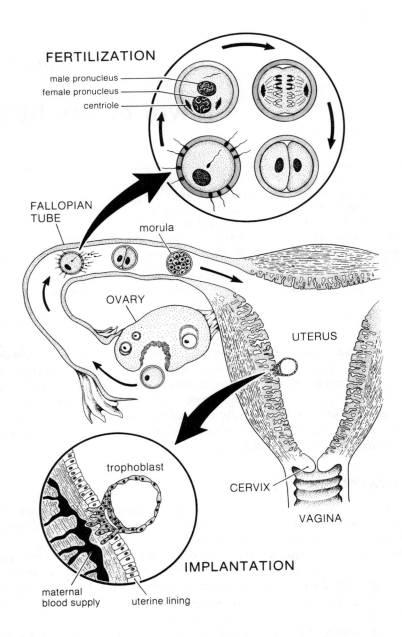

Figure 4.1.   Fertilization and implantation. The ovum or egg is dropped from the ovary into the fallopian tube where it is fertilized by a sperm. The fertilized egg regains its diploid number of chromosomes and starts dividing as it travels toward the uterus. It reaches the uterus after 7 days, and implantation of the embryo then takes place.

mucosal secretions of the vagina and cervix are thinned and easier to penetrate. If intercourse occurs at this time, the sperm have a better chance of reaching the egg and fertilizing it. Once the sperm have pushed through the cervix and into the uterus, a few thousand of them find their way to the correct fallopian tube. The journey is difficult, as they are swimming against the current created by the fallopian tube's **cilia**, the tiny, hairlike protrusions that help push the ova downward.

After the few hundred surviving sperm reach the egg, they poke and push at the egg's outer layer until one breaks through (see Figure 4.1). Why one sperm succeeds where another has failed is unclear. What is known is that once one sperm fertilizes the egg, another sperm cannot penetrate it. The rest of the sperm die within 24 hours.

Once inside the egg, the sperm nucleus quickly detaches from its **flagellum** and edges toward the ovum's nucleus. The two nuclei join, restoring to the fertilized egg the diploid number of 46 chromosomes (see Figure 4.1). Because the egg always contains an X chromosome, if the sperm nucleus also contains an X chromosome, a female (XX) will result. If the sperm carries a Y chromosome, a male (XY) will be produced.

On the rare occasion when two eggs instead of one are released simultaneously from the ovary and are both fertilized within a few days of each other, fraternal twins result. Although the twins share the same environment at the same time, they are as genetically distinct as any two siblings. Identical twins, on the other hand, result from a single fertilized egg that divides by chance into two separate organisms. They share the same environment and the same genetic inheritance. Yet, even they may differ because of external influences during pregnancy. For example, one may be better nourished and larger at birth than the other. The incidence of fraternal twins is 1 in 90 while the incidence of identical twins is 1 in 200 (Strandskov, 1945).

EMBRYOGENESIS

After fertilization, the egg quickly begins to divide, first into two, then four, then eight cells. At this stage, the group of multiplying cells is called the *morula*. By 5 days after conception, the cluster of cells, or **blastocyst**, contains over 50 cells. While all the cells start out as primitive, unspecialized units, they soon develop into three distinct layers: the ectoderm, the mesoderm, and the endoderm. The ectoderm evolves into skin, the spinal cord, and teeth. The mesoderm becomes blood vessels, muscles, and bone, and the endoderm turns into the digestive system, lungs, and urinary tract (Langman, 1975).

Seven days after conception, the *embryo,* appearing as a hollow cluster of cells, reaches the uterus. Only about half of all fertilized eggs survive to this point. When one does survive, it attaches itself to the wall of the uterus, beginning a process called **implantation** (see Figure 4.1). To ensure this process, the embryo produces a hormone, **chorionic gonadotrophin**, which prevents the mother from menstruating and sweeping away the microscopic embryo. The spongy layers of the uterine wall, rich in blood supply, allow the embryo to push its minute roots, or **villi**, alongside the maternal blood vessels that will feed it.

By the third week, a primitive placenta has formed, providing an improved means of supplying nutrition. Now oval-shaped, the embryo is beginning to round up at one end to form the brain (Figure 4.2). The pattern of development is from head to tail, or **cephalocaudal**. Surrounding the embryo is a layer that will form the amniotic sac. Fluid will gradually fill this sac to protect the embryo and keep it from drying out (Moore, 1977).

At the fourth week, the embryo is about half a centimeter long. Yet, its central nervous system is starting to develop, with the **neural tube** folding over to form the spinal cord (see Figure 4.2). The facial structure is also taking shape; six **pharyngeal** arches will join in the center to form lips, palate, and **mandible** or jaw.

The next week, the heart begins to form. It starts out as a U-shaped tube. Seven days later, after undergoing an incredible series of changes, it will be beating about 60 times a minute. Other organs are also experiencing swift changes. During this week, the limb buds become evident (see Figure 4.2). In only 35 days, the embryo has grown from one cell to more than 10,000.

Soon, the embryo begins to take on a more human form. During the second month, the internal body organs start to function. The system of blood vessels expands. The brain grows rapidly. Optic swellings at the side of the **forebrain**

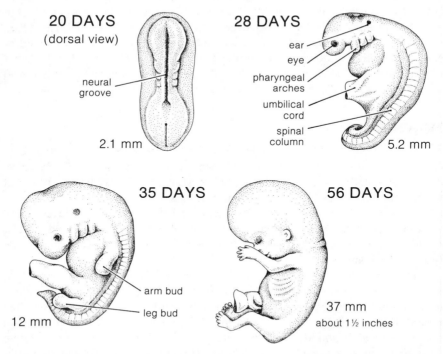

Figure 4.2. Embryogenesis. The changes that take place in the embryo from 3 to 8 weeks after fertilization are enormous. All systems are formed, and the embryo takes on a human fetal appearance. Length increases 20-fold during this time.

become eyes and move toward the center of the face. Eyebrows and the **retina** are evident. The primitive sexual organs are beginning to undergo meiotic division and produce primitive eggs and sperm. The embryo is now about 1½ inches long (Nilsson, 1974).

During this period of development, the changes are so precise and predictable that physicians can tell when certain congenital (birth) defects took place. For example, they know that if a child is born with a cleft palate, the defect occurred between days 35 and 37 of gestation, when the **palatal** arches normally close.

FETAL DEVELOPMENT

By the end of these 2 months, the embryo has become a *fetus* (see Figure 4.2). The next 7 months of fetal development are devoted to the refining and enlarging of the organs and body parts that formed during embryogenesis. In the third month, the fetus, although weighing only about an ounce, is active, kicking, and turning. The amniotic fluid, being produced in greater quantities now, measures approximately 8 ounces. This fluid is constantly recirculated, being swallowed by the fetus and then excreted as urine. During the fourth month, the fetus, weighing about 6 ounces and measuring about 10 inches in length, kicks with authority. This is when the mother usually begins to feel movement, called **quickening**. The heartbeat is also audible.

As growth continues, the placenta assumes more and more importance to the fetus. It acts as a barrier against the penetration of harmful substances and as a remover of waste materials, as well as a source of nutrition from the maternal circulation. It functions as lungs, kidneys, intestine, and liver for the fetus. Hormones produced by the placenta aid in the continuation of the pregnancy and, later, in the production of maternal milk.

Over the fifth and sixth months, refinement of development and growth continue. Fingernails form, and the skin becomes thicker. Muscle control improves, and movements become more purposeful. The fetus startles at loud noises, stretches, and moves about. By the end of the sixth month, the baby weighs about 2 pounds and is roughly 14 inches long. Most infants born at this time survive.

The final 3 months are mainly taken up with weight and height gain. The baby's weight usually increases to around 7 pounds. Length changes from 14 to 19 inches. The baby is so large now that he or she assumes a single position, usually head down, awaiting the termination of the pregnancy. Total reliance on the mother's body for food and protection will soon end.

MATERNAL NUTRITION

During development, the fetus gets all its nutrition from the mother. Adequate supplies of carbohydrates, protein, fat, vitamins, minerals, and water are needed for growth and metabolic maintenance as well as for the differentiation of new organ systems. The fetus, like a parasite, absorbs the nutrition it needs from the mother.

If the mother is malnourished, the main effect on the fetus is low birth weight (Naeye, Blanc, & Paul, 1973b). No increase in malformations or miscarriages seems to result. One study of such malnutrition provides an illustration. In Holland, in 1944, the Dutch organized a transportation strike against the occupying German forces. This limited the shipment of food from the countryside to the cities. Starvation was rampant. Pregnant women were placed on rations that provided only half their nutritional requirements. Yet, although their infants were small in size, they were otherwise well (Smith, 1947). The proportion of stillbirths, newborn deaths, and congenital malformations was no higher than usual. Twenty years later, follow-up studies showed the intellectual functioning of these children to be within normal limits (Stein & Susser, 1975). Thus, they were relatively resistant to the effects of maternal malnutrition. (This problem is discussed further in Chapter 9).

MALFORMATIONS

Although maternal malnutrition leaves the fetus relatively unharmed, other problems during pregnancy can result in severe malformations. Congenital malformations are defined as physical abnormalities of prenatal origin that are present at birth and that severely interfere with the child's normal development (Smith, 1982). Overall, they occur in approximately 3% of all births. These defects can result from genetic problems as well as from maternal infections, drugs, and other environmental teratogens (Kalter & Warkany, 1983).

Genetic Abnormalities

The two most common types of genetic problems are chromosomal abnormalities and single-gene defects, called *inborn errors*.

Chromosomal abnormalities are caused by three mechanisms: nondisjunction, deletion, and translocation (see Chapter 1). Approximately 1 in 500 newborns has such an abnormality. At least one disorder has been associated with virtually each of the 23 pairs of chromosomes (Creasy, Crolla, & Alberman, 1976). Most of the affected children have mental retardation, are short in stature, and unusual in appearance. Some have extra or lost **digits**; others have congenital heart defects.

Abnormalities resulting from single-gene defects can be equally devastating. As noted in Chapter 2, a mistake in decoding the DNA message of a single gene may lead to the production of a malfunctioning hemoglobin or enzyme. One example of this phenomenon is phenylketonuria (PKU). In this disorder, an enzyme necessary for the breakdown of the amino acid, phenylalanine, is not produced. Without this enzyme, phenylalanine accumulates and leads to severe brain damage during childhood. Fortunately, PKU in children can now be treated, and the children may have normal intellectual functioning (see Chapter 8). Unfortunately, if a woman who has PKU becomes pregnant, her fetus is at significant risk for having mental retardation, even though the fetus itself does not have the disorder. Although adults can tolerate high levels of phenylalanine, this substance is extremely toxic to the fetal brain. Pre-liminary results suggest that placing the woman back on the low phenylalanine diet used in her childhood may be successful in preventing mental retardation in her children (Lenke & Levy, 1980; Lipson, Beuhler, Bartley, et al., 1984).

Cell Migration Defects

Some disorders—for example, cleft lip, cleft palate, and spina bifida—do not result from a genetic problem but rather derive from defective cell migration.

Spina bifida can lead to significant disabilities. This incomplete formation of the spinal column occurs in about 3 per 1,000 live births. Instead of the primitive neural plate closing to form a tube, the cell migration is incomplete, and the tube remains open. The spinal nerves cannot grow beyond this **meningomyelocele** (Figure 4.3). Depending on the level of the interruption, nerve connections needed for walking and bowel and bladder control may be disrupted. In addition, hydrocephalus is a frequent

A. NORMAL EMBRYONIC DEVELOPMENT

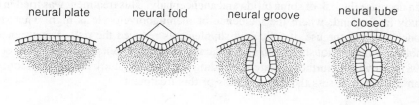

neural plate   neural fold   neural groove   neural tube closed

B. NORMAL SPINE AT BIRTH

C. SPINA BIFIDA

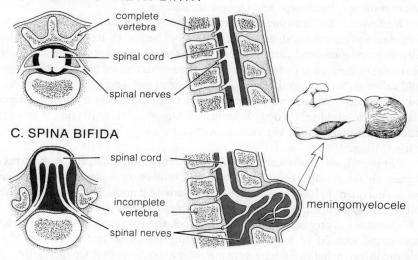

complete vertebra
spinal cord
spinal nerves

spinal cord
incomplete vertebra
spinal nerves
meningomyelocele

Figure 4.3.   Spina bifida. A) The normal formation of the spinal cord during the first month of gestation. B) Complete closure of the neural groove has occurred, and the spinal cord appears normal in cross-section on the left and in longitudinal section on the right. C) Incomplete closure leads to a split spine, spina bifida. As no nerves form below the abnormality, the child is paralyzed from the meningomyelocele downward.

complication because the open spine permits the lower portion of the brain to slip through the cranial vault into the spinal column, interfering with the circulation of the cerebrospinal fluid. This leads to an accumulation of fluid in the ventricles of the brain and enlargement of the head.

At birth, children with spina bifida are at risk for developing **meningitis** because of the open spinal cord. Decisions must be made quickly as to the course of action (Lorber, 1971; Smith & Smith, 1973). The split spine can be surgically repaired, preventing infection; a **shunt** can relieve the hydrocephalus. However, depending on the level of the **lesion**, the child may have normal intelligence but may never be able to walk or control bladder and bowel function.

Even more severe than spina bifida is **anencephaly**, another disorder that involves a lack of closure of the central nervous system. In anencephaly, major portions of the brain and skull are neither formed nor covered. Children with this disorder have profound retardation, and most of them die as newborns. Recently, research has suggested that supplements of the vitamin folic acid during pregnancy can decrease the risk of spina bifida and anencephaly. This treatment was tried in one study in England, where the incidence of meningomyelocele is high. That study concluded that the use of folic acid supplements reduced the risk of recurrence in mothers who previously had an affected child (Smithells, Sheppard, Schorah, et al., 1981). However, further research including a controlled study is needed before one can accurately assess the effectiveness of this treatment.

Teratogens

A teratogen is any agent that causes a defect in the fetus. Teratogens include radiation, drugs, infections, and chronic illnesses.

Radiation Radiation was the first agent shown to cause birth defects, initially in animals and later in survivors of Hiroshima and Nagasaki. Research studies found that a direct relationship existed between the distance a pregnant woman was from the focal point of the atomic bomb explosion in Hiroshima and the amount of damage her child suffered. Women who survived the explosion and were within a half-mile of it had miscarriages. Women who were about 1¼ miles out had a very high incidence of microcephalic children (Wood, Johnson, & Omori, 1967). Beyond 2 miles, the children were born healthy but were shown to have a high incidence of leukemia later in life (Miller, 1968).

No one is absolutely certain how much radiation is harmful to an expectant woman. On the average, people absorb about 2 **millisieverts** (the amount of radiation that is equivalent in biological effect to 100 **rads** of gamma rays) each year. About half of this exposure comes from medical X rays (Figure 4.4).

One study of pregnant women receiving **cobalt** treatment for cancer (up to 5,000 rads) found that 20 of their 75 infants were born with central nervous system abnormalities, including 16 who were microcephalic (Cooper & Cooper, 1966). This study and others have led physicians to be very cautious about their use of X rays in pregnant women. For example, women normally are not permitted to have abdominal X rays more than 2 weeks after their last period. Also, some of the diagnostic tests

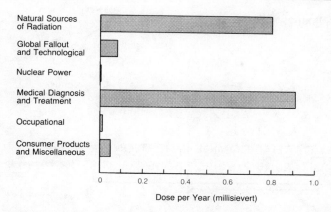

Figure 4.4.   Sources and doses of radiation in everyday life. (From Upton, A.C. [1982, February]. The biological effects of low-level ionizing radiation. *Scientific American, 246*, p. 42; reprinted by permission. Copyright © 1982 by Scientific American, Inc. All rights reserved.)

previously involving X rays, such as the measurement of fetal size, are now done with ultrasound.

Drugs   Drugs are another cause of fetal malformation. Although only a few drugs are highly teratogenic, a larger number may carry some increased risk of malformation. Most teratogenic effects are noted at birth but, in a few instances, the problems appear only in later childhood. Because of the uncertainty over the effects of a number of drugs, most doctors advise pregnant women to refrain, if possible, from taking any medication. Drugs about which teratogenic effects are known include thalidomide, **anticonvulsants**, anticancer drugs, sex hormones, acne medications, antibiotics, alcohol, and tobacco.

Thalidomide   The use of thalidomide for nausea during the first trimester of pregnancy was a common practice in Europe in the late 1950s. The drug was never released in the United States because the Food and Drug Administration has stricter rules about testing for teratogenic side effects. However, after the drug was released in Europe, it apparently had few obvious side effects, and it sold well to expectant mothers. A few years later, in 1961, a number of case reports began appearing in the European literature about a previously rarely reported fetal malformation, phocomelia. Affected children had shortened or missing arms and legs. An **epidemiological** study revealed that all the women with affected children had received thalidomide during their first trimester (McBride, 1961; Taussig, 1962). In addition, a relationship existed between the day of ingestion of the drug and the type of malformation. Taken between 21–35 days after conception, thalidomide resulted in babies born with shortened or missing arms. When expectant mothers took thalidomide between 23–30 days gestation, the children had shortened or missing legs and arms. After the 35th day, no defects occurred (Figure 4.5). Apparently, thalidomide prevented the normal formation of arm and leg buds between days 21–35 (Knapp,

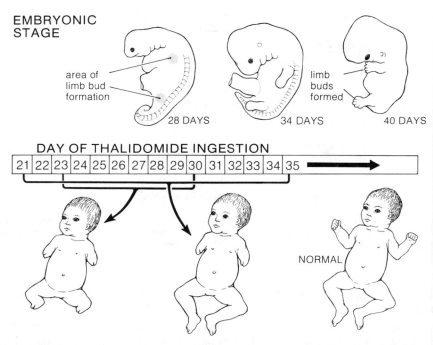

EMBRYONIC STAGE

area of limb bud formation

28 DAYS

limb buds formed

34 DAYS

40 DAYS

DAY OF THALIDOMIDE INGESTION

| 21 | 22 | 23 | 24 | 25 | 26 | 27 | 28 | 29 | 30 | 31 | 32 | 33 | 34 | 35 |

NORMAL

Figure 4.5. Effects of thalidomide at various gestational ages. Phocomelia resulted from ingestion of the drug thalidomide between 21 and 35 days after conception. The extent of the malformation depended on when the ingestion occurred.

Lenz, & Nowack, 1962). However, if the limb buds had already formed, no defects took place.

Anticonvulsants A number of drugs used to treat seizure disorders are thought to be teratogenic (American Academy of Pediatrics, 1979). Infants born to mothers with seizure disorders have been found to have a high incidence of cleft lip and palate (Barry & Danks, 1974). Initially, research focused on whether the seizures or the drugs used to treat them were responsible. The lack of oxygen or vigorous contractions during grand mal seizures might perhaps be the cause. More recent research studies (Hanson & Smith, 1975) have found that 10% of the children of mothers receiving Dilantin, a common anticonvulsant, had an unusual facial appearance and malformed arms and legs. Children born to mothers with epilepsy who were not receiving Dilantin did not have these abnormalities (American Academy of Pediatrics, 1979). Dilantin, therefore, was shown to be a teratogen.

The situation is less clear with other anticonvulsants. Phenobarbital, another frequently used anticonvulsant, has been shown to cause abnormalities in mice. Infant mice born to mothers treated with phenobarbital have smaller brains and more malformations that those born to untreated mice. Whether or not the drug has similar effects on humans is unknown. Two other anticonvulsants, Mysoline and Depakene, may also cause abnormalities. Mysoline has a chemical structure similar to that of phenobarbital and, thus, may carry comparable risks. Research has linked Depakene, or valproate, which is different chemically from other anticonvulsants, to an increased incidence of spina bifida (Bjerkedal, Czeizel, Goujard, et al., 1982). The rest of the anticonvulsants have not been used extensively enough to evaluate their teratogenic potential (Barry & Danks, 1974).

Unfortunately, discontinuing the use of all seizure medications puts a woman at risk for **convulsions** that may harm her or her fetus. At this point, many physicians stop using anticonvulsants in pregnant women who have infrequent seizures. For those who have severe epilepsy, the dosage of the drug is often lowered during the first trimester when the most harm to the fetus would occur.

Chemotherapeutic Agents   Anticancer drugs are harmful to embryos for different reasons than are anticonvulsant drugs. Since cancer cells grow more rapidly than do normal cells, the function of anticancer drugs is to injure or kill these rapidly dividing cells within the tumor. However, in a pregnant woman, the most rapidly dividing cells are those within the developing embryo. As the anticancer drugs can cross the placenta, a high incidence of malformations and miscarriages takes place. In the case of **methotrexate**, a commonly used anticancer drug, the infant's head and skeleton are malformed, as are the eyes and ears (Jick, Holmes, Hunter, et al., 1981). Other chemotherapeutic agents are also thought to lead to fetal malformations. As a result, therapeutic abortion is often suggested if anticancer therapy is needed during the first trimester of pregnancy.

Sex Hormones   In the past, estrogen and progesterone (female sex hormones) were used to prevent miscarriages in mothers who had a history of recurrent miscarriages. A number of malformations followed. The use of progesterone led to enlarged sexual glands in male and female infants. Even more sinister was the effect of DES, an estrogen used primarily in the early 1950s. Many females born to women who took DES during their pregnancies developed vaginal or cervical cancer some 20 years later (Herbst, 1981).

Acne Medication   Recently, studies have found that isotretinoin (Accutane), a vitamin-A product used to treat severe acne, results in **craniofacial** malformations (Rosa, 1983). Therefore, this medication should not be used either on the skin or orally during early pregnancy.

An antibiotic used to treat acne, called tetracycline, also can affect the fetus. Tetracycline leads to the staining of the teeth. Although both primary and permanent teeth do not emerge until much later, they are formed before birth. The defect results from the mixing of the tetracycline with calcium when the teeth are being formed. These stained teeth are at high risk for developing cavities because of defects in the **dentin**. Since many other safe antibiotics are available, pregnant women can easily avoid taking tetracycline.

Alcohol   The most frequently abused drug is alcohol. Its effect on the fetus is devastating. In the body, alcohol breaks down to form acetaldehyde, a highly toxic substance. The interaction of this substance with embryonic tissue probably causes malformations. In chronic alcoholics, the incidence of malformed children is at least 35% (Clarren & Smith, 1978). These infants have an unusual facial appearance with droopy eyelids, congenital heart defects, and are small in size. Most are found to have moderate mental retardation.

The question of the effect on the fetus of moderate or occasional drinking remains unanswered. The spectrum of malformations depends on the amount of alcohol ingested and whether the drinking occurs in binges (Streissguth, Landesman-Dwyer, Martin, et al., 1980). Physicians suggest refraining from drinking during early pregnancy.

Besides alcohol, other drugs such as LSD (McGlothlin, Sparkes, & Arnold, 1970) and heroin (Naeye, Blanc, Leblanc, et al., 1973a) are abused. No evidence indicates that these drugs cause fetal malformations. However, infants born to heroin addicts may suffer severe withdrawal symptoms in the newborn period that can lead to brain damage or death.

Tobacco   The main effect of smoking on the fetus seems to be low birth weight. A woman who smokes two packs a day, for example, will have an infant weighing about 1 pound less than that of a nonsmoker (Johnston, 1981). The number of cigarettes a woman smokes seems to be important. No fetal malformations have been associated with smoking.

Although the above mentioned drugs have been linked to problems in prenatal development, a number of drugs, so far, appear to be harmless. These include aspirin, penicillin, **acetaminophen** (Tylenol), and Benadryl, an **antihistamine** (Jick, Holmes, Hunter, et al., 1981). Also, studies have not found an association between coffee consumption and birth defects (Linn, Schoenbaum, Monson, et al., 1982).

Infections   Besides drugs, intrauterine infections can lead to fetal malformations. Unfortunately, while the placenta acts as a barrier to some harmful substances, it does not prevent the passing of drugs or infectious organisms from the mother to the embryo. A group of infections called TORCH infections all cause similar malformations (Nahmias, 1974). These include **toxoplasmosis** (Wilson, Remington, Stagno, et al., 1980), **syphilis, rubella, cytomegalovirus** (Pass, Stagno, Myers, et al., 1980), and **herpesvirus** (Hanshaw, 1973).

Rubella, or German measles, illustrates this problem (Tartakow, 1965). Before 1969, when a vaccine was developed, rubella epidemics occurred about every 8 years. The disease itself was innocuous. The women would develop a salmon-colored rash and a low-grade fever, both of which went away in a few days. Serious complications in adults rarely followed. Unfortunately, the harm was relegated to the embryo (Table 4.1). Scores of infants were born with blindness, deafness, microcephaly, mental retardation, **cerebral palsy**, and congenital heart defects (Miller, Cradock-Watson, & Pollock, 1982). The virus could be grown from the infants' urine or body tissues for up to 2 years after birth. This placed susceptible women who were nurses or health care workers at risk for contracting rubella.

As with thalidomide, the time of the infection is crucial. If the rubella infection occurs within a month before conception, the mother has a 42% risk of having an affected fetus. Between conception and 12 weeks, 52% of the fetuses develop a full-blown congenital rubella syndrome. Infection after 26 weeks usually results in a normal infant (Sever, Larsen, & Grossman, 1979).

Table 4.1. Pregnancy outcomes of mothers who had congenital rubella

	Age of infection	Percentage of affected infants
Preconception	0–28 days before conception	43
First trimester	0–12 weeks after conception	51
Second trimester	13–26 weeks after conception	23
Third trimester		0

Source: Sever, Hardy, Nelson, et al. (1969).

Since the development of the rubella vaccine, very few new cases of congenital rubella have occurred. This vaccine is given to all children between ages 1 and 2 years; immunity lasts throughout life. Women who have not received the vaccine should be tested for immunity. If they are not immune, they should receive the rubella vaccine before they try to become pregnant. After they are vaccinated, women should avoid becoming pregnant for 2 months (Preblud, Stetler, Frank, et al., 1981).

If a woman is not immune and contracts rubella during the first trimester of her pregnancy, she may be able to have an affected fetus diagnosed by amniocentesis (Daffos, Forestier, Grangeot-Keros, et al., 1984). At 18–20 weeks of gestation, the amniotic fluid can be tested for the presence of IgM, an **immunoglobulin** that the fetus produces to fight the rubella virus. If this substance is present in the fluid, the fetus has been infected. The mother could then decide whether or nor to terminate her pregnancy. As long as this antibody is not present in the fluid, even if the mother has the virus, the fetus is probably unharmed. Overall, in the United States, fewer than 100 children are born with congenital rubella each year (Miller, Cradock-Watson, & Pollock, 1982).

The story for the other TORCH infections is similar to that of rubella. In adults, a cytomegaloviral (CMV) infection might masquerade as a flu or **mononucleosis**-like illness. As many as 30%–60% of pregnant women have **antibodies** against this type of infection, indicating recent exposure (Montgomery, Youngblood, & Medearis, 1972). Between 2 and 20 per 1,000 live-born infants have sustained intrauterine infections from CMV (Pass, Stagno, Myers, et al., 1980). This compares with 0.1–0.5/1,000 for herpes, 0.5–1.0 for toxoplasmosis (Desmonts & Couvreur, 1974), and 0.2–0.5 for nonepidemic rubella (Sever, Larsen, & Grossman, 1979).

Because CMV infections are so widespread, they may be a significant cause of microcephaly and mental retardation. When a CMV infection occurs late in pregnancy, the primary effect is on hearing (Wilson, Remington, Stagno, et al., 1980). Postnatal CMV infections are not associated with any developmental handicaps (Kumar, Nankervis, Jacobs, et al., 1984). The incidence of these infections among pregnant women is so high that scientists are now working to develop a vaccine with the hope it will be as effective as the rubella vaccine (Elek & Stern, 1974).

In addition to the TORCH infections, the virus **varicella**, or chickenpox, has also been associated with fetal malformations. Although chickenpox is common and extremely contagious, the abnormalities it causes are both less severe and less common. Brain development is normal, but the fetus may have limb or facial abnormalities. A vaccine for this virus is now being tested (Arbeter, Starr, Weibel, et al., 1983).

Chronic Illness The most common chronic illness associated with an increased risk of malformations is diabetes. Fetuses of diabetic mothers have an increased incidence of growth delay as well as other complex problems including spina bifida, cardiovascular abnormalities, and malformations of one of the long bones of the leg, the femur (Haust, 1981). The cause is unknown. Well-controlled diabetics are at less risk for producing a child with these disorders than are diabetics under poor control (Pedersen & Molsted-Petersen, 1981).

DEFORMATIONS

So far, this chapter has focused on malformations or birth defects that occur during the first trimester of pregnancy. Deformations, on the other hand, refer to fetal abnormalities produced by uterine constraints during the third trimester. Unlike malformations, deformations are often reversible and are not usually genetically inherited.

A number of deformities result from the fetus simply not having enough room to move in the amniotic sac (Smith, 1982). For example, if the fetus does not have normal kidney function, very little amniotic fluid (most of which is comprised of fetal urine) will be produced. Without the buffering effect of the amniotic fluid, deformities of the chest wall or long bones can take place (Figure 4.6).

With **twinning**, crowding is more likely, and deformities are common. The human uterus was intended to carry one fetus. It may not be able to expand to the point of allowing free movement and kicking of two fetuses. The consequence might be a twisted or deformed foot (club foot) or a misshapen head that has been caught in one position (Clarren & Smith, 1977).

Certain deformities such as bowed legs will correct themselves when the child learns to walk. Orthopedic surgery or the placing of a cast can correct other bony deformities. Thus, deformities are isolated defects usually unassociated with developmental disabilities.

SUMMARY

A multitude of malformations and deformations exist that can create longstanding problems for a child. Of these, deformations are easier to correct. Treatment of malformations, on the other hand, is rather limited, and prevention seems to be the key (Scrimgeour, 1978).

The best protection against the teratogenic effects of drugs and radiation is the

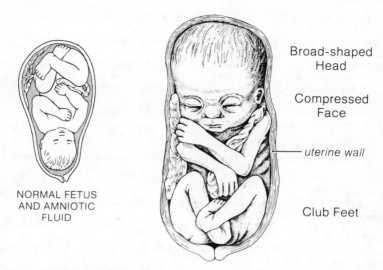

Broad-shaped
Head

Compressed
Face

—— uterine wall

NORMAL FETUS
AND AMNIOTIC
FLUID

Club Feet

Figure 4.6. Deformations. During the third trimester, insufficient amniotic fluid or a lack of fetal movement caused by inadequate room within the uterus may lead to bony deformities, including club foot.

limitation or avoidance of all but essential medications (Wilson, 1973), abstinence from alcohol, and the avoidance of radiation exposure during pregnancy.

To prevent congenital rubella infection, women may be tested for past rubella infection by checking their antibody level. If unprotected, nonpregnant women can be given a vaccine to immunize themselves against a future rubella infection (Krugman & Butz, 1974).

Even though treatment is limited for many of these conditions, it is important to realize that 20 years ago most of the reasons for these malformations were unknown, and prenatal diagnosis was unavailable.

REFERENCES

Aladjem, S., Brown, A.K., & Sureau, C. (Eds.). (1980). *Clinical perinatology* (2nd ed.). Saint Louis: C.V. Mosby Co.

American Academy of Pediatrics Committee on Drugs. (1979). Anticonvulsants and pregnancy. *Pediatrics, 63,* 331–333.

Arbeter, A.M., Starr, S.E., Weibel, R.E., et al. (1983). Live attenuated varicella vaccine: The KMcC strain in healthy children. *Pediatrics, 71,* 307–312.

Barry, J.E., & Danks, D.M. (1974). Anticonvulsants and congenital abnormalities. (Letter). *Lancet, 2,* 48–49.

Bjerkedal, T., Czeizel, A., Goujard, J., et al. (1982). Valproic acid and spina bifida. *Lancet, 2,* 1096.

Bolognese, R.J., Schwarz, R.H., & Schneider, J. (Eds.). (1982). *Perinatal medicine: Clinical management of the high risk fetus and neonate* (2nd ed.). Baltimore: Williams & Wilkins Co.

Charney, E.B., Weller, S.C., Sutton, L.N., et al. (1985). Management of the newborn with myelomeningocele: Time for a decision-making process. *Pediatrics, 75,* 58–64.

Clarren, S.K., & Smith, D.W. (1977). Congenital deformities. *Pediatric Clinics of North America, 24,* 665–677.

Clarren, S.K., & Smith, D.W. (1978). The fetal alcohol syndrome. *New England Journal of Medicine, 298,* 1063–1071.

Cooper, G., Jr., & Cooper, J.B. (1966). Radiation hazards to mother and fetus. *Clinical Obstetrics and Gynecology, 9,* 11–21.

Creasy, M.R., Crolla, J.A., & Alberman, E.D. (1976). A cytogenetic study of human spontaneous abortions using banding techniques. *Human Genetics, 31,* 177–196.

Daffos, F., Forestier, F., Grangeot-Keros, L., et al. (1984). Prenatal diagnosis of congenital rubella. *Lancet, 2,* 1–4.

Desmonts, G., & Couvreur, J. (1974). Congenital toxoplasmosis. A prospective study of 378 pregnancies. *New England Journal of Medicine, 290,* 1110–1116.

DiLiberti, J.H., Farndon, P.A., Dennis, N.R., et al. (1984). The fetal valproate syndrome. *American Journal of Medical Genetics, 19,* 473–481.

Elek, S.D., & Stern, H. (1974). Development of a vaccine against mental retardation caused by cytomegalovirus infection in utero. *Lancet, 1,* 1–5.

Elwood, J.M. (1983). Can vitamins prevent neural tube defects? *Canadian Medical Association Journal, 129,* 1088–1092.

Hanshaw, J.B. (1973). Herpesvirus hominis infections in the fetus and the newborn. *American Journal of Diseases of Children, 126,* 546–555.

Hanson, J.W., & Smith, D.W. (1975). The fetal hydantoin syndrome. *Journal of Pediatrics, 87,* 285–290.

Haust, M.D. (1981). Maternal diabetes mellitus—effects on the fetus and placenta. *Monographs in Pathology, 22,* 201–285.

Herbst, A.L. (1981). Clear cell adenocarcinoma and the current status of DES-exposed females. *Cancer, 48,* 484–488.

Jick, H., Holmes, L.B., Hunter, J.R., et al. (1981). First-trimester drug use and congenital disorders. *Journal of the American Medical Association, 246,* 343–350.

Johnston, C. (1981). Cigarette smoking and the outcome of human pregnancies: A status report on the consequences. *Clinical Toxicology, 18,* 189–209.

Kalter, H., & Warkany, J. (1983). Medical progress. Congenital malformations: Etiologic factors and their role in prevention. *New England Journal of Medicine, 308,* 424–431.

Knapp, K., Lenz, W., & Nowack, E. (1962). Multiple congenital abnormalities. *Lancet, 2,* 725.

Krugman, S., & Butz, S.L. (1974). Rubella immunization: A 5-year progress report. *New England Journal of Medicine, 290,* 1375–1376.

Kumar, M.L., Nankervis, G.A., Jacobs, I.B., et al. (1984). Congenital and postnatally acquired cytomegalovirus infections: Long-term follow-up. *Journal of Pediatrics, 104,* 674–679.

Langman, J. (1975). *Medical embryology: Human development—normal and abnormal* (3rd ed.). Baltimore: Williams & Wilkins Co.

Lenke, R.R., & Levy, H.L. (1980). Maternal phenylketonuria and hyperphenylalaninemia. An international survey of the outcome of treated and untreated pregnancies. *New England Journal of Medicine, 303,* 1202–1208.

Linn, S., Schoenbaum, S.C., Monson, R.R., et al. (1982). No association between coffee consumption and adverse outcomes of pregnancy. *New England Journal of Medicine, 306,* 141–145.

Lipson, A., Beuhler, B., Bartley, J., et al. (1984). Maternal hyperphenylalaninemia fetal effects. *Journal of Pediatrics, 104,* 216–220.

Lorber, J. (1971). Results of treatment of myelomeningocele. An analysis of 524 unselected cases, with special reference to possible selection for treatment. *Developmental Medicine and Child Neurology, 13,* 279–303.

McBride, W.G. (1961). Thalidomide and congenital abnormalities. *Lancet, 2,* 1358.

McGlothlin, W.H., Sparkes, R.S., & Arnold, D.O. (1970). Effect of LSD on human pregnancy. *Journal of the American Medical Association, 212,* 1483–1487.

McLaughlin, J.F., Shurtleff, D.B., Lamers, J.Y., et al. (1985). Influence of prognosis on decisions regarding the care of newborns with myelodysplasia. *New England Journal of Medicine, 312,* 1589–1594.

Miller, E., Cradock-Watson, J.E., & Pollock, T.M. (1982). Consequences of confirmed maternal rubella at successive stages of pregnancy. *Lancet, 2,* 781–784.

Miller, E., Hare, J.W., Cloherty, J.P., et al. (1981). Elevated maternal Hemoglobin A1c in early pregnancy and major congenital anomalies in infants of diabetic mothers. *New England Journal of Medicine, 304,* 1331–1334.

Miller, R.W. (1968). Effects of ionizing radiation from the atomic bomb on Japanese children. *Pediatrics, 41*, 257–270.

Milunsky, A., Graef, J.W., & Gaynor, M.F., Jr. (1968). Methotrexate induced congenital malformations. *Journal of Pediatrics, 72*, 790–795.

Montgomery, R., Youngblood, L., & Medearis, D.N., Jr. (1972). Recovery of cytomegalovirus from the cervix in pregnancy. *Pediatrics, 49*, 524–531.

Moore, K.L. (1977). *The developing human* (2nd ed.). Philadelphia: W.B. Saunders Co.

Naeye, R.L., Blanc, W., Leblanc, W., et al. (1973a). Fetal complications of maternal heroin addiction: Abnormal growth, infections, and episodes of stress. *Journal of Pediatrics, 83*, 1055–1061.

Naeye, R.L., Blanc, W., & Paul, C. (1973b). Effects of maternal nutrition on the human fetus. *Pediatrics, 52*, 494–503.

Nahmias, A.J. (1974). The TORCH complex. *Hospital Practice, 9*, 65–72.

Nilsson, L. (1974). *Behold man*. Boston: Little, Brown & Co.

Pass, R.F., Stagno, S., Myers, G.J., et al. (1980). Outcome of symptomatic congenital cytomegalovirus infection: Results of long-term longitudinal follow-up. *Pediatrics, 66*, 758–762.

Pedersen, J.F., & Molsted-Petersen, L. (1981). Early fetal growth delay detected by ultrasound marks increased risk of congenital malformation in diabetic pregnancy. *British Medical Journal, 283*, 269–271.

Preblud, S.R., Stetler, H.C., Frank, J.A., et al. (1981). Fetal risk associated with rubella vaccine. *Journal of the American Medical Association, 246*, 1413–1417.

Quilligan, E.J., & Kretchmer, N. (Eds.). (1980). *Fetal and maternal medicine*. New York: John Wiley & Sons.

Rosa, F.W. (1983). Teratogenicity of isotretinoin. *Lancet, 2*, 513.

Scrimgeour, J.B. (Ed.). (1978). *Towards the prevention of fetal malformations*. Edinburgh: Edinburgh University Press.

Sever, J.L., Hardy, J.B., Nelson, K.B., et al. (1969). Rubella in the collaborative perinatal research study. *American Journal of Diseases of Children, 118*, 123–132.

Sever, J.L., Larsen, J.W., Jr., & Grossman, J.H. III. (1979). *Handbook of perinatal infections*. Boston: Little, Brown & Co.

Slone, D., Siskind, V., Heinonen, O.P., et al. (1976). Aspirin and congenital malformations. *Lancet, 1*, 1373–1375.

Smith, C.A. (1947). Effects of maternal undernutrition upon the newborn infant in Holland (1944–1945). *Journal of Pediatrics, 30*, 229–243.

Smith, D.W., with assistance of Jones, K.L. (1982). *Recognizable patterns of human malformation: Genetic, embryologic, and clinical aspects* (3rd ed.). Philadelphia: W.B. Saunders Co.

Smith, G.K., & Smith, E.D. (1973). Selection for treatment in spina bifida cystica. *British Medical Journal, 4*, 189–197.

Smithells, R.W., Sheppard, S., Schorah, C.J., et al. (1981). Apparent prevention of neural tube defects by periconceptional vitamin supplementation. *Archives of Disease in Childhood, 56*, 911–918.

Stein, Z., & Susser, M. (1975). The Dutch famine, 1944–45, and the reproductive process. I. Effects or six indices at birth. *Pediatric Research, 9*, 70–76.

Stevenson, R.E. (1977). *The fetus and newly born infant: Influences of the prenatal environment*. St. Louis: C.V. Mosby Co.

Strandskov, H.H. (1945). Plural birth frequencies in the total, the "white," and "colored" U.S. population. *American Journal of Physical Anthropology, 3*, 49–57.

Streissguth, A.P., Landesman-Dwyer, S., Martin, J.C., et al. (1980). Teratogenic effects of alcohol in humans and laboratory animals. *Science, 209*, 353–361.

Tartakow, I.J. (1965). The teratogenicity of maternal rubella. *Journal of Pediatrics, 66*, 380–391.

Taussig, H.B. (1962). Thalidomide—A lesson in remote effects of drugs. *American Journal of Diseases of Children, 104*, 111–113.

Upton, A.C. (1982). The biological effects of low-level ionizing radiation. *Scientific American, 246*, 41–49.

Wilson, C.B., Remington, J.S., Stagno, S., et al. (1980). Development of adverse sequelae in children born with subclinical congenital Toxoplasma infection. *Pediatrics, 66*, 767–774.

Wilson, J.G. (1973). Present status of drugs as teratogens in man. *Teratology, 7*, 3–15.

Wood, J.W., Johnson, K.G., & Omori, Y. (1967). *In utero* exposure to the Hiroshima atomic bomb. An evaluation of head size and mental retardation: Twenty years later. *Pediatrics, 39*, 385–392.

Chapter 5

Having a Baby
The Birth Process

Upon completion of this chapter, the reader will:
—know the stages of labor and how long each lasts
—be able to identify and characterize the maternal factors that cause problems during labor and delivery
—be aware of the infant factors that cause problems during labor and delivery
—know the preventive and monitoring measures that help ensure safer deliveries

---

Approximately 266 days after conception, a complex series of events leads to the birth of an infant. It is remarkable that so much is known about the developing fetus, yet so little is understood about the process of labor. By an as yet unidentified mechanism, the mother's immune system tolerates the fetus and allows it to remain inside her and grow. Then, when it is time for the child to be born, another directive tells the mother's body to reject the fetus, and labor begins.

Whatever triggers the process, about 85% of women deliver within 7 days on either side of their due date (called the **estimated date of confinement** or **EDC**). This date is calculated by counting back 3 months from the first day of the last menstrual period and adding 7 days. For example, a pregnant woman whose last period began on March 8 would be due around December 15. About this date, she would begin the early stages of labor.

LABOR

The first stage of labor starts with fairly mild contractions, which may be confused with the **Braxton-Hicks** contractions that occur throughout pregnancy. Within hours, however, the contractions become stronger, last longer, and are more frequent. This prolonged stage, often lasting from 12 to 30 hours, allows time for the baby's head to get molded into position for delivery.

To understand this better, it is important to go back a bit in fetal development. By the sixth month, in about 90% of the cases, the baby has settled head first into the mother's pelvis. It is unlikely the baby will shift further. This is called the **vertex position**. At this time, the mother's bony pelvic girdle is closed, making it difficult for the fetus to proceed further down the birth canal. The extended period of time during the first stage of labor allows for the gradual molding of the baby's head to fit the birth canal, the spreading of the pelvic bones, and the opening of the cervix.

During the second stage, the baby's head pushes through the birth canal and appears at the vaginal opening. The cervix becomes fully dilated during this stage, which usually lasts about an hour.

The third stage, lasting about 10–15 minutes, ends with the complete expulsion, or birth, of the newborn (Sciarra, 1977). The infant's nose and mouth are immediately suctioned and, in 9 out of 10 cases, the mother is presented with a ruddy-cheeked, screaming, healthy baby. But what of the remaining 10%?

PROBLEMS DURING LABOR AND DELIVERY

Problems during labor and delivery may rest with either the mother or the infant (Table 5.1). However, maternal factors present the majority of problems.

Maternal Factors

Infants of disadvantaged, teenage, and middle-age women are at the greatest risk (Babson & Clarke, 1978). Often, the disadvantaged or teenage pregnant woman has received little prenatal care. Her nutrition may also have been inadequate during pregnancy. The combination of these factors increases her chances of having premature labor and of producing an infant who is small in size (Zuckerman, Walker, Frank, et al., 1984). The mother over 35 years of age and the teenage mother also have a greater likelihood of developing **toxemia** and of having placental

Table 5.1.   Number of perinatal deaths per 1,000 births in the United States by cause

Cause	Stillbirths	Infants 0–28 days old
Maternal infection	2.0	41.0
Abruptio placenta	2.5	1.3
Placenta previa	0.3	0.5
Congenital malformations	1.1	2.3
Rh incompatibility	1.1	0.4
Umbilical cord compression	1.1	0.2
Birth trauma	0.1	0.5
Incompetent cervix	0.1	0.1
Cesarean section	0.0	0.3
Diagnosis unknown	4.9	2.5

Source: Naeye (1977).

insufficiency; this increases their baby's chance of having a low birth weight because of intrauterine growth retardation.

Infants of women with chronic diseases, such as diabetes, hypertension, or thyroid disease, also have more complications. In addition, maternal infections increase the chances for problems. Finally, women with obstetrical problems such as an incompetent cervix, uterine fibroids, or a previous **placenta previa** (see discussion later in this chapter) tend to have repeated troubles in labor and delivery.

Chronic Maternal Illness Probably the most worrisome chronic illness is diabetes (White, 1965). Uncontrolled diabetes leads to a very high rate of prematurity and stillbirths. Even with good control, through the use of diet, drugs, or insulin, there are a number of significant risks to the infant of a diabetic mother. First, diabetic mothers are prone to toxemia (see discussion later in this chapter). Second, their infants are born large in size, but with immature body organs because they often are born prematurely. Lastly, because the fetal pancreas has been overproducing insulin to supply both the mother and the infant, the amount of insulin in the baby remains high after birth and results in a low blood sugar level, or **hypoglycemia** (Ayromlooi, Zervoudakis, & Sadaghat, 1973).

Infants of women with other chronic illnesses, such as thyroid disease (Ayromlooi, Zervoudakis, Sadaghat, 1973), kidney disease, heart disease, and hypertension, seem to have fewer problems. However, these children still run the risks associated with being born small in size because of prematurity or growth retardation.

Acute Maternal Illness Chapter 4 described some of the effects of maternal infections on the developing embryo. At the time of labor and delivery, a maternal infection presents different problems. Bacterial or viral infections can no longer cause malformations, but they can be transmitted from the mother to the relatively immune-deficient newborn, sometimes with fatal results.

An example of this is the *herpesvirus* infection of the vagina. Vaginal herpes is characterized by blisters and oozing lesions in the vagina. Treatment of this infection with the anti-viral drug, Acyclovir, has been successful in most cases (Mindel, Adler, Sutherland, et al., 1982). Infants born to mothers with untreated herpes are at risk for developing the infection which can spread throughout the body, causing death in about 60% of affected infants (Kibrick, 1980). Of the survivors, half will have significant neurological deficits.

Unfortunately, Acyclovir is less effective in treating **systemic** herpes in the newborn than in treating vaginal herpes. Therefore, to try to protect the baby from contracting the virus, the obstetrician will take the precaution of delivering the baby by cesarean section.

While viral infections are usually contracted during delivery, bacterial infections more commonly develop during the first week of life. One of the most feared is group B streptococcal **sepsis** (Franciosi, Knostman, & Zimmerman, 1973). *Sepsis* is the term used to describe a bacterial infection spread by the blood throughout the body. It may also be called *blood poisoning*. The mortality rate from sepsis ranges from 10% to 50%, depending on what organism causes the infection and how early it is detected and treated. If an infant has symptoms of an infection—for example, lethargy, an unstable temperature, and poor feeding—the pediatrician will place him or her on **intravenous** antibiotics for a few days. Blood cultures are obtained and, if an infection is confirmed, treatment continues for 1 to 3 weeks.

Toxemia Toxemia, or pregnancy-induced hypertension, may develop slowly or come about very quickly. This syndrome, consisting of high blood pressure, **edema**, and protein in the urine, is experienced more often by teenage and middle-age women. About 10% of these women develop toxemia at some time during the second and third trimesters of pregnancy (Hellman & Pritchard, 1971). Bedrest and medication can lower the blood pressure, reduce the edema, and prevent seizures. Yet, the risk of prematurity and of low birth weight remains. Uncontrolled toxemia leads to a high incidence of stillbirths. In these cases, the obstetrician may be forced to induce labor or to perform a cesarean section even if the infant is premature.

Placenta Previa and Abruptio Placenta Normally, the placenta is attached high up in the uterus. In placenta previa, the placenta is implanted low in the uterus and lies over the cervical opening (Figure 5.1). The more extensive the overlay, the greater is the risk of bleeding as the cervix opens. If the amount of bleeding is extensive, it may imperil fetal circulation and lead to brain damage or death.

As with toxemia, placenta previa commonly occurs during the final months of pregnancy. During that time, it is the most common cause of vaginal hemorrhage. Although the incidence during pregnancy is low, being 1/200 pregnancies, the fetal mortality rate is high, 15% (Naeye & Tafari, 1983). Placenta previa is more common in women over 35 and in women who have had many previous pregnancies. Women who have had placenta previa once will have about a 6% chance of recurrence during subsequent pregnancies. The cause of placenta previa is unclear. Some physicians

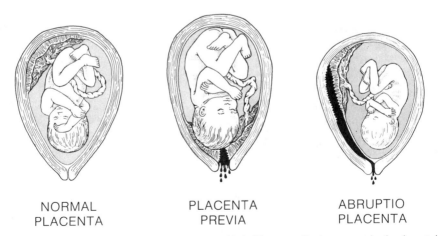

NORMAL PLACENTA   PLACENTA PREVIA   ABRUPTIO PLACENTA

Figure 5.1. A normal placenta is located in the upper third of the uterus. In placenta previa, the placenta is abnormally placed so that it lies over the cervical opening. During labor, as the cervix dilates, the placenta tears and bleeding occurs. In abruptio, a normally placed placenta becomes partially separated from the uterine wall in the second or third trimester, and bleeding results.

speculate that it may relate to defective uterine blood supply as a result of uterine inflammation or **atrophy**. In these conditions, the placenta must branch out to get adequate nutrition and thus may extend its "roots" over the cervical opening.

Women with placenta previa in the second trimester are advised to get plenty of bedrest so that they can carry the fetus as long as possible. A cesarean section is frequently performed when it is determined the fetus is mature enough to survive outside the uterus (Crenshaw, Jones, & Parker, 1973). If the baby were born vaginally, the opening of the cervix during labor might burst the overlying blood vessels and lead to severe blood loss.

While placenta previa is a condition involving the abnormal placement of the placenta in the uterus, **abruptio placenta** involves a precipitous detachment of a normally placed placenta (see Figure 5.1). This happens during the second or third trimester. Although abruptio placenta occurs in only about 1/500 pregnancies, the fetal mortality rate is close to 50%. This condition most commonly occurs in women with toxemia, in women who carry fetuses with short umbilical cords, or in women who have undergone physical **trauma** such as a car accident (Crosby, 1974). Unlike placenta previa, age does not seem to be a factor, although multiple previous pregnancies do increase the risk (Niswander, Friedman, Hoover, et al., 1966a).

Symptoms of an abruption include profuse vaginal bleeding, decreased fetal heart sounds, and a tightly contracted uterus. The baby will die unless removed immediately. The mother also may go into shock due to a loss of blood.

Dystocia Besides the problems of infection, toxemia, and placental placement, structural abnormalities of the uterus or pelvis, called **dystocia**, may cause premature or prolonged labor with detrimental effects on the fetus.

The most common bony abnormality is *cephalopelvic disproportion* (CPD), meaning the maternal pelvis is too small to allow passage of the baby's head. This leads to labor that does not progress normally. To determine if CPD exists, an obstetrician may permit a short "trial of labor" before a decision is made to proceed with a spontaneous delivery, or to use forceps, or to perform a cesarean section. This avoids the risk of brain damage to the infant caused by the lack of oxygen that might occur during such a prolonged labor (Niswander, 1983).

In another structural problem, **uterine fibroid tumors** may take up space in the uterus and lead to placenta previa. They may also interfere with the normal position of the fetus (head first) so that a breech position (backside first) results.

In addition, in rare cases, a woman may have a double-chambered, or **bicornuate**, uterus (Figure 5.2). This may also impede fetal growth and influence the labor process.

An *incompetent cervix* is an equally serious problem that may cause prematurity and miscarriage (Willson, Carrington, & Ledger, 1983). This term refers to a cervix that dilates during the second trimester of pregnancy; it is incapable of staying closed properly until term is reached. To allow the woman to carry her child the complete 9 months, an incompetent cervix may be closed temporarily with a **suture**. The woman may also need to remain in bed for the rest of the pregnancy.

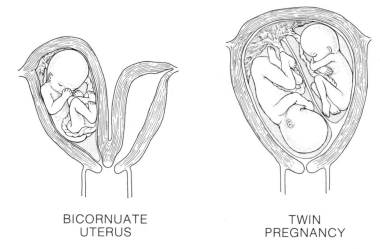

BICORNUATE UTERUS   TWIN PREGNANCY

Figure 5.2.   Two causes of fetal crowding and growth disturbance are a bicornuate uterus and twin pregnancy. Note that the second twin to be born is often smaller than the first and is in a breech position.

Infant Factors

The most common infant factors affecting labor and delivery are breech delivery, birth defects, multiple pregnancies, and prolapsed umbilical cord.

   Breech Delivery   In a breech delivery, the baby is born backside first instead of head first. This presents a problem because the baby's head is the widest part. When a baby is born head first, or in the vertex position, the head is gradually molded during labor to fit the narrow pelvic opening. In a breech birth, the backside comes through without difficulty, but the baby's head may get stuck. A prolonged labor and brain damage to the baby may result (Brenner, Bruce, & Hendricks, 1974). Therefore, when a baby is breech, and a difficult delivery is anticipated, a physician will often perform a cesarean section.

   Birth Defects   Certain intrinsic abnormalities in the fetus may lead to problems with labor and delivery. For example, an infant who has **osteogenesis imperfecta**, an inherited birth defect causing brittle bones, may suffer multiple fractures or even die of a skull fracture during the birth process. Another example is the child with congenital hydrocephalus. The hydrocephalus itself may cause brain damage. In addition, the enlarged head may make vaginal delivery impossible. If this is not recognized quickly, the baby may suffer further injury from **hypoxia**, lack of oxygen.

   A number of other defects can lead to the death of an infant, even without an abnormal labor. Five percent of stillborn infants have been found to have a major chromosomal abnormality (Valdes-Dapena & Arey, 1970). These infants may have malformations of the heart, lungs, and brain that are incompatible with survival.

   Brain abnormalities, unassociated with chromosomal problems, may also lead to the newborn's death. One of these is anencephaly. In anencephaly, the **cortex** of the brain is missing, and the infant rarely survives for long after birth.

Multiple Pregnancies Multiple pregnancies present a problem that is unrelated to either fetal or maternal abnormalities. Human beings, as is true of other two-breasted mammals, are designed to produce a single offspring from a pregnancy. When a woman is carrying more than one fetus, the uterine space is crowded, and problems can develop.

Twins account for about 1% of all births. The major complications associated with twins are prematurity, toxemia, and difficult deliveries. About 40% of the time, the second twin is lying in a breech position at the time of delivery (Cameron, 1968) (see Figure 5.2). This contrasts with single pregnancies where only 3% of the babies are in a breech position. The first twin gets out rapidly and without distress. Twin B, however, must wait a turn and then come out backward without proper molding of the head. As already discussed above, this increases the risk of brain injury.

Prolapsed Umbilical Cord Besides the already-mentioned problems associated with multiple pregnancies, the likelihood of a prolapsed umbilical cord is also higher in twins than in single pregnancies. This happens when the umbilical cord is below the fetus and precedes the fetus down the birth canal (Niswander, Friedman, Hoover, et al., 1966c). This can result in a blockage of the flow of blood through the cord to the child and may lead to brain damage. Prolapsed cord is considered to be a surgical emergency and requires an immediate cesarean section.

PREVENTIVE MEASURES

Based on this chapter's description, the process of labor and delivery seems extremely risky and unpredictable. However, it is important to remember that this chapter has concentrated on 10% of the deliveries; the remaining 90% proceed smoothly. Furthermore, certain preventive and monitoring measures now exist that have reduced the risk of stillbirths from a rate of 2.5% to that of 1.2% over the past 20 years. The major procedures include amniocentesis, ultrasound, uterine monitoring devices, fetal scalp electrodes, and cesarean section.

Amniocentesis

The most common uses of amniocentesis were discussed in Chapter 3. However, the procedure is also valuable during the final trimester of pregnancy to assess the maturity of the fetus and to determine the presence of Rh incompatibility.

Fetal maturity is assessed by measuring two chemicals present in the amniotic fluid, **lecithin** (L) and **sphingomyelin** (S) (Amenta & Silverman, 1983). These two chemicals are necessary to produce **surfactant**, the compound needed to keep the newborn infant's lungs expanded and functioning properly. Researchers have found that the ratio of concentration of these two chemicals (called the L/S ratio) changes as the infant approaches maturity. Measuring these two chemicals enables the physician to estimate lung maturity. Since the most common problem of premature infants is respiratory distress syndrome (RDS), which is caused by immature lungs, the ability to evaluate lung maturity is extremely useful. If the L/S ratio is more than 2:1, the infant should be near term, and the lungs should be maturing. Lower ratios indicate immature lungs and a greater risk for RDS (Figure 5.3).

Another group of infants for whom this is especially valuable is infants of diabetics. As stated earlier, these infants are large for their gestational age. Thus, the uterine size may appear to be at full term when the infant is actually premature. By measuring the L/S ratio in the amniotic fluid of the mother, a decision about when to deliver the baby can be made, and the risk of prematurity is decreased.

Although amniocentesis now has many functions, it was initially used to determine Rh incompatibility (Walker & Jennison, 1962). It was discovered that **bilirubin**, a yellow pigment, is present in the amniotic fluid of Rh− women who are carrying sensitized Rh+ children (see Chapter 6). This pigment accumulates when there is a breakdown of a large number of red blood cells. High levels of bilirubin indicate that the fetus is very **anemic** and at risk for brain damage or death before birth. By repeatedly measuring the amount of bilirubin present in the amniotic fluid, the physician can tell if the baby is seriously ill and can then perform an intrauterine blood transfusion, if necessary, to correct the anemia and preserve the child (Liley, 1965). The physician may also need to consider early delivery of the child and treatment with exchange blood transfusions.

Besides amniocentesis, other prenatal diagnostic tools such as fetoscopy, discussed in Chapter 3, and **amnioscopy** can be useful during labor. In amnioscopy, the physician can look through the amniotic membrane to see the infant.

Ultrasound

Ultrasound has taken the place of X rays in the monitoring of fetal development, primarily because the sound waves used in ultrasound do not appear to be hazardous

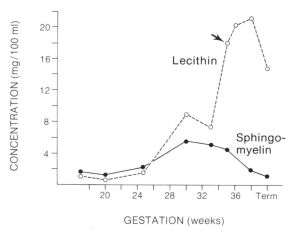

Figure 5.3.   Concentration of lecithin (L) and sphingomyelin (S) in the amniotic fluid. Note that at 34–35 weeks, the L/S ratio is more than 2:1, indicating that adequate surfactant is being produced. Respiratory distress syndrome (RDS) is less likely to develop after this stage, and a safe delivery is possible. (From Gluck, L., Kulovich, M.V., Borer, R.C., et al. [1971]. Diagnosis of the respiratory distress syndrome by amniocentesis. *American Journal of Obstetrics and Gynecology, 109,* 440; reprinted by permission.)

to the infant, whereas the safety of radiation is less certain (Thompson, 1974). One example is the use of ultrasound to visualize two skulls in a twin pregnancy rather than using an abdominal X ray to see two sets of fetal parts (Figure 5.4). Ultrasound is also used to identify placental placement (normal, previa, or abruptio), to monitor the growth of the fetus, to determine the gender of the fetus, and to diagnose congenital anomalies.

Monitoring Uterine Contractions and Fetal Heart Rate

Amniocentesis and ultrasound are tools used prior to labor. Once labor begins, the uterine contractions can be monitored.

With each uterine contraction, physiological changes occur in the fetus. This is indicated by changes in the fetal heart rate which can be recorded. The contractions begin in the cervix and move upward, eventually reaching the **fundus uteri**, or top of the uterus. When a contraction starts, the infant's heart rate begins to decrease. A severe slowing of the heart rate, called **bradycardia**, and its prolonged duration show that the infant is in distress. The monitoring is done by placing a probe on the mother's abdomen. This permits the simultaneous recordings of the uterine muscle contractions and the fetal heart rate (Figure 5.5). Normally, during each contraction, the fetal heart rate drops about 25%, from approximately 160 to 120 beats per minute. As the contraction subsides, the rate returns to normal (Schwarcz, Belizan, Cifuentes, et al., 1974).

When certain problems with the labor exist—for example, an abruptio placenta—the pattern of decline and return of the fetal heart rate is different. In

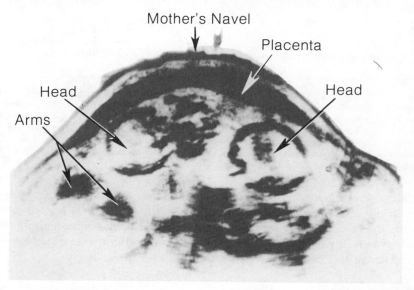

Figure 5.4. Ultrasound of a pregnant woman carrying twins. This is a cross-section view through the maternal abdomen. The two fetal heads and the placenta lie just under the uterine wall. Fetal arms are also defined. (Courtesy of Dr. Roger Sanders, The Johns Hopkins Hospital, Baltimore.)

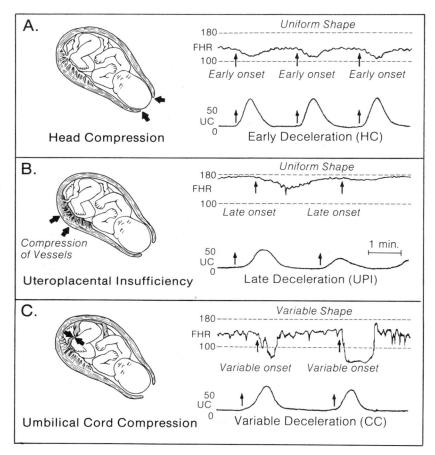

Figure 5.5. Fetal monitoring. A) Early deceleration of the heart rate is a normal accompaniment to uterine contractions during labor. It results from compression of the fetal head. B) Late heart deceleration occurs if the placental blood vessels are abnormally pressed together during the end of the uterine contraction. C) Variable deceleration of the heart. This abnormal finding of early, mid, and late deceleration suggests compression and obstruction of the umbilical cord circulation during labor. (UC, uterine contraction; FHR, fetal heart rate, beats/minute.) (Redrawn with permission from: Hon, E. [1968]. *An atlas of fetal heart rate patterns.* New Haven, CT: Harty.)

abruptio, the heart rate decline occurs late during the contraction and lasts longer. With umbilical cord compression, the decline in the heart rate is profound, prolonged, and occurs at various times during the contractions. By recognizing these problems early, a physician may regulate the labor or perform a cesarean section to prevent severe loss of oxygen to the fetus.

Fetal Scalp Electrode

Another recent technique is the use of a fetal scalp electrode. When a woman is in the second stage of labor, the infant's head appears in the birth canal. At this time, a fetal scalp electrode can be placed just under the skin of the baby's scalp. The electrode measures the fetal heart rate more directly.

Cesarean Section

The cesarean operation has been mentioned throughout this chapter as a means of saving the child when problems arise. However, it is overused. Of all deliveries, 50% are spontaneous vaginal ones, 25% require the use of forceps, and 25% are done by cesarean section (Niswander, 1981). Since only about 10% of pregnancies are threatened by the problems discussed in this chapter, some cesarean sections are done for less important reasons, such as the convenience of the mother or the physician. Even the previously followed rule of performing repeated cesarean sections once a mother had one delivery by cesarean is now in question. Many obstetricians will permit a trial of labor in a woman who had a previous cesarean section.

It should be stressed that a cesarean section for fetal distress is lifesaving; other uses are less well justified. Certain risks exist with cesarean sections, both to the infant and to the mother. First, infants delivered by cesarean section under general anesthesia are more lethargic than are those delivered vaginally (Fisher & Paton, 1974). Second, respiratory distress is more likely. This is because the infant does not undergo the first stage of labor during which the uterine contractions squeeze most of the fluid from the fetal lungs. Thus, infants delivered by cesarean section have "wet lungs." For the mother, the problems include the risk of anesthesia, possible infection, and bleeding. Taking these possible complications into account, the infant mortality rate due to cesarean section delivery is 0.3/1,000, a small but not insignificant number.

SUMMARY

The period of labor and delivery is a critical one for the normal development of the infant. Complications can result from such divergent sources as toxemia, cephalopelvic disproportion, and placenta previa or from the existence of twins, hydrocephalus, or congenital malformations. All these complications may lead to premature delivery, intrauterine growth retardation, or inadequate circulation of blood and oxygen during delivery. The impact of such complications can be severe and long-lasting. Fully half of all cases of cerebral palsy are attributable to birth injury and prematurity. However, frequently the cause of the disability is unclear. In some cases, the pregnancy and labor go well, but the child still suffers injury. While new fetal monitoring techniques aid in decreasing the risk of birth injuries, additional public health measures, including improved prenatal care of teenage and disadvantaged women, are needed to ensure the health of pregnant women and their infants.

REFERENCES

Amenta, J.S., & Silverman, J.A. (1983). Amniotic fluid lecithin, phosphatidylglycerol, L/S ratio, and foam stability test in predicting respiratory distress in the newborn. *American Journal of Clinical Pathology, 79*, 52–64.

Ayromlooi, J., Zervoudakis, I.A., & Sadaghat, A. (1973). Thyrotoxicosis in pregnancy. *American Journal of Obstetrics and Gynecology, 117,* 818–823.

Babson, S.G., & Clarke, N.G. (1978). Relationship between infant death and maternal age. *Journal of Pediatrics, 103,* 391–393.

Brenner, W.E., Bruce, R.D., & Hendricks, C.H. (1974). The characteristics and perils of breech presentation. *American Journal of Obstetrics and Gynecology, 118,* 700–712.

Cameron, A.H. (1968). The Birmingham twin survey. *Proceedings of the Royal Society of Medicine, 61,* 229–234.

Crenshaw, C., Jr., Jones, D.E., & Parker, R.T. (1973). Placenta previa: A survey of twenty years experience with improved perinatal survival by expectant therapy and cesarean delivery. *Obstetrical and Gynecological Survey, 28,* 461–470.

Crosby, W.M. (1974). Trauma during pregnancy: Maternal and fetal injury. *Obstetrical and Gynecological Survey, 29,* 683–699.

Fisher, D.E., & Paton, J.B. (1974). The effect of maternal anesthetic and analgesic drugs on the fetus and newborn. *Clinical Obstetrics and Gynecology, 17,* 275–287.

Franciosi, R.A., Knostman, J.D., & Zimmerman, R.A. (1973). Group B streptococcal neonatal and infant infections. *Journal of Pediatrics, 82,* 707–718.

Gluck, L., Kulovich, M.V., Borer, R.C., et al. (1971). Diagnosis of the respiratory distress syndrome by amniocentesis. *American Journal of Obstetrics and Gynecology, 109,* 440–445.

Hardy, J.B., Welcher, D.W., Stanley, J., et al. (1978). Long-range outcome of adolescent pregnancy. *Clinical Obstetrics and Gynecology, 21,* 1215–1232.

Hellman, L.M., & Pritchard, J.A. (Eds). (1971). *Williams obstetrics* (14th ed.). New York: Appleton-Century-Crofts.

Hon, E. (1968). *An atlas of fetal heart rate patterns.* New Haven, CT: Harty.

Jouppila, P., Kauppila, A., Koivisto, M., et al. (1975). Twin pregnancy. The role of active management during pregnancy and delivery. *Acta Obstetrica et Gynecologica Scandinavica, Suppl. 44,* 13–20.

Kauppila, A., Jouppila, P., Koivisto, M., et al. (1975). Twin pregnancy. A clinical study of 335 cases. *Acta Obstetrica et Gynecologica Scandinavica, Suppl. 44,* 5–12.

Kibrick, S. (1980). Herpes simplex infection at term. What to do with mother, newborn, and nursery personnel. *Journal of the American Medical Association, 243,* 157–160.

Koivisto, M., Jouppila, P., Kauppila, A., et al. (1975). Twin pregnancy. Neonatal morbidity and mortality. *Acta Obstetrica et Gynecologica Scandinavica, Suppl. 44,* 21–29.

Lemons, J.A., & Jaffe, R.B. (1973). Amniotic fluid lecithin-sphingomyelin ratio in the diagnosis of hyaline membrane disease. *American Journal of Obstetrics and Gynecology, 115,* 233–237.

Liley, A.W. (1965). The use of amniocentesis and fetal transfusion in erythroblastosis fetalis. *Pediatrics, 35,* 836–847.

Mindel, J.A., Adler, M.W., Sutherland, S., et al. (1982). Intravenous acyclovir treatment for primary genital herpes. *Lancet, 1,* 697–700.

Naeye, R.L. (1977). Causes of perinatal mortality in the U.S. Collaborative Perinatal Project. *Journal of the American Medical Association, 238,* 228–229.

Naeye, R.L., & Tafari, N. (1983). *Risk factors in pregnancy and diseases of the fetus and newborn.* Baltimore: Williams & Wilkins Co.

Nilsson, L. (1978). *A child is born.* New York: Dell Books.

Niswander, K.R. (Ed.). (1981). *Obstetrics: Essentials of clinical practice* (2nd ed.). Boston: Little, Brown & Co.

Niswander, K.R. (Ed.). (1983). *Manual of obstetrics: Diagnosis and therapy* (2nd ed.). Boston: Little, Brown & Co.

Niswander, K.R., Friedman, E.A., Hoover, D.B., et al. (1966a). Fetal morbidity following potentially anoxigenic obstetric conditions. I. Abruptio placentae. *American Journal of Obstetrics and Gynecology, 95,* 838–845.

Niswander, K.R., Friedman, E., Hoover, D., et al. (1966b). Fetal morbidity following potentially anoxigenic obstetric conditions. II. Placenta previa. *American Journal of Obstetrics and Gynecology, 95,* 846–852.

Niswander, K.R., Friedman, E., Hoover, D., et al. (1966c). Fetal morbidity following potentially anoxigenic obstetric conditions. 3. Prolapse of the umbilical cord. *American Journal of Obstetrics and Gynecology, 95,* 853–859.

Ryan, G.M., Jr., & Schneider, J.M. (1978). Teenage obstetric complications. *Clinical Obstetrics and Gynecology, 21,* 1191–1197.

Schwarcz, R.L., Belizan, J.M., Cifuentes, J.R., et al. (1974). Fetal and maternal monitoring in spontaneous labors and in elective inductions. A comparative study. *American Journal of Obstetrics and Gynecology, 120,* 356–362.

Sciarra, J.J. (Ed). (1977). *Gynecology and obstetrics.* Hagerstown, MD: Harper & Row.

Thompson, H.E. (1974). Evaluation of the obstetric and gynecologic patient by the use of diagnostic ultrasound. *Clinical Obstetrics and Gynecology, 17,* 1–25.

Tucker, S.M. (1978). *Fetal monitoring and fetal assessment in high risk pregnancy.* St. Louis: C.V. Mosby Co.

Valdes-Dapena, M.A., & Arey, J.B. (1970). The causes of neonatal mortality: An analysis of 501 autopsies on newborn infants. *Journal of Pediatrics, 77,* 366–375.

Walker, A.H., & Jennison, R.F. (1962). Antenatal prediction of haemolytic disease of newborn. Comparison of liquor amnii and serological studies. *British Medical Journal, 5313,* 1152–1156.

White, P. (1965). Pregnancy and diabetes, medical aspects. *Medical Clinics of North America, 49,* 1015–1024.

Willson, J.R., Carrington, E.R., & Ledger, W.J. (1983). *Obstetrics and gynecology* (7th ed.). St. Louis: C.V. Mosby Co.

Zuckerman, B.S., Walker, D.K., Frank, D.A., et al. (1984). Adolescent pregnancy: Biobehavioral determinants of outcome. *Journal of Pediatrics, 105,* 857–863.

Chapter 6

The First
Weeks of Life

Upon completion of this chapter, the reader will:
—understand the significance of the Apgar score
—know the physiological changes that take place immediately after birth
—comprehend the reasons why infections may be devastating to a newborn
—be able to enumerate he basic components of the body's immune system
—be aware of the various kinds of intracranial hemorrhages newborns suffer and the significance of each
—know why jaundice occurs
—understand the cause of and problems associated with Rh incompatibility
—be familiar with the reason why hypoglycemia occurs and its possible consequences for a newborn

---

Karen has given the last push, and Michael's torso emerges from the birth canal. Life outside the womb has begun. On examination at 1 minute, the obstetrician notes that Michael has a heart rate of 120 beats per minute and good respiratory effort. He has some flexion of his extremities, but no active movement. His cry is vigorous. While his body is pink, his arms and legs are blue. The Apgar score at 1 minute is 8 (Table 6.1). The baby is fine. At 5 minutes, Michael has made more progress. He is moving about, and his entire body has become pink. The 5-minute Apgar score is 10. Karen, relieved and pleased, smiles contentedly.

Marie, on the other hand, is having difficulty delivering her son, David. She has just undergone an emergency cesarean section because of an abruptio placenta. She has lost a great deal of blood and needed several blood transfusions. David is delivered quickly but, at 1 minute of age, he is limp and blue with no heartbeat or respiratory effort. The Apgar score is 0. Immediately, a tube is placed down David's windpipe, and he is artificially ventilated. Another tube is inserted into one of the blood vessels in the baby's umbilical cord, and the heart is stimulated with intravenous **glucose** and **Adrenalin**. After a few minutes, the baby is somewhat pink, the heart rate is 80, and spontaneous breathing has tentatively started. He has begun to

Table 6.1. The Apgar scoring system

	Points			Score			
				1 minute		5 minutes	
	0	1	2	Michael	David	Michael	David
Heart rate	Absent	<100	>100	2	0	2	1
Respiratory effort	Absent	Slow, irregular	Normal respiration; crying	2	0	2	1
Muscle tone	Limp	Some flexion	Active motion	1	0	2	1
Gag reflex	No response	Grimace	Sneeze; cough	2	0	2	1
Color	Blue all over; pale	Blue extremities	Pink all over	1	0	2	1
			Totals	8	0	10	5

move his extremities. The 5-minute Apgar score is 5 (see Table 6.1). The doctors breathe a sign of relief, knowing, however, that the effects of their efforts will not be known completely for many months. Years ago, David would have been stillborn.

APGAR SCORE

Michael and David have both survived. However, their risk of having a developmental disability is different. Their Apgar scores reflect this difference. This scale, developed by Dr. Virginia Apgar, measures the effect of various complications of labor and delivery on the newborn infant. It ranges from 0 to 10 and is taken at 1 minute and 5 minutes after birth. A low Apgar score generally indicates that the child is more likely to have a disability. One study reported that of 99 children who had Apgar scores below 4, 12% later developed multiple handicaps, including cerebral palsy, mental retardation, and seizures; 80% developed normally. In addition, 73% of all the children later diagnosed as having cerebral palsy had 5-minute Apgar scores above 6 (Nelson & Ellenberg, 1981; Paneth & Fox, 1983). Thus, the predictive ability of the Apgar score is questionable. Even so, it is safe to say that David is more likely to have developmental problems than Michael and will need close follow-up. Yet, David still has a good chance to develop normally.

PHYSIOLOGICAL CHANGES AT BIRTH

As the Apgar score illustrates, many changes take place in the first few moments after birth. The most important ones involve the respiratory and circulatory systems. Other changes include the infant's ability to regulate temperature and to absorb nutrients.

For the infant, the first breath is the most difficult because the lungs are collapsed and waterlogged. An extremely strong force must be exerted to open the air pockets, the **alveoli**, to permit the adequate exchange of air. The first cry increases the pressure enough to open the alveoli. The alveoli remain open even when air is expelled because of the action of a chemical mentioned in the previous chapter, called *surfactant*. It is a lack of surfactant that places premature infants at risk for developing respiratory distress syndrome (discussed in Chapter 7).

Equally important are the changes in the circulatory system. During fetal life, a number of vital organs are bypassed because the placenta takes care of **oxygenation** and **detoxification**. At birth, these bypasses must cease so the infant can function independently. The three most important bypasses are the *foramen ovale,* the *ductus arteriosus,* and the *ductus venosus.* The first two take blood around the unexpanded lungs, while the third transports blood around the fetal liver.

To understand how the first two bypasses work, it is important to know something about the normal flow of the postnatal circulation. The heart has four chambers: the right and left **atria**, or upper chambers, and the right and left ventricles, or lower chambers. Normally, the blood brought to the heart by the vena cava, one of the body's main veins, flows from the right atrium to the right ventricle. It is then carried by the **pulmonary** artery to the lungs, where it is oxygenated. The pulmonary veins later return the blood to the left atrium. The oxygenated blood then passes to the left ventricle and out to the body via the **aorta**, the body's primary artery, thus completing the cycle (Figure 6.1).

In the fetus, an opening called the foramen ovale permits much of the blood to flow directly from the right to the left atria, bypassing the right ventricle and the lungs (Figure 6.1). The blood that does not pass through the foramen ovale flows to the right ventricle and pulmonary artery. However, it is then short-circuited from entering the collapsed lungs by the ductus arteriosus. This bypass diverts the blood flow from the pulmonary artery into the aorta. Again, the lungs are bypassed.

With the first breath, a series of muscle contractions is initiated in the wall of the ductus arteriosus, forcing it to close. In addition, a flap folds over and covers the foramen ovale as the pulmonary artery allows more blood to flow through the lungs. The closure of these two bypasses must take place for proper oxygenation of the blood to occur. Usually, these bypasses have shut down by the time the infant is a few days old, and the adult circulatory pattern has been established.

The third bypass involves the umbilical circulation. Normally, the liver serves as a processor of wastes in our bodies. In the fetus, however, the umbilical vessels bypass the liver, and the placenta acts as the purifier of toxic products. A small

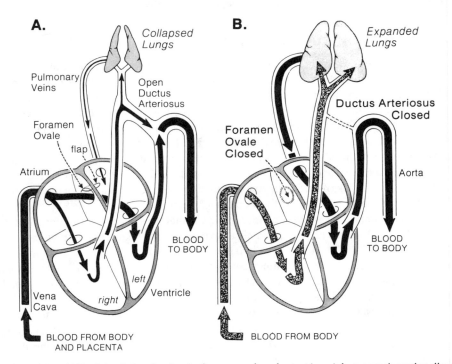

Figure 6.1.   A) Fetal circulation showing the foramen ovale and patent (open) ductus arteriosus that allow the blood flow to bypass the unexpanded lungs. B) Adult circulation. The fetal bypasses close off with expansion of the lungs.

channel, the ductus venosus, accomplishes this detour around the liver (Figure 6.2). After birth, it closes off along with an umbilical vein and two arteries. Venous blood then passes through the liver and is cleansed on its way back to the heart.

In addition to the closing of these three bypasses, the baby must begin to establish temperature regulation. This is very difficult because the newborn has a large surface area and little fatty tissue to protect him- or herself against temperature loss. This explains the necessity of incubators or of warm swaddling of the newborn.

Since the placental circulation is no longer available to provide nutrition, becoming adept at feeding is another change needed in the newborn. The infant must develop a strong suck and **rooting** response to seek and obtain nourishment either from the mother's breast or the bottle.

CAUSES OF ILLNESS AND DEATH IN NEWBORNS

Once an infant is born, the risk of death occurring during the first month of life is only about 1 in 1,000. Causes of death range from severe congenital malformations to infections (Kulkarni, Hall, Rhodes, et al., 1978) (Figure 6.3).

The incidence of serious illness in the newborn is about 1 in 100. Newborns have few ways of indicating severe illness. They stop feeding, become irritable, lethargic, and floppy. The pediatrician runs through a short list of possible diagnoses including infection, intracranial hemorrhage, jaundice, hypoglycemia, inborn errors of metabolism (see Chapter 8), and congenital anomalies (e.g., heart disease). Early and appropriate treatment may help to avoid severe developmental disabilities in the

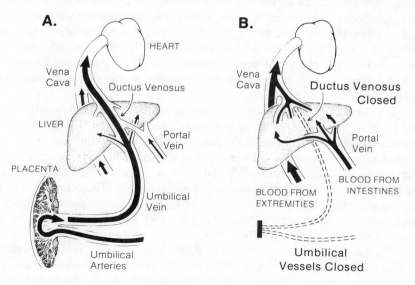

Figure 6.2.   A) Fetal circulation. The blood from the umbilical vein bypasses the liver through the ductus venosus. B) Adult circulation. The umbilical vein ceases to function and the ductus venosus closes. Now blood from the body passes through the liver where it is cleansed.

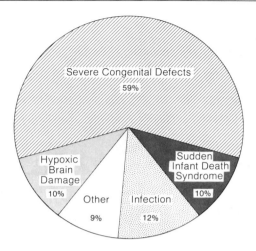

Figure 6.3. Causes of death during the first month of life. In the United States, the neonatal mortality rate is about 1 in 1,000 births. (From National Center for Health Statistics, 1978.)

infant (Falkner, 1977). However, some problems, such as intracranial hemorrhage and congenital defects, are not treatable.

Infections

Because it is so easily treated, the first concern of the pediatrician is the possibility of *sepsis,* or a generalized bacterial infection. Occurring in about 1 in 500 newborns, such infections are diagnosed by taking a blood sample and culturing it for bacteria. Before antibiotics were available, more than 90% of newborn infants with sepsis died; now, under 20% do (Krugman & Gershon, 1975). However, the frequency of such infections has increased recently because more very low birth weight infants are surviving, and these children are more susceptible to infection than are full-term infants.

In newborns, the bacteria causing these infections are different from the bacteria that cause sepsis in older children and adults (Harris & Polin, 1983). Some of the bacteria that attack newborns are the same ones that harmlessly exist as part of the vaginal, skin, or gastrointestinal **flora** in older children. The problem for newborns is that they lack a completely developed defense or immune system. Older children have a series of defense mechanisms against infection. These include the skin, mucous secretions, B and T **lymphocytes**, **phagocytes**, and the complement system. While newborns have some of these defenses, they are seriously lacking in others (Coen, Grush, & Kauder, 1969).

The first line of defense against infection is the skin. It provides a protective covering and prevents the entrance of bacteria or viruses into the bloodstream. If this covering is removed, such as occurs in third degree burns, the likelihood of sepsis greatly increases. The infant's skin covering, though thinner than an older person's, is adequate.

The next wall of defense is the mucous secretions. Saliva and the secretions of the **trachea**, or windpipe, prevent bacteria from stagnating and growing in the inviting warmth and moistness of the body. Also, these secretions contain antibodies that attack the bacteria before they can reach the bloodstream. Children with a disease such as cystic fibrosis, which is associated with a decrease in these secretions, have an increased risk of severe infections. The secretions in the newborn do not contain enough antibodies.

Involved in another step in immunity are the B and T cells. B cells are specific lymphocytes, or white blood cells, that produce the major antibody groups, immunoglobulins G, A, and M, in response to bacterial infections. These antibodies attach themselves to bacteria to form complexes that can then be engulfed by the phagocytes, bacteria-swallowing white cells. Newborns do not produce enough of these antibodies until about 6 months of age. Before that age, they must rely on the immunoglobulins transmitted from the mother during fetal life. In addition, the infant will receive small amounts of immunoglobulin A if breast-fed. These are not found in infant formulas.

The products of B cells are principally bacteria fighters, whereas T cells combat viral infections. The newborn lacks both B and T cells, so that both bacterial and viral infections, such as herpes, can cause life-threatening illness. Sufficient amounts of T cells are produced after the first few months of life, so the risk to the baby diminishes over time (Gotoff, 1974).

The final armament in the body's defense mechanism is the complement system. This consists of a cascade of components produced in the body that, among other things, attracts the phagocytes to the area of infection. They act like a ZIP code, directing the immune responses of the body. Both these chemicals and phagocytes are inadequate in the newborn.

Since the newborn is deficient in so much of the body's immune system, it is understandable that infection in the neonate can be devastating. Infections can be contracted either through the placenta (congenital rubella), the maternal vagina (herpes), or by contamination of the amniotic fluid during a difficult delivery (beta streptococcus or *strep*). Because of the ease with which newborns are infected, infants whose mothers have had premature rupture of their amniotic membranes are carefully observed for signs of infection. Finally, newborns may contract infections from other infants or staff in the nursery (Knittle, Eitzman, & Baer, 1975).

Early diagnosis and treatment of infection is essential, for, if untreated, it can spread rapidly through the infant's body. Twenty years ago, the predominant organism affecting newborns was **E. coli** bacteria; now, beta *strep* is the main problem (Baker, Barrett, Gordon, et al., 1973).

To provide adequate treatment, the specific organism must first be identified. When the question of sepsis arises, blood cultures are obtained, and the infant is placed on intravenous antibiotics. Usually, the infant's condition improves within 2 to 3 days. Since antibiotics only destroy bacteria, they have no effect in fighting viral infections such as herpes. Most infants suffering from bacterial infections will recover without significant complications. However, if the infection spreads to the coverings of the brain, causing meningitis, the mortality rate rises to 30%–60%. In addition, many of those infants who survive meningitis are left with severe neurological deficits (Feigin, 1983; Fitzhardinge, Kazemi, Ramsay, et al., 1974).

Intracranial Hemorrhage

Besides infections, newborns may have **intracranial** hemorrhages. These may result from an intrauterine stroke, a birth injury to the head, or a lack of oxygen during a prolonged labor (Brown, Purvis, Forfar, et al., 1974). Many infants, especially premature babies, have a small amount of bleeding but do not suffer any long-term consequences. Larger bleeds, on the other hand, may result in severe brain damage or death. Two signs of an intracranial hemorrhage are decreased alertness and poor feeding. Further testing must be done to determine whether a hemorrhage has, in fact, occurred.

The kinds of hemorrhages range from minor extracranial bleeds, called **cephalohematomas**, to intracranial hemorrhages, called **subarachnoid, subdural**, and **intracerebral**.

After birth, many babies have a large swelling on the back of the head, a cephalohematoma (Figure 6.4). This collection of blood under the skin is caused by trauma to the blood vessels in the scalp during delivery. The incidence is 2.5%, and the prognosis is excellent.

While the cephalohematoma carries an excellent prognosis, the intracranial bleeds may affect significantly the child's neurological development. The *dura mater* and *arachnoid mater* are two of the three fibrous layers surrounding and protecting the brain and spinal cord; the other layer is the *pia mater* (see Figure 6.4). Each has blood vessels running beneath it. During uterine contractions, the fetal head with-

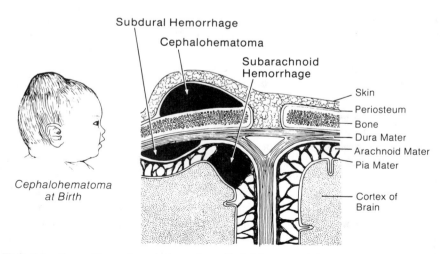

Figure 6.4. Types of hemorrhages in the newborn. Cephalohematoma is frequent, and the child with this problem has a good prognosis. Subdural and subarachnoid hemorrhages carry a more guarded prognosis.

stands tremendous pressure. Since the skull bones have not fused, the brain is compressible. Increased pressure on the head, therefore, may lead to increased brain pressure. If the delivery is prolonged, the oxygen supply is inadequate, and circulation is impaired. This combination of lack of circulation and increased intracranial pressure can lead to brain damage. The blood vessels are also affected, especially those below the dura. A subdural hemorrhage can then occur and may lead to cerebral palsy or death. Surgical drainage of the hemorrhage is often lifesaving. The mechanism and treatment for a subarachnoid hemorrhage is similar.

Equally serious is the intracerebral hemorrhage. A combination of high blood pressure and hypoxia may damage the blood vessels surrounding the ventricles of the brain (Horbar, Pasnick, McAuliffe, et al., 1983; Thorburn, Lipscomb, Stewart, et al., 1982). In full-term infants, these vessels are more resistant to damage. In premature babies, the vessels are fragile and more susceptible to disruption (Tarby & Volpe, 1982). Bleeding starts in the ventricles (an **intraventricular** hemorrhage) and may also move into the surrounding brain tissue. The blood count, or **hematocrit**, may drop, and seizures may begin. Confirmation of an intracerebral hemorrhage is made with the use of a CT scan (Figure 6.5) or with ultrasound (Figure 6.6), allowing

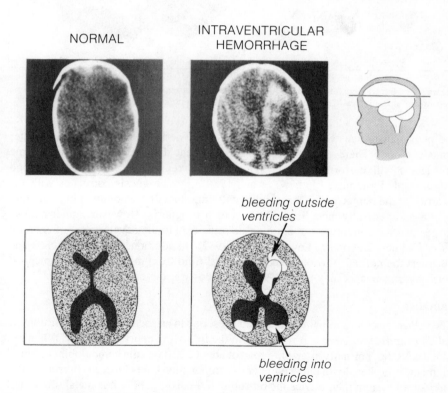

Figure 6.5.   Intraventricular hemorrhage as shown on a CT scan.

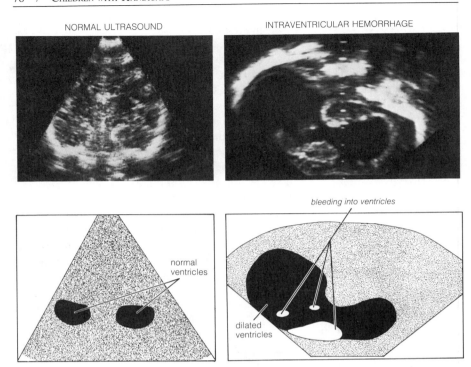

NORMAL ULTRASOUND   INTRAVENTRICULAR HEMORRHAGE

bleeding into ventricles

normal
ventricles

dilated
ventricles

Figure 6.6. Intraventricular hemorrhage as shown on an ultrasound. (Courtesy of Dr. Roger Sanders, Department of Radiology, The Johns Hopkins Hospital, Baltimore.)

the physician to see whether the ventricles, and perhaps the surrounding tissue, contain blood. There is no effective way to treat this problem, although some physicians will perform repeated spinal taps to remove the accumulated blood (Mantovani, Pasternak, Mathew, et al., 1980). The prognosis correlates with the severity of the hemorrhage. Small intraventricular bleeds are common in premature infants and generally have little effect on their prognosis. However, larger hemorrhages that have involved the brain tissue often lead to the development of cerebral palsy (Palmer, Dubowitz, Levene, et al., 1982). In addition, if the blood clots and obstructs the normal flow of the cerebrospinal fluid from the ventricle to the spinal cord, hydrocephalus may result (Palmer, Dubowitz, Levene, et al., 1982).

Jaundice

The yellow discoloration of the body and eyes, due to an accumulation of bilirubin, is called **jaundice** or *icterus*. It results from the following course of events: When red blood cells die, normally after a life span of about 120 days, the hemoglobin, or blood pigment, is broken down into a number of components. One of these is bilirubin. The circulatory system then carries the bilirubin to the liver. There it is metabolized and neutralized in a process called *conjugation*. Bilirubin can accumulate when too many red blood cells break down or when there is a blockage in conjugation (Cashore & Stern, 1982).

While jaundice is generally a sign of severe liver disease in the adult, it may be quite innocuous in a newborn infant. Usually, jaundice in infants is due to the immaturity of the enzyme system necessary for conjugation of bilirubin. The infant may become yellow-tinged at 2 to 3 days of age and ordinarily returns to a normal color by 1 week of age, without therapy. The bilirubin level is usually below 10–15 **milligrams** (mg) per 100 **milliliters** (ml). If jaundice persists, placement of the baby under fluorescent lights, which aid in conjugation, leads to a drop to normal in the bilirubin level (Valkeakari, Anttolainen, Aurekoski, et al., 1981).

A modest elevation in the bilirubin level has little effect on the developing infant. However, a marked increase above 20 mg/100 ml in a full-term infant may pose a serious threat to the child. The most severe cause of **hyperbilirubinemia** is Rh incompatibility in which a massive breakdown of red blood cells leads to jaundice (Kandall, Saldana, & Gastner, 1975). The Rh factor is a minor blood group attached to the four major blood types: A, B, AB, and O. Thus, a person may be ORh− or ORh+, ARh−, or ARh+, and so on.

Incompatibility of the Rh blood groups between mother and father may have disastrous consequences for the fetus. For this to happen, the mother must be Rh− and the father and the fetus must be Rh+. Problems develop in the following way: While the fetal and maternal circulatory systems are separate, an occasional fetal blood cell gets into the maternal circulation. The mother's immune system recognizes the baby's red cells as being foreign and begins to destroy the fetus's red blood cells. This may cause the fetus to become severely anemic.

In the past, many infants died *in utero* and those who survived suffered brain damage and had cerebral palsy, a high-frequency hearing loss, paralysis of the upward gaze, and discoloration of the teeth. This clinical syndrome is called **kernicterus** (Oski & Naiman, 1982).

Over the years, treatment of Rh incompatibility changed from a palliative approach to a preventive one. Initially, in the 1950s, intrauterine blood transfusions were given to save these children. Around the 26th week of gestation, a needle was inserted through the uterus into the fetal abdominal cavity, and a transfusion of red blood cells was then given. The red blood cells were absorbed into the fetal circulation and improved the anemia. Several transfusions were required, and they were not without risk to the fetus (Liley, 1965). Once born, the babies needed repeated exchange transfusions to lower the bilirubin level. Very slowly, donor blood was infused, and the infant's blood was removed. Over a period of an hour, 80% of the infant's blood could be replaced by healthy adult blood (McKay, 1964).

More recently, the effort has tended toward prevention. A drug, RhoGAM, has made this possible. RhoGAM is a gamma globulin (antibody) injection given to Rh− women after delivery or miscarriage of an Rh+ infant (Clarke, 1968). It works by blocking the formation of antibodies in the mother's circulation. Subsequent Rh+

infants will then be born without this anemia. This treatment has resulted in the virtual disappearance of kernicterus and a marked decrease in the need for exchange transfusions.

Incompatibility of the major blood groups may still result in jaundice, but this is usually a far less severe problem than Rh incompatibility and generally resolves with treatment under fluorescent lights.

Hypoglycemia

At birth, infants are suddenly faced with the need to supply their own energy requirements for maintenance of their body temperature, muscle activity, and blood sugar regulation. The concentration of blood sugar in the newborn is about half that in adults. If the infant suffers **asphyxia** during birth, he or she is forced to use a mechanism called *anaerobic* (without air) *metabolism* to produce energy. This is a very wasteful form of metabolism that uses up the stored sugar. Since the ability to produce sugar is impaired, the blood sugar level drops significantly (Finer, Robertson, Peters, et al., 1983). This condition is called *hypoglycemia*. The child may appear lethargic, jittery, and may have intermittent breathing (**apnea**) or seizures. If sugar is quickly given intravenously, neurological problems rarely result. However, if the hypoglycemia is prolonged and uncorrected, it may lead to permanent brain damage. This complication is far more likely to take place in infants of diabetic mothers and premature or small-for-dates infants than in full-term infants (Haworth & Vidyasager, 1971).

The infant of the diabetic mother presents an interesting example of the problem of altered metabolism (Cowett & Schwartz, 1983). Since the pancreas of the diabetic mother does not produce insulin, the fetal pancreas overproduces insulin to compensate. Insulin takes care of two functions: 1) lowering of blood sugar, and 2) the laying down of fatty tissue. Because of the overproduction of insulin, infants of diabetic mothers appear obese and have enlarged body organs from an increase in fat content. This is further complicated because they are often born prematurely. After birth, the **islet cells** of the pancreas continue to overproduce insulin. This results in a precipitous fall in the blood sugar level, which is often difficult to control. The insulin production falls off within a week or two, so the infant will fare well if providing oral glucose has been successful in maintaining normal blood sugar levels during the first days of life (Koivisto, Blanco-Sequeiros, & Krause, 1972).

Although hypoxia and maternal diabetes are the most common causes of low blood sugar in the newborn, they are not the only ones. Sepsis, congenital heart disease, brain hemorrhage, and drug withdrawal (Olofsson, Buckley, Andersen, et al., 1983) are also associated with hypoglycemia. In these cases, the primary determinant of prognosis is the condition predisposing the infant to hypoglycemia rather than the hypoglycemia itself.

In addition, mineral imbalances may lead to symptoms that simulate hypoglycemia. Most common are deficiencies in calcium and magnesium (Tsang, 1972; Tsang, Chen, Hayes, et al., 1974). Again, if these disorders are diagnosed early, they can usually be corrected with an intravenous feeding of the deficient mineral.

Congenital Defects

Congenital defects are the other major causes of developmental disabilities and death in the newborn period. The various genetic and chromosomal abnormalities that may affect fetal development were discussed in Chapter 4. Some are lethal and result in spontaneous abortions. With others, the children are born but are more susceptible to such problems as intracranial hemorrhage, jaundice, hypoglycemia, and infection. For example, spina bifida leads to a greater likelihood of developing meningitis and sustaining further brain damage. Thus, when an infant has problems as a newborn and later is diagnosed as having developmental disabilities, it may be unclear whether the newborn's difficulties caused the disabilities or whether the pre-existing congenital defects brought about the problems during the newborn period.

SUMMARY

The first month of life is a critical period in the infant's development. Many metabolic and physical changes take place to enable the child to cope with the new environment outside the protection of the womb. Because these changes are so momentous and rapid, many abnormalities may occur. Some—for example, hypoglycemia—are usually correctable if identified early. Others, such as hypoxia, can best be handled preventively, with fetal monitoring and early delivery. Still others, such as some congenital malformations, cannot be treated. For those who suffer brain damage, the extent of their problems may not be known for several months. Overall, 99.9% of all newborns survive the first month of life, and the vast majority will grow up to be normal.

REFERENCES

Autio-Harmainen, H., Rapola, J., Hoppu, K., et al. (1983). Causes of neonatal deaths in a pediatric hospital neonatal unit. An autopsy study of a ten-year period. *Acta Paediatrica Scandinavica, 72,* 333–337.

Avery, G.B. (1981). *Neonatology: Pathophysiology and management of the newborn* (2nd ed.). Philadelphia: J.B. Lippincott Co.

Baker, C.J., Barrett, F.F., Gordon, R.C., et al. (1973). Suppurative meningitis due to streptococci of Lancefield group B: A study of 33 infants. *Journal of Pediatrics, 82,* 724–729.

Blanc, W.A. (1961). Pathways of fetal and early neonatal infection. Viral placentitis, bacterial and fungal chorioamnionitis. *Journal of Pediatrics, 59,* 473–496.

Brown, J.K., Purvis, R.J., Forfar, J.O., et al. (1974). Neurological aspects of perinatal asphyxia. *Developmental Medicine and Child Neurology, 16,* 567–580.

Brown, R.J.K., & Valman, H.B. (1979). *Practical neonatal paediatrics* (4th ed.). Boston: Blackwell Scientific.

Cashore, W.J., & Stern, L. (1982). Neonatal hyperbilirubinemia. *Pediatric Clinics of North America, 29,* 1191–1203.

Clarke, C.A. (1968). Prevention of rhesus iso-immunisation. *Lancet, 2,* 1–7.

Coen, R., Grush, O., & Kauder, E. (1969). Studies of bactericidal activity and metabolism of the leukocyte in full-term neonates. *Journal of Pediatrics, 75,* 400–406.

Cowett, R.M., & Schwartz, R. (1983). The infant of the diabetic mother. *Pediatric Clinics of North America, 29,* 1213–1231.

Falkner, F.T. (1977). *Fundamentals of mortality risks during the perinatal period and infancy.* New York: S. Karger.

Feigin, R.D. (1983). Neonatal meningitis: Problems and prospects. *Hospital Practice, 18*, 175–179.

Finer, N.N., Robertson, C.M., Peters, K.L., et al. (1983). Factors affecting outcome in hypoxic-ischemic encephalopathy in term infants. *American Journal of Diseases of Children, 137*, 21–25.

Fitzhardinge, P.M., Kazemi, M., Ramsay, M., et al. (1974). Long-term sequelae of neonatal meningitis. *Developmental Medicine and Child Neurology, 16*, 3–8.

Gotoff, S.P. (1974). Neonatal immunity. *Journal of Pediatrics, 85*, 149–154.

Harris, M.C., & Polin, R.A. (1983). Neonatal septicemia. *Pediatric Clinics of North America, 30*, 243–258.

Haworth, J.C., & Vidyasager, D. (1971). Hypoglycemia in the newborn. *Clinical Obstetrics and Gynecology, 14*, 821–839.

Horbar, J.D., Pasnick, M., McAuliffe, T.L., et al. (1983). Obstetric events and risk of periventricular hemorrhage in premature infants. *American Journal of Diseases of Children, 137*, 678–681.

Jenista, J.A. (1983). Perinatal herpesvirus infections. *Seminars in Perinatology, 7*, 9–15.

Kandall, S., Saldana, L., & Gastner, L.M. (1975). Hemolytic disease of the newborn. In H.F. Conn (Ed.). *Current Therapy Edition 27*. Philadelphia: W.B. Saunders Co.

Kendall, N., & Woloshin, H. (1952). Cephalhematoma associated with fracture of skull. *Journal of Pediatrics, 41*, 125–132.

Knittle, M.A., Eitzman, D.V., & Baer, H. (1975). Role of hand contamination of personnel in the epidemiology of gram-negative nosocomial infections. *Journal of Pediatrics, 86*, 433–437.

Koivisto, M., Blanco-Sequeiros, M., & Krause, U. (1972). Neonatal symptomatic and asymptomatic hypoglycaemia: A followup study of 151 children. *Developmental Medicine and Child Neurology, 14*, 603–614.

Krugman, S., & Gershon, A.A. (Eds.) (1975). *Infections of the fetus and the newborn infant: Proceedings*. New York: Symposium by the New York University Medical Center and the National Foundation-March of Dimes.

Kulkarni, P., Hall, R.T., Rhodes, P.G., et al. (1978). Postneonatal infant mortality in infants admitted to a neonatal intensive care unit. *Pediatrics, 62*, 178–183.

Liley, A.W. (1965). The use of amniocentesis and fetal transfusion in erythroblastosis fetalis. *Pediatrics, 35*, 836–847.

McKay, R.J., Jr. (1964). Current status of use of exchange transfusion in newborn infants. *Pediatrics, 33*, 763–767.

Mantovani, J.F., Pasternak, J.F., Mathew, O.P., et al. (1980). Failure of daily lumbar punctures to prevent the development of hydrocephalus following intraventricular hemmorrhage. *Journal of Pediatrics, 97*, 278–281.

National Center for Health Statistics. (1978). *Hospital handbook on birth registration and fetal death reports*. Hyattsville, MD: U.S. Department of Health, Education & Welfare.

Nelson, K.B., & Ellenberg, J.H. (1981). Apgar scores as predictors of chronic neurologic disability. *Pediatrics, 68*, 36–44.

Oh, W. (Ed.). (1982). Symposium on the newborn. *Pediatric Clinics of North America, 29*, 1055–1299.

Olofsson, M., Buckley, W., Andersen, G.E., et al. (1983). Investigation of 89 children born by drug-dependent mothers. I. Neonatal course. *Acta Paediatrica Scandinavica, 72*, 403–406.

Oski, F.A., & Naiman, J.L. (1982). *Hematologic problems in the newborn* (3rd ed). Philadelphia: W.B. Saunders Co.

Palmer, P., Dubowitz, L.M., Levene, M.I., et al. (1982). Developmental and neurological progress of preterm infants with intraventricular hemorrhage and ventricular dilatation. *Archives of Disease in Childhood, 57*, 748–753.

Paneth, N., & Fox, H.E. (1983). The relationship of Apgar score to neurologic handicaps: A survey of clinicians. *Obstetrics and Gynecology, 61*, 547–550.

Rabe, E.F. (1967). Subdural effusions in infants. *Pediatric Clinics of North America, 14*, 831–850.

Rementeria, J.L. (Ed.). (1977). *Drug abuse in pregnancy and neonatal effects*. St. Louis: C.V. Mosby Co.

Schinazi, R.F., & Prusoff, W.H. (1983). Antiviral agents. *Pediatric Clinics of North America, 30*, 77–92.

Schneider, M. (1983). Neonatal cranial ultrasound. *Pediatric Annals, 12*, 133, 135, 138–139.

Sell, E.J. (1980). *Follow-up of the high risk newborn—a practical approach*. Springfield, IL: Charles C Thomas.

Tarby, T.J., & Volpe, J.J. (1982). Intraventricular hemorrhage in the premature infant. *Pediatric Clinics of North America, 29*, 1077–1104.

Thorburn, R.J., Lipscomb, A.P., Stewart, A.L., et al. (1982). Timing and antecedents of periventricular haemorrhage and of cerebral atrophy in very preterm infants. *Early Human Development, 6*, 221–238.

Tsang, R.C. (1972). Neonatal magnesium disturbances. *American Journal of Diseases of Children, 124,* 282–293.

Tsang, R.C., Chen, I., Hayes, W., et al. (1974). Neonatal hypocalcemia in infants with birth asphyxia. *Journal of Pediatrics, 84,* 428–433.

Valkeakari, T., Anttolainen, I., Aurekoski, H., et al. (1981). Follow-up study of phototreated fullterm newborns. *Acta Paediatrica Scandinavica, 70,* 21–25.

Volpe, J.J. (1981). *Neurology of the newborn.* Philadelphia: W.B. Saunders Co.

Chapter 7

Born Too Soon, Born Too Small

Upon completion of this chapter, the reader will:
—know the difference between the premature infant and the small for gestational age infant
—recognize some of the causes of prematurity
—be able to identify some of the distinguishing physical characteristics of the premature infant
—understand the complications and illnesses associated with prematurity
—be aware of the methods used to care for the premature and the small for gestational age infant

---

Infants born too soon or too small are at risk for a number of problems. First, they have more difficulty than usual in adapting to the postnatal environment because their body organs may be less mature. Second, their growth potential may be restricted. Finally, as newborns, they may suffer a number of biochemical and physical disturbances that place them at a greater risk for brain damage than normal. This chapter addresses the problems of low birth weight infants and discusses some new forms of medical management that have improved their prognosis.

DEFINITIONS

A *premature infant* is defined as a child born at or before the 36th week of gestation, 1 month before the estimated date of confinement. A small for gestational age (SGA) infant, on the other hand, refers to a newborn whose weight is below the 10th percentile for the gestational age (Lubchenco, 1976). For example, a baby born at 35 weeks gestation who weighs 5 pounds, or 2,250 grams, would be considered premature but appropriate in size for the gestational age; this weight falls at the 25th percentile for this age. However, if this infant were born at term weighing the same 5 pounds, he or she would be small for gestational age. At 40 weeks gestational age, the 10th percentile for weight is 5½ pounds, or 2,500 grams (Figure 7.1). SGA babies are sometimes also called *dysmature* or small-for-dates.

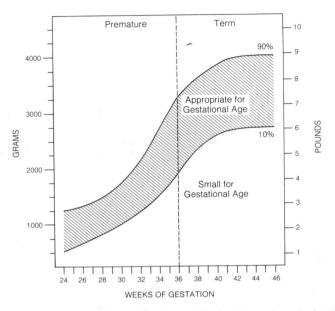

Figure 7.1.   Newborn weight chart by gestational age. The shaded area between the 10th and 90th percentiles represents infants who are appropriate for gestational age. Weight below the 10th percentile makes an infant small for gestational age. Prematurity is defined as an infant born before 36 weeks gestation. (From Lubchenco, L.O. [1976]. *The high risk infant*. Philadelphia: W.B. Saunders Co.; reprinted by permission.)

Although both premature and SGA infants have higher rates of illness and death as newborns than full-term infants, the complications for these two groups are somewhat different. Problems associated with prematurity are discussed here first.

CAUSES OF PREMATURITY

A number of maternal factors increase the likelihood of a premature delivery. Although premature deliveries account for only 2% of all deliveries, 20% of adolescent pregnancies result in such births (Block, Saltzman, & Block, 1981; Goldberg & Craig, 1983). Why this happens is not completely clear, but physicians presume the immature uterus of the adolescent is more susceptible to early contractions than that of an older woman (Zuckerman, Alpert, Dooling, et al., 1983). Women who have had many previous pregnancies, whose cervical muscles are weak, or who are carrying twins also run a greater risk of delivering prematurely. In addition, women who develop an infection during the third trimester or who have chronic illnesses such as diabetes have premature infants more often (Niswander & Gordon, 1972). An early rupture of the membranes may also precipitate prematurity (Lubchenco, 1976). Finally, certain malformations or injuries to the fetus may lead to a premature birth.

PHYSICAL AND DEVELOPMENTAL
CHARACTERISTICS OF PREMATURE INFANTS

Several physical and neurodevelopmental characteristics distinguish the premature infant from the full-term infant (Druzin, 1983). Dubowitz, Dubowitz, and Goldberg (1970) developed a scoring system that takes into account these findings and enables physicians to confirm the mother's dates or to arrive at the gestational age when the mother's dates are unknown (Figure 7.2).

NEUROMUSCULAR MATURITY

NEUROMUSCULAR MATURITY SIGN	SCORE 0	1	2	3	4	5	RECORD SCORE HERE
POSTURE							
SQUARE WINDOW (WRIST)	90°	60°	45°	30°	0°		
ARM RECOIL	180°		100°-180°	90°-100°	<90°		
POPLITEAL ANGLE	180°	160°	130°	110°	90°	<90°	
SCARF SIGN							
HEEL TO EAR							

TOTAL NEUROMUSCULAR MATURITY SCORE

PHYSICAL MATURITY

PHYSICAL MATURITY SIGN	SCORE 0	1	2	3	4	5	RECORD SCORE HERE
SKIN	gelatinous red, transparent	smooth pink, visible veins	superficial peeling, &/or rash few veins	cracking pale area rare veins	parchment deep cracking no vessels	leathery cracked wrinkled	
LANUGO	none	abundant	thinning	bald areas	mostly bald		
PLANTAR CREASES	no crease	faint red marks	anterior transverse crease only	creases ant. 2/3	creases cover entire sole		
BREAST	barely percept.	flat areola no bud	stippled areola, 1-2mm bud	raised areola, 3-4mm bud	full areola 5-10mm bud		
EAR	pinna flat, stays folded	sl. curved pinna; soft with slow recoil	well-curv. pinna; soft but ready recoil	formed & firm with instant recoil	thick cartilage ear stiff		
GENITALS (Male)	scrotum empty no rugae		testes descending, few rugae	testes down good rugae	testes pendulous deep rugae		
GENITALS (Female)	prominent clitoris & labia minora		majora & minora equally prominent	majora large, minora small	clitoris & minora completely covered		

Reference
Ballard JL, Novak KK, Driver M: A simplified score for assessment of fetal maturation of newly born infants. *J Pediatr* 95:769-774, 1979. Reprinted by permission of Dr Ballard and Journal of Pediatrics.

TOTAL PHYSICAL MATURITY SCORE

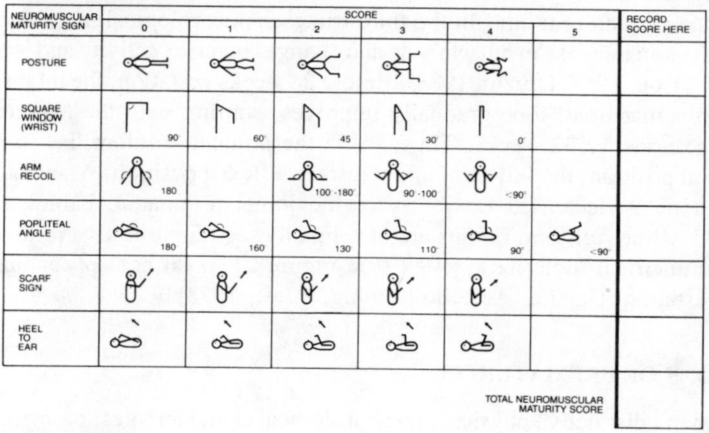

SCORE
Neuromuscular _____
Physical _____
Total _____

MATURITY RATING

TOTAL MATURITY SCORE	GESTATIONAL AGE (WEEKS)
5	26
10	28
15	30
20	32
25	34
30	36
35	38
40	40
45	42
50	44

GESTATIONAL AGE (weeks)
By dates _____
By ultrasound _____
By score _____

Figure 7.2. Scoring system to assess newborn infants. The score for each of the neuromuscular and physical signs is added together to obtain a score called the total maturity score. Gestational age is determined from this score. (From Ballard, J.L., Novak, K.K., & Driver, M. [1979]. A simplified score for assessment of fetal maturation of newly born infants. *Journal of Pediatrics, 95,* 770; reprinted by permission.)

The main characteristics that distingush a premature infant are the presence of body hair, a reddish skin color, and the absence of skin creases, ear cartilage, and breast buds. Premature infants have fine hair, or lanugo, over the entire body; this is lost by 38 weeks gestation. Also, the very premature infant lacks skin creases on the soles of the feet; these develop after 32 weeks. Skin color is ruddier because the blood vessels are closer to the surface, and the skin appears translucent. Finally, breast buds and cartilage in the ear lobe do not appear until around the 34th week of gestation (Figure 7.3).

Besides physical characteristics, differences in neurological development are also evident in the premature infant. In the third trimester, neurological maturation principally involves an increase in muscle tone and changes in reflex activity and joint mobility (Amiel-Tison, 1968; Druzin, 1983). Before 28 weeks gestation, the infant is very floppy. After that time, tone gradually improves, starting with the legs and moving up to the arms by 32 weeks. Thus, while the premature infant lies in an extended, rag-doll position, the full-term infant rests in a flexed position. Associated with increased tone is decreased flexibility of the joints. Premature babies are "double-jointed," while full-term infants are not. Finally, certain primitive reflexes such as the asymmetrical tonic neck reflex (see Figure 21.3) do not appear until 30–32 weeks gestation (Capute, Accardo, Vining, et al., 1978).

COMPLICATIONS OF PREMATURITY

In addition to having distinctive physical and neurological characteristics, premature infants face an increased risk of complications in the newborn period compared to

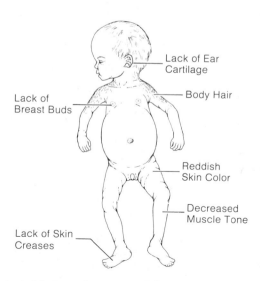

Figure 7.3.   Typical physical features of a premature infant.

full-term infants. Among these problems are *respiratory distress syndrome, patent ductus arteriosus,* periodic breathing or *apnea,* and *biochemical abnormalities.*

Respiratory Distress Syndrome

Approximately 20% of all premature infants develop respiratory distress syndrome (RDS), sometimes called *hyaline membrane disease,* during their first week of life. The extent of prematurity affects the incidence of this disorder. For example, less than 10% of the babies born between 34 and 36 weeks develop RDS, while over 60% of babies born at less than 32 weeks gestation do (Schaffer, Avery, & Taeusch, 1984).

Typically, the infant's breathing appears normal at birth, but he or she begins to have grunting respirations within a few hours. The baby starts using the abdominal muscles to help breathe, but the lungs don't expand properly. If this continues, the baby needs extra oxygen or has to be ventilated artificially. The cause of this problem is as follows: Normally, the first breaths of a newborn open the alveoli, or air pockets, of the lungs. The alveoli are coated with surfactant, a chemical that normally then prevents them from closing. But some premature babies do not produce enough surfactant to keep the alveoli open, so they collapse after each breath. The more premature the infant, the less surfactant is produced. Thus, the very premature infant has the greatest risk of developing respiratory distress syndrome. A recent study found that treating such infants with surfactant before they took their first breath improved their respiratory condition and reduced the amount of artificial ventilation that they needed (Enhorning, Shennan, Possmayer, et al., 1985). An X-ray film of the child's chest has a "ground glass" or white appearance. The collapsed alveoli are dense and look white on the film. This contrasts with normal lung expansion where the chest is filled with air that is translucent and appears black on the X-ray film (Figure 7.4).

For years, physicians have known that infants with respiratory distress syndrome need to be treated with oxygen. Yet, in the initial treatment of these infants, an error was made. Too high a concentration of oxygen was used. This caused an unanticipated complication, called *retinopathy of prematurity* (ROP) or *retrolental*

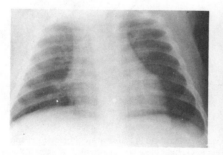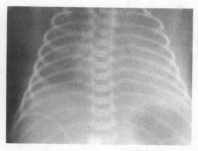

Figure 7.4.   Chest X rays of a normal newborn (left) and of a premature infant with respiratory distress syndrome (RDS) (right). Note the "white out" of lungs caused by the collapse of alveoli in RDS.

fibroplasia, an eye problem leading to detachment of the retina and blindness (Hittner, Godio, Speer, et al., 1983; Patz, 1984; Porat, 1984). Many of the surviving premature infants born in the 1940s and 1950s were left blind. Now, lower levels of oxygen are used, and the infants' eyes are checked by an **ophthalmologist** while they are in the nursery. In addition, some controversial evidence suggests that vitamin E supplements may reduce the risk of developing retrolental fibroplasia (Hittner, Godio, Speer, et al., 1983).

Another innovation that has helped these infants is the use of positive end expiratory pressure (PEP). Before 1970, about half of all the premature infants who developed RDS died from it. Now less than 10% of these infants die. With PEP, an artificial respirator is adapted to apply a constant pressure to the alveoli, keeping them open at all times and allowing an effective exchange of oxygen and carbon dioxide. Before the use of PEP, enough oxygen was supplied to the lungs, but because the alveoli remained collapsed, an inadequate exchange of oxygen occurred between the alveoli and the pulmonary blood vessels (Figure 7.5). Since the blood was not sufficiently oxygenated, there remained the possibility of damage to the brain and other organs that became depleted of oxygen.

In terms of future intellectual development, the prognosis for children who suffer RDS is reassuring. Although the prognosis varies with the gestational age and weight of the infant, overall the risk for severe developmental delay is less than 15% (Rothberg, Maisels, Bagnato, et al., 1983).

Patent Ductus Arteriosus

The **vascular** changes that occur after birth were discussed in Chapter 6. One of these changes is the closing of the ductus arteriosus, which connects the pulmonary artery and the aorta during fetal life. However, in premature infants, this closure may not

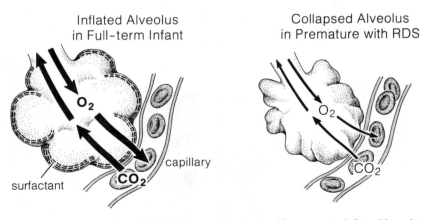

Inflated Alveolus in Full-term Infant

Collapsed Alveolus in Premature with RDS

O_2

O_2

capillary

surfactant

CO_2

CO_2

Figure 7.5.   Schematic drawing of alveoli in a normal newborn and in a premature infant with respiratory distress syndrome (RDS). Note that the inflated alveolus is kept open by surfactant. Oxygen moves from the alveolus to the red blood cells in the pulmonary capillary. Carbon dioxide moves in the opposite direction. This exchange is much less efficient when the alveolus is collapsed. The result is hypoxia.

take place after birth. The normal constriction of muscle fibers that leads to closure is stimulated by increased oxygen intake following birth. In the premature infant with RDS, the oxygen level in the blood simply does not become high enough to stimulate this closing (Thibeault, Emmanouilides, Nelson, et al., 1975). Thus, besides poor ventilation, the infant must cope with a patent, or open, ductus arteriosus. If this duct remains open, it can lead to heart failure. About 20% of the babies who weigh less than 2,000 grams at birth have this complication.

To close the ductus, medical or surgical methods are normally used. The drug **indomethacin** causes the muscles of the arterial wall to contract (Peckham, Miettinen, Ellison, et al., 1984). However, it also carries the risks of decreasing urine output and increasing bleeding. An alternate approach is performing surgery to tie off the duct (Peckham, Miettinen, Ellison, et al., 1984). Surgery also places the infant at an increased risk.

Apnea

Another problem for the premature infant is the immaturity of his or her central nervous system. The **brain stem** area of the central nervous system controls respiratory efforts. Not only does the premature infant have difficulty moving air into the lungs, but he or she also often forgets to breathe. This is called *apnea*. The more premature the infant, the more serious is this problem. Furthermore, those infants who have suffered brain damage because of other newborn complications are more likely to have apnea. To treat apnea, a drug, theophylline (related to **caffeine**), which stimulates respiration, is often used. Rocker beds that also activate breathing may be used for infants who do not respond to drug therapy (Korner, Guilleminault, Van den Hoed, et al., 1978). Persistent apnea may be a bad prognostic sign. It may indicate that the child has suffered some brain damage, or it may be a precursor of sudden infant death syndrome (SIDS).

Sudden infant death syndrome occurs more commonly in premature babies than in full-term infants (Brady & Gould, 1983). In this illness, a previously healthy child is found dead in the crib during the first year of life. Unfortunately, no preventive treatment exists (Naeye, 1980). Those premature infants who have persistent apneic episodes are sent home with an apnea monitor that sounds an alarm if the baby stops breathing (Spitzer & Fox, 1984). The parents are also trained to give artificial resuscitation (see Appendix D). This has helped parents to intervene during episodes of respiratory arrest and to improve their child's chances for survival (Spitzer & Fox, 1984).

Besides interfering with proper breathing, an immature central nervous system also hinders adequate nutritional intake. Many premature infants do not suck or swallow effectively and must be fed by stomach tube or intravenously. Using this approach, these infants can continue to gain adequate weight.

Biochemical Abnormalities

In addition to problems unique to premature babies, these infants are also more susceptible to the same problems experienced by full-term infants during the newborn period, including jaundice, intracerebral hemorrhage (Gaither, 1982), hypo-glycemia, and hypothermia. For example, since prematures can develop *kernicterus* at lower levels of bilirubin than the full-term infant, treatment for an elevation in bilirubin is begun earlier. *Hypoglycemia* is also more common, because prematures have smaller reserves of glucose than their full-term counterparts. Thus, symptoms of hypoglycemia, including lethargy, vomiting, and seizures, may occur. These symptoms are avoided by providing early feedings, administering intravenous glucose, and monitoring blood glucose levels. Finally, loss of heat, caused by inadequate insulation with fatty tissues, places the premature baby at risk for **hypothermia**; this is why incubators are used in the hospital to warm the infants.

SMALL FOR GESTATIONAL AGE INFANTS

The SGA infant is one who is small in size for his or her gestational age. These infants may be either premature or full-term.

Women who come from lower socioeconomic environments more often have infants who are small for gestational age. Physicians speculate that this may result from inadequate nutritional intake during pregnancy. Also, this condition is more common in infants of women with chronic illnesses and in women over 40 years of age. Older women tend to have SGA infants because the blood supply to their placentas is not sufficient to provide adequate nutrition to the fetus (Scott & Jordan, 1972).

Small for gestational age infants have many of the same problems as premature infants. However, they are spared one complication; they rarely get respiratory distress syndrome (Lee, Eidelman, Tseng, et al., 1976). It seems the prenatal stresses that interfere with normal intrauterine growth also stimulate the production of surfactant. However, they do suffer from hypothermia, **hypocalcemia**, and hypo-glycemia. Furthermore, even with proper nutrition, these infants tend to remain short and underweight throughout their lives (Starfield, Shapiro, McCormick, et al., 1982; Vohr & Oh, 1983). Also, the incidence of developmental disabilities is higher in this group of infants compared to babies whose weight is appropriate for their gestational age (Allen, 1984; Parkinson, Wallis, & Harvey, 1981). Full-term SGA babies are more likely to have learning disabilities (see Chapter 20) and attention deficit disorder (Chapter 19); premature SGA babies are, in addition, at an increased risk for mental retardation and cerebral palsy (Allen, 1984).

MEDICAL CARE OF THE LOW BIRTH WEIGHT INFANT

The best treatment for the low birth weight infant is prevention. Health officials hope that their efforts in the areas of education and nutrition for adolescent mothers will lead to fewer premature deliveries (Block, Saltzman, & Block, 1981; Goldberg & Craig, 1983). Improved control of chronic illnesses in pregnant women should also decrease this number. For women who are at risk for having low birth weight infants, it is best to deliver in a setting that has a newborn intensive care unit (NICU), even if this requires moving a woman in labor.

Once born, these infants are immediately placed under a heater to stabilize body temperature. If RDS is evident, the baby is either given oxygen or is **intubated** and mechanically ventilated. The heart and respiratory rates are constantly monitored. Blood samples are taken and tested for glucose, calcium, bilirubin, **acid-base balance**, and **electrolyte** levels. Intravenous fluids are given to compensate for any biochemical imbalances. If the bilirubin level starts to rise, the baby is placed under fluorescent lights. In the rare instance where the level rises rapidly, the infant may receive an exchange blood transfusion. If signs of infection such as lethargy and poor feeding develop, the blood is checked, and intravenous antibiotics are usually started. If the baby experiences episodes of apnea, he or she either receives medication or is placed on a rocker bed to stimulate normal breathing.

Usually, the baby's condition stabilizes within a few weeks. By then, adequate nutrition is possible and growth begins. The RDS subsides, and the child no longer needs the respirator. The jaundice abates. The baby starts maintaining his or her temperature, and the biochemical levels become normal. The baby is then transferred from the NICU to an intermediate care unit, where he or she will feed and grow. The baby is discharged when able to feed from a nipple, maintain his or her temperature outside the isolette, and continue to grow well. Usually, the baby weighs between 1,800 and 2,500 grams (4 to 5.5 pounds) when leaving the hospital.

A CASE HISTORY

Sarah was the 32-week product of a 14-year-old adolescent. The mother had received no prenatal care and arrived at the emergency room in labor, with her membranes already ruptured. Upset and screaming, she was taken to the labor room. Over the next 24 hours, her cervix dilated no further. A decision was made to deliver the baby by cesarean section. The surgery went well, and Sarah weighed 1,800 grams at birth, an appropriate weight for her gestational age. She breathed spontaneously and was active. Her 5-minute Apgar score was 8.

Within 4 hours, however, problems arose. Sarah began to breathe rapidly in an attempt to get air, and her chest X ray showed evidence of RDS. She was intubated and placed on a ventilator. The next day, her bilirubin level began to rise. She was treated with fluorescent lights, and the bilirubin level stabilized and gradually began to fall.

Because she was too weak to suck properly, Sarah was fed with a **nasogastric tube**. When she was 5 days old, an X ray showed that the RDS was resolving. The tube in her throat was removed on the seventh day. Then, another problem developed—apnea. Every 5 or 10 minutes, Sarah would forget to breathe, and the shrill alarm of the respiratory monitor would ring. Touching her with a finger usually made her gulp a breath of air, and she would begin to breathe again. She was placed on theophylline and, within a few days, the episodes of apnea became less frequent. Sarah was then transferred out of the intensive care unit and went home at 6 weeks of age, weighing 2,200 grams. At the time of her discharge, she followed objects visually, was alert to the sound of a bell, and appeared to be an active, healthy premature baby. Sarah's mother had received training on how to care for her and, although very young, she was quite competent and loving.

PROGNOSIS

Over the past 20 years, the progress in neonatology (the care of newborns) has been just short of phenomenal. In 1960, more than 70% of the infants who weighed less than 1,500 grams at birth and more than 90% of those who weighed less than 1,000 grams died during the newborn period (Figure 7.6). Of those who survived, about one-half had severe retardation as well as cerebral palsy; another one-fourth were moderately affected. Less than 20% of the surviving infants were normal. Now, about 70% of the infants who weigh less than 1,500 grams are surviving, as well as about half of the infants who weigh less than 1,000 grams. Of both groups of infants, about 25% have developmental disabilities (Budetti, Barrand, McManus, et al., 1981). Even many infants weighing less than 2 pounds (900 grams) are surviving and doing well. In one recent study, 30% of the infants who weighed 500–1,000 grams

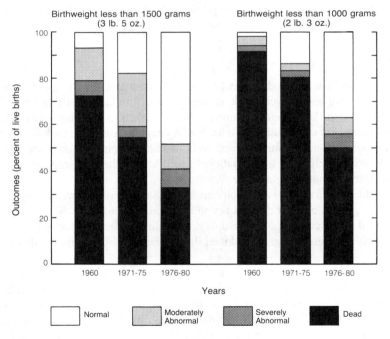

Figure 7.6. The changing outcome for premature infants from 1960–1980. Infants weighing less than 1,500 grams had a mortality rate of over 70% in 1960, about 55% in the early 1970s, and around 30% in the late 1970s. In 1960, approximately 75% of the surviving infants had developmental disabilities compared to about 25% in 1980. Similar improvement in prognosis was seen in infants who weighed less than 1,000 g. (From Budetti, P., Barrand, N., McManus, P., et al. [1981]. *The costs and effectiveness of neonatal intensive care,* p. 38. Washington, DC: Office of Technology Assessment, U.S. Government Printing Office.)

survived; over half of these survivors had no handicaps. The rest of them had various degrees of mental retardation and cerebral palsy; in addition, 3% were deaf and 3% were blind (Bennett, Robinson, & Sells, 1983; Kitchen, Ford, Orgill, et al., 1984; Ment, Scott, Ehrenkranz, et al., 1982). Infants who were both premature and small for gestational age fared the worst.

As the incidence of cerebral palsy in premature infants due to **anoxia**, or lack of oxygen, has decreased (Franco & Andrews, 1977; Rothberg, Maisels, Bagnato, et al., 1983), the concern about development has turned more toward learning disabilities and attention deficit disorder (Nickel, Bennet, & Lamson, 1982). By 2 years of age, premature infants should have caught up to full-term infants, in both their physical and developmental achievement.

SUMMARY

For premature infants, different complications lead to different prognoses. Complications consistent with a good developmental prognosis include RDS, hyperbilirubinemia, hypoglycemia, and hypocalcemia. Those associated with a poorer prognosis include intraventricular hemorrhage (Gaither, 1982; Krishnamoorthy, Shannon, DeLong, et al., 1979; Tarby & Volpe, 1982), sepsis, and periodic apnea. Even though an increased risk of developmental disabilities exists with these complications, many of the children still do well. With improved prenatal care and an increased number of NICUs, the prognosis for low birth weight infants should continue to improve (Kulkarni, Hall, Rhodes, et al., 1978).

REFERENCES

Allen, M.C. (1984). Developmental outcome and followup of the small for gestational age infant. *Seminars in Perinatology, 8,* 123–156.
Amiel-Tison, C. (1968). Neurological evaluation of the maturity of newborn infants. *Archives of Disease in Childhood, 43,* 89–93.
Anwar, M., Kadam, S., Hiatt, I.M., et al. (1985). Serial lumbar punctures in prevention of post-hemorrhagic hydrocephalus in preterm infants. *Journal of Pediatrics, 107,* 446–450.
Avery, M.E., Fletcher, B.D., & Williams, R.G. (1981). *The lung and its disorders in the newborn infant* (4th ed.). Philadelphia: W.B. Saunders Co.
Ballard, J.L., Novak, K.K., & Driver, M. (1979). A simplified score for assessment of fetal maturation of newly born infants. *Journal of Pediatrics, 95,* 769–774.
Bennett, F.C., Robinson, N.M., & Sells, C.J. (1983). Growth and development of infants weighing less than 800 grams at birth. *Pediatrics, 71,* 319–323.
Block, R.W., Saltzman, S., & Block, S.A. (1981). Teenage pregnancy. *Advances in Pediatrics, 28,* 75–98.
Brady, J.P., & Gould, J.B. (1983). Sudden infant death syndrome: The physician's dilemma. *Advances in Pediatrics, 30,* 635–672.
Brazelton, T.B. (1984). *Neonatal behavioral assessment scale* (2nd ed.). Philadelphia: J.B. Lippincott Co.
Budetti, P., Barrand, N., McManus, P., et al. (1981). *The costs and effectiveness of neonatal intensive care.* Washington, D.C.: Office of Technology Assessment, U.S. Government Printing Office.
Caputo, A.J., Accardo, P.J., Vining, E.P.G., et al. (1978). *Primitive reflex profile.* Baltimore: University Park Press.
Druzin, M.L. (1983). Methods of determining fetal maturity. *Pediatric Annals, 12,* 18–22.

Dubowitz, L.M., Dubowitz, V., & Goldberg, C. (1970). Clinical assessment of gestational age in the newborn infant. *Journal of Pediatrics, 77,* 1–10.

Dubowitz, L.M., Levene, M.I., Morante, A., et al. (1981). Neurologic signs in neonatal intraventricular hemorrhage: A correlation with real-time ultrasound. *Journal of Pediatrics, 99,* 127–133.

Enhorning, G., Shennan, A., Possmayer, F., et al. (1985). Prevention of neonatal respiratory distress syndrome by tracheal instillation of surfactant: A randomized clinical trial. *Pediatrics, 76,* 145–153.

Franco, S., & Andrews, B.F. (1977). Reduction of cerebral palsy by neonatal intensive care. *Pediatric Clinics of North America, 24,* 639–649.

Gaither, J.L. (1982). The effects of intraventricular hemorrhage on Bayley developmental performance in preterm infants. *Seminars in Perinatology, 6,* 305–316.

Gesell, A., & Amatruda, C.S., joint authors; Knobloch, H., & Pasamanick, B. (Eds.). (1974). *Gesell and Amatruda's developmental diagnosis: The evaluation and management of normal and abnormal neuropsychologic development in infancy and early childhood* (3rd ed). Hagerstown, MD: Harper & Row.

Goldberg, G.L., & Craig, C.J. (1983). Obstetric complications in adolescent pregnancies. *South African Medical Journal, 64,* 863–864.

Hack, M., Caron, B., Rivers, A., et al. (1983). The very low birth weight infant: The broader spectrum of morbidity during infancy and early childhood. *Journal of Developmental and Behavioral Pediatrics, 4,* 243–249.

Hittner, H.M., Godio, L.B., Speer, M.E., et al. (1983). Retrolental fibroplasia: Further clinical evidence and ultrastructural support for efficacy of vitamin E in the preterm infant. *Pediatrics, 71,* 423–432.

Kitchen, W., Ford, G., Orgill, A., et al. (1984). Outcome of infants with birth weights 500 to 999 gm: A regional study of 1979 and 1980 births. *Journal of Pediatrics, 104,* 921–927.

Klaus, M.H., & Fanaroff, A.A. (1979). *Care of the high risk neonate* (2nd ed.). Philadelphia: W.B. Saunders Co.

Klaus, M., & Kennell, J. (1982). Interventions in the premature nursery: Impact on development. *Pediatric Clinics of North America, 29,* 1263–1273.

Klein, N., Hack, M., Gallagher, J., et al. (1985). Preschool performance of children with normal intelligence who were very low-birth-weight infants. *Pediatrics, 75,* 531–537.

Korner, A.F., Guilleminault, C., Van den Hoed, J., et al. (1978). Reduction of sleep apnea and bradycardia in preterm infants on oscillating water beds: A controlled polygraphic study. *Pediatrics, 61,* 528–533.

Krishnamoorthy, K.S., Shannon, D.C., DeLong, G.R., et al. (1979). Neurologic sequelae in the survivors of neonatal intraventricular hemorrhage. *Pediatrics, 64,* 233–237.

Kulkarni, P., Hall, R.T., Rhodes, P.G., et al. (1978). Postneonatal infant mortality in infants admitted to a neonatal intensive care unit. *Pediatrics, 62,* 178–183.

Lee, K.S., Eidelman, A.I., Tseng, P.I., et al. (1976). Respiratory distress syndrome of the newborn and complications of pregnancy. *Pediatrics, 58,* 675–680.

Lubchenco, L.O. (1976). *The high risk infant.* Philadelphia: W.B. Saunders Co.

McCormick, M.C. (1985). The contribution of low birth weight to infant mortality and childhood morbidity. *New England Journal of Medicine, 312,* 82–90.

Ment, L.R., Scott, D.T., Ehrenkranz, R.A., et al. (1982). Neonates of less than or equal to 1250 grams birth weight: Prospective neurodevelopmental evaluation during the first year post-term. *Pediatrics, 70,* 292–296.

Naeye, R.L. (1980). Sudden infant death. *Scientific American, 242,* 56–62.

Nickel, R.E., Bennet, F.C., & Lamson, F.N. (1982). School performance of children with birth weights of 1,000 g or less. *American Journal of Diseases of Children, 136,* 105–110.

Niswander, K.R., & Gordon, M. (1972). *The women and their pregnancies.* Philadelphia: W.B. Saunders Co.

Parkinson, C.E., Wallis, S., & Harvey, D. (1981). School achievement and behaviour of children who were small-for-dates at birth. *Developmental Medicine and Child Neurology, 23,* 41–50.

Patz, A. (1984). Current concepts of the effect of oxygen on the developing retina. *Current Eye Research, 3,* 159–163.

Peckham, G.J., Miettinen, O.S., Ellison, R.C., et al. (1984). Clinical course to 1 year of age in premature infants with patent ductus arteriosus: Results of a multicenter randomized trial of indomethacin. *Journal of Pediatrics, 105,* 285–291.

Philipp, C. (1984). The relationship between social support and parental adjustment to low-birthweight infants. *Social Work, 29,* 547–550.

Porat, R. (1984). Care of the infant with retinopathy of prematurity. *Clinics in Perinatology, 11*, 123–151.

Rothberg, A.D., Maisels, M.J., Bagnato, S., et al. (1983). Infants weighing 1,000 grams or less at birth: Developmental outcome for ventilated and nonventilated infants. *Pediatrics, 71*, 599–602.

Scarpelli, E.M., Auld, P.A.M., & Goldman, H.S. (Eds.) (1978). *Pulmonary disease of the fetus, newborn, and child.* Philadelphia: Lea & Febiger.

Schaffer, A.J., Avery, M.E., & Taeusch, H.W. (1984). *Schaffer's diseases of the newborn* (5th ed.). Philadelphia: W.B. Saunders Co.

Scott, J.M., & Jordan, J.M. (1972). Placental insufficiency and the small-for-dates baby. *American Journal of Obstetrics and Gynecology, 113*, 823–832.

Sever, J.L., Larsen, J.W., & Grossman, J.H. (1979). *Handbook of perinatal infections.* Boston: Little, Brown & Co.

Shapiro, S., McCormick, M.C., Starfield, B.H., et al. (1983). Changes in infant mortality associated with decreases in neonatal mortality. *Pediatrics, 72*, 408–415.

Spitzer, A.R., & Fox, W.W. (1984). Sudden infant death syndrome (SIDS). Guidelines for averting tragedy. *Postgraduate Medicine, 75*, 125–133, 137–138.

Starfield, B., Shapiro, S., McCormick, M., et al. (1982). Mortality and morbidity in infants with intrauterine growth retardation. *Journal of Pediatrics, 101*, 978–983.

Tarby, T.J., & Volpe, J.J. (1982). Intraventricular hemorrhage in the premature infant. *Pediatric Clinics of North America, 29*, 1077–1104.

Thibeault, D.W., Emmanouilides, G.C., Nelson, R.J., et al. (1975). Patent ductus arteriosus complicating the respiratory distress syndrome in premature infants. *Journal of Pediatrics, 86*, 120–126.

Vohr, B.R., & Oh, W. (1983). Growth and development in preterm infants small for gestational age. *Journal of Pediatrics, 103*, 941–945.

Zuckerman, B., Alpert, J.J., Dooling, E., et al. (1983). Neonatal outcome: Is adolescent pregnancy a risk factor? *Pediatrics, 71*, 489–493.

Chapter 8

Mutant Genes, Missing Enzymes
PKU and Other Inborn Errors

Upon completion of this chapter, the reader will:
—understand what is meant by inborn errors of metabolism
—know the differences between a number of these disorders, including PKU, maple syrup urine disease, and hyperammonemia
—know which of these disorders have newborn screening tests
—be aware of the disorders in this group that are treatable and those for which there is no treatment
—recognize the different types of treatment for some of these disorders

---

For us to receive adequate nutrition, the food we eat must be broken down into fats, proteins, and carbohydrates and then metabolized. This conversion is carried out by enzymes that also work to maintain **homeostasis**, that is, the control of functions as diverse as blood sugar levels, blood pressure, and rate of growth.

Approximately 1 in 5,000 children is born deficient in an important regulatory enzyme. These children have what are called inborn errors of metabolism, disorders that are inherited as Mendelian traits, usually autosomal recessive ones. Most of these disorders can now be detected prenatally once a mother is known to be at risk (see Chapter 3). Inborn errors are a relatively recently classified group of diseases. One of the first, *phenylketonuria,* or PKU, was described by Følling in 1934 (Stanbury, Wyngaarden, Frederickson, et al., 1983). Most of the others have been identified since 1955, and about five new disorders are recognized each year (McKusick, 1983).

In the past, many of these disorders led to severe mental retardation or early death. Recently, the combination of early diagnosis and better treatment has improved the prognosis. Nonetheless, a number of these disorders remain resistant to known methods of treatment.

This chapter focuses on these inborn errors. Rather than providing an exhaustive discussion of each disorder, it uses examples of different inborn errors to explain some of the newer diagnostic and therapeutic approaches. Therapeutic methods include: 1) dietary restriction of a toxic material, as in PKU and maple syrup urine disease, 2) diversion therapy around an enzyme block, as in congenital hyperammonemia, 3) provision of a deficient compound, as in **hypothyroidism**, 4) enzyme replacement therapy, as in Gaucher's disease and Hurler's syndrome, 5) organ transplantation, as in **glycogen** storage disease, and 6) **megavitamin** supplementation, as in methylmalonic aciduria.

NEWBORN SCREENING

Before treatment is possible, diagnosis is necessary. Because the toxic accumulation of substances causes progressive brain damage, early diagnosis, preferably in the newborn period, is crucial. PKU is the classic example. Occurring with a frequency of 1 in 14,000, PKU presents no symptoms in infancy (Stanbury, Wyngaarden, Frederickson, et al., 1983). However, if diagnosis is delayed beyond the first few months of life, the child will have multiple disabilities, including severe retardation, hyperactivity, and seizures, even if he or she is later treated (Partington & Laverty, 1978).

The brain damage in PKU results from a buildup of *phenylalanine*. Normally, much of the phenylalanine we ingest is used for growth of bone and tissue. The enzyme, phenylalanine hydroxylase, breaks down the remaining phenylalanine and eliminates it in the form of other nontoxic substances. In classic PKU, phenylalanine is not broken down because the production of this enzyme is deficient. Therefore, the phenylalanine starts to accumulate in the blood and the brain shortly after birth. Before birth, the excessive phenylalanine from the fetus passes across the placental membrane, where it is metabolized by the normal maternal enzyme. This is also the case with many other inborn errors. The children appear normal at birth, but, soon after, the toxins begin to collect.

This problem has spawned the need for a newborn screening test for PKU and other inborn errors of metabolism. In 1959, Dr. Robert Guthrie developed such a test at the University of Buffalo (Guthrie, 1972). Now this test and other related tests for congenital hypothyroidism, **galactosemia, homocystinuria**, and maple syrup urine disease are routinely performed on all babies prior to discharge from the newborn nursery. To perform the test, a few drops of blood are taken following a heel stick and are placed on filter paper. The blood sample is sent to the state health department, where staff can identify a positive test before a child is 2 weeks old (Figure 8.1). Then, confirmation of the diagnosis and early treatment, which for PKU means a phenylalanine-restricted diet, can be started. Treatments are also available for the other disorders that can be detected by newborn screening. However, it is important to remember that these screening tests determine only a few of the many possible causes of mental retardation. These are not general tests for mental retardation as some have come to believe.

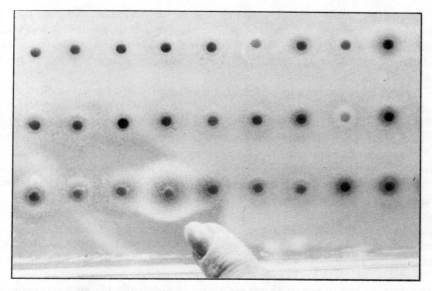

Figure 8.1. PKU spot test. Blood spots are placed in a culture medium containing bacteria that require large amounts of phenylalanine for growth. The finger points to the one blood spot containing excessive bacterial growth. The child who gave this blood has PKU.

TREATMENT

Dietary Restriction

Treatment for PKU is straightforward. Because phenylalanine accumulates and leads to brain damage, the child should be placed on a phenylalanine-restricted diet. As an infant, a child with PKU receives a special formula containing only small amounts of phenylalanine and normal amounts of other essential amino acids (Koch, Shaw, Acosta, et al., 1970). As the child grows, he or she can eat only small quantities of high-protein food such as meats, cheeses, and poultry, but is allowed normal amounts of fruits, vegetables, and other low-protein food. This diet is not too difficult to enforce when a child is young. However, by the time the child reaches 5 or 6 years of age and is more aware of other good tasting food and peer pressure to eat certain food, it is harder to maintain the diet. Food stealing often becomes a problem.

Because of these difficulties, the question has been asked whether it would be safe to discontinue the diet when a child reaches 6 years of age, when most brain growth has been completed. Studies suggest that the IQ scores in PKU patients who stop therapy after 6 years of age do not decrease (Holtzman, Welcher, & Mellits, 1975). Yet, a matched group of children who were maintained on the diet past this age actually experienced a modest increase in IQ scores between 6 and 8 years, so that the difference in the scores between the two groups became statistically significant (Koch, Azen, Friedman, et al., 1982). Thus, most metabolic specialists believe that the diet should be continued indefinitely (Brunner, Jordan, & Berry, 1983).

Even in the ideally treated PKU children, some deficits remain. Although the IQ scores of these children fall in the normal range, they are significantly lower than those of their parents (Dobson, Williamson, Azen, et al., 1977). Also, the incidence of attention deficit disorder, hyperactivity, and learning disabilities is higher in these children than in the normal population.

Despite these concerns, it is clear that, when started in infancy, the diet yields remarkable results. A study at the University of Toronto (Hanley, Linsao, & Netley, 1971) showed the difference in IQ scores between children treated within the first month of life compared to their siblings who were treated later in life (Table 8.1). The children who were treated early had IQ scores around 100 while those treated later in infancy scored between 20 and 40.

Besides PKU, another disorder responsive to dietary restriction therapy is *maple syrup urine disease*. It is much less common than PKU, occurring in about 1 in 120,000 infants (Stanbury, Wyngaarden, Frederickson, et al., 1983). Also, acute symptoms develop in the newborn period that, if undetected, lead to brain damage or death. Affected infants vomit, are lethargic, and may become comatose. In addition, their urine has an unusual sweet odor reminiscent of maple syrup, hence the name of the disease. This disorder is caused by the accumulation of three amino acids—valine, leucine, and isoleucine—that are not being metabolized properly. Treatment consists of a diet restricted in all three of these amino acids. It is a diet that is much more difficult to balance and, so, the children's health is more fragile. Similar to juvenile diabetics, these children often begin vomiting and become lethargic during infections or dietary indiscretions. While treatment has been lifesaving, it has been less successful in preventing brain damage than the treatment for PKU.

Diversion Therapy

Equally devastating is a group of inborn errors called the *congenital hyper-ammonemias*. Occurring in about 1 in 30,000 children, these disorders result from a child's inability to tolerate a normal protein intake. When protein is broken down into its component amino acids, ammonia, a **neurotoxin**, is released. Normally, the

Table 8.1. Results of treating PKU diagnosed at various stages

	Age at diagnosis (months)				
	0–2	2–6	6–12	12–24	24+
Number of cases	38	6	11	19	20
IQ scores:					
90+	27	0	0	1	2
80–89	6	3	0	2	1
70–79	4	1	3	2	0
Under 70	1	2	8	14	17
Mean IQ	93.5	71.6	54.5	55.5	40.8

Source: Hanley, W.B., Linsao, L.S., & Netley, C. (1971). The efficiency of dietary therapy for phenylketonuria. *Canadian Medical Association Journal, 104,* 1089; reprinted by permission.

ammonia is converted into a nontoxic product called **urea** through the five enzyme steps in the urea cycle. The urea is then excreted in the urine. If any one of these five enzymes is deficient, ammonia will accumulate and cause symptoms similar to those described for maple syrup urine disease. A problem with treating these disorders through diet restriction is that the degree of protein restriction required to prevent an accumulation of the ammonia is incompatible with normal growth or prolonged survival. In the past, fewer than 15% of these patients treated with protein-restricted diets survived to 1 year of age (Shih, 1976).

A novel approach has been the use of two drugs, sodium benzoate and sodium phenylacetate, to sop up the accumulating ammonia and convert it into nontoxic products that can be excreted in the urine. In this way, a detour around the metabolic block is provided. Using this method, over 90% of the affected children have lived longer than one year (Batshaw, Brusilow, Waber, et al., 1982). Unfortunately, many of these children have already suffered brain damage before treatment as a result of neonatal coma (Batshaw, 1984; Msall, Batshaw, Suss, et al., 1984). Since no neonatal screening test for these disorders exists, early diagnosis must rely on the acumen of the physician.

Provision of the Deficient Compound

Unlike hyperammonemia, *congenital hypothyroidism* is a disorder with a slow progression and an available newborn screening test. Untreated, a lack of the thyroid hormone thyroxine leads to **cretinism**. Children with this condition are small, floppy, and have severe mental retardation. Occurring in 1 in 6,000 children, hypothyroidism is one of the most common inborn errors of metabolism. Treatment using a thyroid **extract** has been available for over a century. However, newborn screening has only existed for the past 10 years (Dussault, Coulombe, Laberge, et al., 1975). Early diagnosis now permits early treatment with the deficient hormone. This effectively corrects the metabolic disorder, and children treated in the first months of life develop normally.

Gene Replacement Therapy

Theoretically, the most effective form of therapy for an inborn error of metabolism would be the replacement of the defective gene or of the deficient enzyme. As mentioned in Chapter 2, each chromosome contains thousands of genes that direct, among other things, the production of enzymes. In inborn errors of metabolism, a mutation or structural abnormality within the gene causes either the production of a nonfunctional enzyme or no enzyme at all. If one could insert the normal gene into the affected person, it should produce the normal enzyme and cure the inborn error.

Part of the reason no one has yet tried this approach is because such a treatment involves a very complicated process (Anderson, 1984). First, one must identify which gene is deficient. Then, the DNA composition of the gene must be defined. The gene must then be synthesized and attached to a carrier, usually a virus, that would enter the person's body. Finally, the gene must find its way to the specific body organ where it is needed and be normally regulated so that it is active when necessary and inactive at other times.

To date, some of these problems have been solved, and gene replacement has been done in some animal experiments. Researchers have identified the DNA patterns of many genes by using gene-splicing techniques (see Chapter 3); this means that many genes can be synthesized. Also, a way of inserting the gene using certain viruses called **retroviruses** has been developed. However, the safety and effectiveness of this approach is as yet undetermined.

In mice, this approach was used in an experiment in which fertilized mouse eggs were injected with the gene for rat growth hormone (Palmiter, Norstedt, Gelinas, et al., 1983). (Figure 8.2a) (Growth hormone controls weight and height growth.) The mice that developed from these eggs grew to be twice as large as their littermates by adolescence (Figure 8.2b) and were found to be producing the rat growth hormone.

A somewhat different approach has been used to reactivate the gene that controls the production of hemoglobin in sickle cell anemia. In Chapter 2, it was mentioned that sickle cell anemia involves a mutation of the gene for hemoglobin, the blood pigment. Instead of producing normal hemoglobin (HgbA), a defective hemoglobin (HgbS) is made. A significant amount of this HgbS makes the red blood cell look sickle-shaped and causes it to be more fragile than normal. This means that increased numbers of red blood cells are destroyed, and the person develops severe anemia.

Another hemoglobin, HgbF, is normally present during fetal life. After birth, the production of this hemoglobin usually stops. However, by adding the drug Azacytidine, this fetal hemoglobin gene is reactivated. The product of this gene, HgbF, then dilutes the defective HgbS and improves the anemia (Dover, Charache,

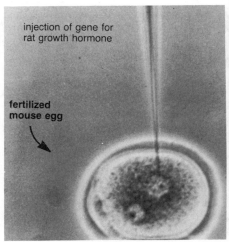
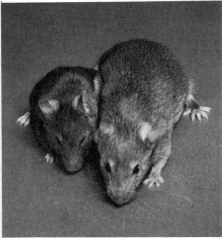

injection of gene for rat growth hormone

fertilized mouse egg

Figure 8.2. a) Microscopic photograph of fertilized mouse egg being injected with a rat gene. b) The mouse on the left is normal. The mouse on the right was injected with rat growth hormone as an embryo and is twice normal size. (Photograph of mice from cover of *Science, 222* (Nov. 18, 1983); reprinted by permission. Copyright © 1983 by American Association for the Advancement of Science.)

Boyer, et al., 1983). Unfortunately, this drug also appears to be **carcinogenic**, so its use is restricted to patients with life-threatening disease. However, the idea of turning genes on or off is an exciting one that may have great therapeutic potential for the future.

Enzyme Replacement Therapy

In treating inborn errors of metabolism, enzyme replacement therapy has been tried, although unsuccessfully, for Gaucher's disease and Hurler's syndrome. Gaucher's disease is a progressive, neurological disorder that causes mental retardation and early death in children. Currently, no effective treatment for this disorder exists. However, the deficient enzyme is readily recovered from placental tissue. Attempts were made to infuse the enzyme directly into affected patients (Brady, Pentchev, Gal, et al., 1974). Although the enzyme level increased for a short period of time, the body soon recognized it as being a foreign protein. The body's immune response was then triggered, and the enzyme was quickly inactivated.

For the treatment of Hurler's syndrome, bone marrow transplantation was tried (Hobbs, Hugh-Jones, Barrett, et al., 1981). (Physicians have previously used this procedure to treat leukemia.) Hurler's syndrome is a progressive, neurological disorder. Children with this syndrome have enlarged livers and spleens and unusual looking faces. In addition, these children have vision and hearing impairments. They usually die by adolescence (Stanbury, Wyngaarden, Frederickson, et al., 1983). Attempts to treat this syndrome with bone marrow transplantation have involved injecting bone marrow obtained from a relative who had normal activity of the enzyme iduronidase. Following the bone marrow transplantation, the enzyme levels were found to increase, and the size of the liver and spleen decreased. However, the neurological damage continued to progress. The enzyme produced by the transplanted cells did not cross the blood-brain barrier, so it could not enter the brain and metabolize the accumulating toxic material.

Organ Transplantation

A more successful approach, with a different disease, has been the use of liver transplantation in treating children with *glycogen storage disease* (Malatack, Finegold, Iwatsuki, et al., 1983). This disease causes hypoglycemia (low blood sugar) and enlargement of the liver. However, no neurotoxins accumulate and, thus, no progressive brain damage takes place. The problem is the inability to turn glycogen, the stored form of glucose, back into sugar under fasting conditions. Because of this problem, children with this disease require almost constant feedings of starch or sugar to maintain normal blood sugar levels (Stanbury, Wyngaarden, Frederickson, et al., 1983). However, following liver transplantation, patients have retained normal glucose levels for years (Malatack, Finegold, Iwatsuki, et al., 1983). While this has been a successful form of treatment, liver transplantation is a very serious operation, and significant health risks are associated with it. Yet, it has been lifesaving for a number of children.

Megavitamin Therapy

For some inborn errors, treatment may involve an enhancement of the deficient enzyme, not a replacement of it. Such is the case for some children with *methylmalonic aciduria*. Clinically, this disease resembles maple syrup urine disease with episodes of vomiting, lethargy, and coma that begin in infancy. Once a diagnosis is made, supplements of vitamin B_{12} are begun. In about half the affected children, the metabolic disturbance is greatly improved (Rosenberg, 1976), and the children develop normally. The other half require dietary restriction similar to that used in treating maple syrup urine disease. The use of megavitamin therapy for the treatment of this disorder has been effective, but it is important to keep in mind that the much-touted use of megavitamin therapy for other disorders, ranging from mental retardation to schizophrenia, has no scientific basis (Smith, Spiker, Peterson, et al., 1984).

SUMMARY

Although all of the inborn errors of metabolism described in this chapter are rare, their consequences are often disastrous. Therapy, in the form of severe dietary restrictions, works for many of these disorders. However, in some instances, the therapy itself can lead to malnutrition. Also, children with these disorders must often continue therapy for the rest of their lives, something difficult to do. In rare instances, megavitamin therapy may yield benefits. And, in all cases, for therapy to succeed at all, it must be started early in life. Researchers continue to look for new therapeutic strategies for these diseases, focusing on gene and enzyme replacement and the use of detours around the blocked pathways. Eventually, safer and more effective therapy may become available.

REFERENCES

Anderson, V.E., & Siegel, P.S. (1976). Behavioral and biochemical correlates of diet change in phenylketonuria. *Pediatric Research, 10,* 10–17.

Anderson, W.F. (1984). Prospects for human gene therapy. *Science, 226,* 401–409.

Batshaw, M.L. (1984). Hyperammonemia. *Current Problems in Pediatrics, 14,* 6–69.

Batshaw, M.L., Brusilow, S., Waber, L., et al. (1982). Treatment of inborn errors of urea synthesis: Activation of alternative pathways of waste nitrogen synthesis and excretion. *New England Journal of Medicine, 306,* 1387–1392.

Brady, R.O., Pentchev, P.G., Gal, A.E., et al. (1974). Replacement therapy for inherited enzyme deficiency. Use of purified glucocerebrosidase in Gaucher's disease. *New England Journal of Medicine, 291,* 989–993.

Brunner, R.L., Jordan, K.M. & Berry, H.K. (1983). Early-treated phenylketonuria: Neuropsychologic consequences. *Journal of Pediatrics, 102,* 831–835.

Dobson, J.C., Williamson, M.L., Azen, C., et al. (1977). Intellectual assessment of 111 four-year-old children with phenylketonuria. *Pediatrics, 60,* 822–827.

Dover, G.J., Charache, S.H., Boyer, S.H., et al. (1983). 5-Azacytidine increases fetal hemoglobin production in a patient with sickle cell disease. *Progress in Clinical and Biological Research, 134,* 475–488.

Dussault, J.H., Coulombe, P., Laberge, C., et al. (1975). Preliminary report on a mass screening program for neonatal hypothyroidism. *Journal of Pediatrics, 86,* 670–674.

Guthrie, R. (1972). Mass screening for genetic disease. *Hospital Practice, 7,* 93–106.

Hanley, W.B., Linsao, L.S., & Netley, C. (1971). The efficiency of dietary therapy for phenylketonuria. *Canadian Medical Association Journal, 104,* 1089–1091.

Hobbs, J.R., Hugh-Jones, K., Barrett, A.J., et al. (1981). Reversal of clinical features of Hurler's disease and biochemical improvement after treatment by bone-marrow transplantation. *Lancet, 2,* 709–712.

Holtzman, N.A., Welcher, D.W., & Mellits, E.D. (1975). Termination of restricted diet in children with phenylketonuria: A randomized controlled study. *New England Journal of Medicine, 293,* 1121–1124.

Koch, R., Azen, C.G., Friedman, E.G., et al. (1982). Preliminary report on the effects of diet discontinuation in PKU. *Journal of Pediatrics, 100,* 870–875.

Koch, R., Shaw, K.N., Acosta, P.B., et al. (1970). An approach to management of phenylketonuria. *Journal of Pediatrics, 76,* 815–828.

McKusick, V.A. (1983). *Mendelian inheritance in man: Catalogs of autosomal, dominant, autosomal recessive, and X-linked phenotypes* (6th ed.). Baltimore: Johns Hopkins University Press.

Malatack, J.J., Finegold, D.N., Iwatsuki, S., et al. (1983). Liver transplantation for type I glycogen storage disease. *Lancet, 1,* 1073–1075.

Msall, M., Batshaw, M.L., Suss, R., et al. (1984). Neurologic outcome in children with inborn errors of urea synthesis. Outcome of urea-cycle enzymopathies. *New England Journal of Medicine, 310,* 1500–1505.

Palmiter, R.D., Norstedt, G., Gelinas, R.E., et al. (1983). Metallothionein—Human GH fusion genes stimulate growth of mice. *Science, 222,* 809–814.

Partington, M.W., & Laverty, T. (1978). Long term studies of untreated phenylketonuria. I. Intelligence or mental ability. *Neuropaediatrie, 9,* 245–254.

Rosenberg, L.E. (1976). Vitamin-responsive inherited metabolic disorders. *Advances in Human Genetics, 6,* 1–74.

Shih, V.E. (1976). Hereditary urea-cycle disorders. In S. Grisol'ia, R. B'aguena, & F. Mayor (Eds.), *The urea cycle.* New York: John Wiley & Sons.

Smith, G.F., Spiker, O., Peterson, C.P., et al. (1984). Use of megadoses of vitamins with minerals in Down syndrome. *Journal of Pediatrics, 105,* 229–234.

Stanbury, J.B., Wyngaarden, J.B., Frederickson, D.S., et al. (Eds.). (1983). *The metabolic basis of inherited disease* (5th ed.). New York: McGraw-Hill Book Co.

Chapter 9

Good Nutrition, Poor Nutrition

Upon completion of this chapter, the reader will:

—know the major food groups and what problems occur if children are deficient in any of them

—be aware of the function of vitamins and minerals, as well as the results of their deficiency

—understand the problems of lead poisoning

—know the effects of malnutrition on children, including its effect on brain development

—recognize the complications associated with obesity

—be able to evaluate the merits of various diets, including vegetarian, mega-vitamin, organic foods, and macrobiotic diets.

Most of us have heard the expression "You are what you eat." This statement highlights the importance of good nutrition, significant to all of us but especially to infants and children, whose growth rate and development are most rapid. To grow well, children need an appropriate mixture of fats, carbohydrates, protein, vitamins, water, and minerals. The optimal caloric distribution of fats, carbohydrates, and protein is: 30% from fat; 55% from carbohydrates; and 15%–20% from protein (Fomon, Haschke, Ziegler, et al., 1982). These nutrients are metabolized or burned up in our bodies to produce energy, the unit of measurement of which is the calorie. The number of calories one needs to eat depends on body size, the amount of physical activity, and the rate of growth. Children, with a high growth rate and activity, need up to 100 calories per kilogram (kg) of body weight each day, while adults require only 30 calories per kilogram (U.S. National Research Council, 1980; Wait, Blair, & Roberts, 1969). (Keep in mind that one kilogram equals 2.2 pounds.)

This chapter explores the nutritional requirements of children, especially children with handicaps, along with the effects of certain nutritional deficiencies. Also examined are various diets including traditional ones, such as breast-feeding, and nontraditional ones, such as vegetarian, organic, megavitamin, and macrobiotic diets.

GROWTH DURING CHILDHOOD

Normally, a newborn loses weight during the first week of life and then gains about 25–35 grams per day for several months (Table 9.1). By 4 to 6 months of age, the birth weight has doubled and, by 12 months, it has tripled. After this, weight gain slows to about 5 pounds a year until approximately 9 to 10 years of age, when the adolescent growth spurt begins (Smith, 1977).

Height moves at a slower pace, increasing by 50% during the first year of life and doubling by 4 years of age. When a child reaches 13 years of age, his or her height has usually tripled (Smith, 1977). Normal growth curves for height, weight, and head circumference (Hamill, Drizd, Johnson, et al., 1977) are included at the end of this chapter on pages 126–128. Since children with handicaps often have a decreased growth potential, it is especially important to monitor their weight and height.

Besides height and weight gain, the brain grows rapidly during the first year of life. Head circumference increases by 1–3 centimeters a month, and brain weight doubles by 2 years of age (Karlberg, Engstrom, Lichtenstein, et al., 1968) (Table 9.2). At this age, the number of nerve cells is in the adult range, and further growth mainly takes place in the form of increased cell size and intercellular connections.

MALNUTRITION

To grow normally, a child must have an adequate nutritional intake. Malnutrition remains the leading cause of infant illness and death in underdeveloped countries (Maclean & Graham, 1982). Although cases of severe malnutrition are rare in this country, an inadequate diet is not uncommon in certain segments of our population, including the impoverished, the food faddists, and children with developmental disabilities. Signs of malnutrition include poor height and weight gain, a decrease in fatty tissue, muscle wasting, reduced rate of growth in head circumference, and an increased susceptibility to infections.

There are two major forms of malnutrition: one involves severe protein deficiency and is called *kwashiorkor*. The other, *marasmus,* is characterized by a protein-calorie insufficiency. Kwashiorkor is exemplified by the "pot-bellied" starving infants in Africa. However, health practitioners may also observe this condition in

Table 9.1. Growth during childhood

Age	Weight gain (g/day)	Height gain (mm/day)
0–3 mo.	25–35	1.1
3–6 mo.	15–20	0.7
6–12 mo.	10–13	0.5
1–6 yr.	5–8	0.2
7–10 yr.	5–11	0.15

Source: Fomon, Haschke, Ziegler, et al. (1982).

Table 9.2.   Increase in head circumference

Age (months)	Head circumference increase (cm/month)
0–1	3.0
1–3	3.0
3–6	3.0
6–9	2.0
9–12	1.0
12–18	1.6
18–24	1.0
24–36	1.0

Source: Karlberg, Engstrom, Lichtenstein, et al. (1968).

children with chronic diseases such as cystic fibrosis and in those with certain inborn errors of metabolism who require protein-restricted diets.

Marasmus, on the other hand, has a spectrum of clinical manifestations, ranging from "failure to thrive" to malnutriton. In its mildest form, "failure to thrive" involves an inadequate food intake for normal weight gain. Yet, the affected child may continue to grow taller at a fairly normal rate. If he or she eats less, growth in both height and weight is diminished. The child will appear thin and wasted and will act irritable and listless. When measured, the amount of **subcutaneous** fat and muscle is decreased. Children with handicaps are at an increased risk for "failure to thrive." By taking ongoing measurements of height, weight, and the thickness of the skin, physicians can readily monitor these children's growth.

One much disputed aspect of malnutrition is its effect on brain growth (Winick, 1979). The question is whether maternal malnutrition during pregnancy influences the growth of the fetus. Studies of the effects of the famine in Holland during World War II on prenatal development (see Chapter 4) suggested that although the birth weight of newborns was decreased, head circumference and intellectual functioning were not affected (Stein & Susser, 1975). Such findings make sense because it is known that the brain, in comparison to other body organs, is affected last during periods of inadequate nutrition. Taking this into account and considering the small nutritional needs of the fetus compared to those of the mother, one might expect malnutrition to have little effect on fetal brain growth (Hurley, 1980).

After birth, however, no such protection exists (Galler, Ramsey, & Solimano, 1984). One study evaluating this phenomenon was done after the Korean War. A number of Korean War orphans were monitored after placement in foster homes in the United States (Winick, 1979). The physical and intellectual development of all the children fell within normal limits during later childhood. However, the infants who were well nourished during the first 6 months of life had significantly higher IQs than those who had been malnourished. As the first year of life is the period of the most rapid brain growth (Winick, 1979), it seems logical that infantile malnutrition would place the child at increased risk for future learning disabilities and attention deficit disorder.

OBESITY

The opposite of malnutrition is obesity, which can be equally devastating. The classic example among children with handicaps is the Prader-Willi syndrome. Children with this syndrome have moderate retardation and are extremely obese. During sleep, they may have apneic episodes that can be life-threatening (Bray, Dahms, Swerdloff, et al., 1983).

In addition to those children with Prader-Willi, children with Down syndrome, muscular dystrophy, cerebral palsy, and other developmental disorders that cause decreased activity are also more likely to become obese. For children with cerebral palsy, obesity may limit their mobility in that it will make them more difficult to transport. Obesity also places individuals at increased risk for heart disease, hypertension, and diabetes.

Thus, physicians must be careful to identify excessive weight gain early and then to institute a weight reduction program. Such a program should involve physical exercise as well as a nutritious, well-balanced, calorie-restricted diet. A nutritionist is of great help in instituting such a program and may use computer programs, such as Nutriquest II, to design an adequate diet. Behavior modification is equally important to maintain weight reduction. The child must be taught to eat only at meals, to eat slowly, and not to steal food. Also, parents should not use food as a reinforcer for accomplishments or good behavior.

NUTRIENTS AND THEIR DEFICIENCIES

To be adequately nourished, one must, as stated earlier, receive the proper quantity of proteins, fats, carbohydrates, and water, as well as smaller amounts of vitamins and minerals.

Proteins, Fats, and Carbohydrates

Proteins, contained in such foods as cheese, meat, eggs, and fish (Table 9.3), are broken down in the digestive tract into amino acids and nitrogen. Amino acids are involved in the synthesis of new tissue, hormones, enzymes, and antibodies; nitrogen is needed to keep existing tissue healthy (Suskind, 1981). There are nine essential

Table 9.3.   Foods commonly consumed by children that are good sources of protein

Food	Portion size	Protein content (g)	Caloric content
Pasteurized cheese	1 oz.	6.5	107
Scrambled egg	2 med.	11.6	65
Chicken sandwich	1	14.3	245
Submarine sandwich	1	13.7	450
Fish sticks	4 sticks	16.6	176
Hamburger	1	13.3	257
Milk, whole	1 cup	8.0	150

Source: Bowes, Church, Pennington, et al. (1984).

amino acids from which all other nonessential amino acids are made. The quality of a specific protein is measured by the completeness of its essential amino acid content. For example, milk is a complete protein in that it contains all of the essential amino acids. Cereal, on the other hand, is incomplete. A lack of protein in our diets can lead to a reduction in growth rate as well as a failure to develop normal secondary sexual characteristics, such as pubic hair and breast tissue. An increased incidence of infections and poor digestion, due to deficiencies of certain enzymes, may also result from protein malnutrition (Shils & Goodhart, 1980).

While proteins are primarily involved in body growth and tissue maintenance, fats mainly produce energy. Fats in food consist primarily of **triglycerides**, which are either saturated or unsaturated. Animal fats also contain cholesterol. Fats yield 9 calories per gram, whereas carbohydrates and proteins yield only 4 calories per gram. Foods high in fats include ice cream, nuts, and potato chips (Table 9.4). In addition to providing energy, fats give food its good taste and make us feel full. This is why dieting on a low-fat diet tends to leave one always feeling hungry. When we eat fat, most of it is burned as fuel. However, some of its also goes to make vitamins, and some aids in producing tissue.

Recently, much controversy has surrounded the issue of whether diets high in cholesterol or unsaturated fats are unhealthy. Increased risks of heart disease and hypertension have been a major concern. It is clear that individuals with some rare enzyme deficiencies are at risk from high cholesterol or unsaturated fat diets. However, whether such a diet has an adverse effect on children's health is uncertain.

Table 9.4. Foods commonly consumed by children that are high in fat content

Food	Portion size	Fat content (g)	Caloric content
French vanilla ice cream	1 cup	23.8	349
Chocolate milk shake	12 oz.	8.4	326
Cream of chicken soup	1 can	14.9	235
Butter	1 tsp.	4.0	36
Whipping cream	1 T.	4.6	44
Peanut butter	6 T.	47.8	576
Potato chips	3½ oz.	39.8	568
Bologna	1 slice	8.2	88
Sausage	1 patty	12.0	150
French fries	3½ oz.	8.4	220
Hot dog	1	23.9	291
Bacon	1 slice	4.2	65
Gravy	4 T.	14.0	164
Chocolate chip cookie	1	3.3	52
Doughnut	1	4.7	122

Source: Bowes, Church, Pennington, et al. (1984).

Similar to fatty foods, foods high in carbohydrates (Table 9.5) are also used as fuel and provide energy as glucose for brain metabolism. Carbohydrates can also be stored in muscles as glycogen and released as needed (American Academy of Pediatrics, 1979). There are two classes of carbohydrates: simple sugars and complex carbohydrates. Lactose, the sugar in milk, and sucrose, table sugar, are examples of simple sugars. They are rapidly absorbed and quickly available for use as energy. Polysaccharides, or complex carbohydrates, are present in cereals, grains, potatoes, and corn. These starches are broken down more slowly into simple sugars and fibers.

Vitamins

Although children need large quantities of fats, proteins, and carbohydrates for normal growth, they require only minute amounts of vitamins. Vitamins are mainly used as cofactors in chemical reactions and activate, or catalyze, the reactions without being used up themselves. Also, the body can store vitamins so that a deficiency does not become evident until weeks or months after the malnutrition has begun. In the

Table 9.5. Foods commonly consumed by children that are rich in carbohydrates

Food	Portion size	Carbohydrate content (g)	Caloric content
Coca-Cola	12 oz.	36.0	129
Jelly beans	10	16.7	66
Milk chocolate (candy bar)	1 bar	25.2	271
Apple Jacks cereal	1 cup	25.5	109
Cheerios	1 cup	17.6	97
Spaghetti with tomato sauce	1 serving	38.5	220
Chocolate cake (Hostess)	1 bar	24.2	160
Strawberry shortcake	1 serving	61.2	399
Jell-O	½ cup	23.5	97
Popsicle, twin pop	1 bar	23.7	95
Chocolate pudding	½ cup	37.1	219
Pancakes and syrup	2	89.0	472
Apple	1 med.	21.7	81
Banana	1 med.	33.3	127
Corn	1 ear	21.0	100
Popcorn	1½ cups	16.0	81
Bagel	1	28.0	165
Bread	1 slice	12.0	62
Orange juice	1 cup	26.0	110
Gum	1 stick	2.0	9
Tomato	1 large	9.4	44

Source: Bowes, Church, Pennington, et al. (1984).

United States, most processed foods are supplemented with vitamins. For example, milk is fortified with vitamin D, vitamin A, and riboflavin, and infant formulas are supplemented with all the essential vitamins. Because of these additives, a normal child over 3 months of age receives at least twice the daily requirement for vitamins in his or her regular food intake (Table 9.6). However, a child with handicaps who does not eat well may need a vitamin supplement. In this instance, the most important vitamins would be A, B complex, C, and D.

Vitamin A   Vitamin A, or retinol, is essential for the light-sensitive reaction of the rods in the eye. The rods are nerve cells involved in black-and-white vision, and they are responsible for our ability to see in the dark. A deficiency in vitamin A leads to night blindness. On the other hand, the administration of too much vitamin A, a possibility with the use of retinol in treating severe acne, can lead to a skin rash, **anorexia**, bone pain, and mildly increased brain pressure (American Academy of Pediatrics, 1971a). Sources of vitamin A include breast milk and fortified cow's milk, liver, carrots, sweet potatoes, greens, peaches, and apricots.

Vitamin B Complex   The vitamin B complex contains a number of different elements (American Academy of Pediatrics, 1979). One of these, B_1, or thiamine, functions as a cofactor in carbohydrate metabolism. Pork, legumes, and nuts are good sources of thiamine. A lack of thiamine leads to a condition called **beri-beri** (Williams, 1961). While extremely uncommon in this country, beri-beri is still a major problem in underdeveloped countries. Children with this condition have congestive heart failure, edema, and neurological abnormalities. Unlike vitamin A, an excess of thiamine is nontoxic because it is excreted in the urine.

Another B complex vitamin, B_6, or pyridoxine, aids in the metabolism of certain amino acids. This vitamin is also essential for the adequate functioning of the central nervous system. A deficiency in vitamin B_6 can lead to seizures, anemia, skin rash, and nerve damage. Adequate amounts of it are found in whole grains, liver, and potatoes (American Academy of Pediatrics, 1979).

The final B vitamin to be considered, vitamin B_{12}, or cyanocobalamin, is vital for the functioning of both the bone marrow and the nerve cells. It is also a cofactor in a number of enzyme reactions. This vitamin is contained in most animal products, including milk and eggs. Deficiencies are rare except among strict vegetarians.

A more common problem associated with a lack of vitamin B_{12} is pernicious anemia, which is due to an inadequate absorption of this vitamin from the digestive tract. This happens either because there is insufficient secretion of a chemical substance in the stomach, called intrinsic factor, or as a result of damage to the lining of some part of the small intestine. An adult suffering from this disorder develops anemia and progressive neurological symptoms. Treatment consists of administering B_{12} by injection, thus bypassing the defective digestive tract. Vitamin B_{12} has also been used to treat some inborn errors of metabolism (see Chapter 8).

Vitamin C   The much-hailed vitamin C, or ascorbic acid, is needed to form collagen, the connective tissue in tendons and in the walls of blood vessels. It also aids in the metabolism of iron. Scurvy is the condition caused by vitamin C deficiency (Hodges, Baker, Hood, et al., 1969). Its symptoms include irritability, leg pain,

Table 9.6. Recommended daily allowances

| Age (years) | Minerals | | | | | Vitamins | | | | | |
	Sodium (mg/kg/day)	Potassium (mg/kg/day)	Calcium (mg)	Iron (mg)	A (i.u.)	Thia-mine (mg)	Ribo-flavin (mg)	Nico-tinic acid (mg)	C (mg)	D (i.u.)
Infants:										
0–1	23 to 57.5	39 to 97.5	500 to 600	1 per kg	1500	0.4	0.6	6	30	400
Children:										
1–3	57.5	97.5	400	8	2000	0.5	0.8	9	40	400
3–6	46.0	78.0	to	10	2500	0.6	1.0	11	50	400
6–9	34.5	58.5	500	12	3500	0.8	1.3	14	60	400
Boys:										
9–12	34.5	58.5	10–15 yr 600 to 700	15	4500	1.0	1.4	16	70	400
12–15	34.5	58.5		15	5000	1.2	1.8	20	80	400
15–18	34.5	58.5	16–19 yr 500 to 600	15	5000	1.4	2.0	22	80	400
Girls:										
9–12	34.5	58.5	10–15 yr 600 to 700	15	4500	0.9	1.3	15	80	400
12–15	34.5	58.5		15	5000	1.0	1.5	17	80	400
15–18	34.5	58.5	16–19 yr 500 to 600	15	5000	0.9	1.3	15	70	400

Source: U.S. National Research Council (1980).

116

swollen gums, and hemorrhaging. While the disease was quite common during the early exploration of the New World in the 16th century, it is extremely unusual now. Citrus fruits furnish us with large amounts of vitamin C and protect against scurvy.

The other use of vitamin C is much more controversial. Linus Pauling's suggestion that megadoses (1–5 grams per day) of vitamin C can prevent the common cold has stirred great debate (Pauling, 1976). Since this theory was published, a number of carefully controlled studies have shown that the use of vitamin C has, at best, a minimal effect on the severity and duration of the symptoms of a cold (Miller, Nance, Norton, et al., 1977). Furthermore, megadoses of vitamin C may have adverse effects. For instance, such doses interfere with the absorption of vitamin B_{12} and may lead to B_{12} deficiency (Herbert & Jacob, 1974). Also, long-term use of such large doses of vitamin C leads to a decrease of this vitamin in the blood. This may explain why a number of infants born to mothers who took 400 mg of vitamin C daily throughout pregnancy developed scurvy (Cochrane, 1965). On the basis of these findings, the American Academy of Pediatrics (1979) suggests caution in substantially exceeding the recommended daily allowance of vitamin C for children.

Vitamin D   For people to have healthy bones, vitamin D is necessary. It is involved in the absorption of calcium from the gut as well as in the mobilization of calcium from bone (Haussler, 1974). Sunlight is the best natural source of vitamin D (Loomis, 1967). Another good source is cow's milk and infant formulas because they are supplemented with it. Breast milk is a poor source, so breast-fed infants may need to take vitamin D supplements if they do not receive enough exposure to sunlight. Whole-grain cereals, vegetables, and fruits all contain negligible amounts of vitamin D.

A lack of vitamin D causes rickets (Harrison & Harrison, 1979). Signs of rickets include bumps along the rib cartilage, called a **rachitic rosary**, an enlargement of the **anterior fontanel** (the soft spot in the skull), **scoliosis**, and abnormalities in the long bones and pelvis (Figure 9.1). Treatment consists of the oral administration of large doses of vitamin D. Black children are more likely to develop rickets than white children, because their skin absorbs less ultraviolet light from the sun, the main source of vitamin D.

Some anticonvulsants, especially the combination of phenobarbital and Dilantin, actually interfere with the utilization of vitamin D. Although the deficit infrequently causes symptoms of rickets (Hahn, Hendin, Scharp, et al., 1975), research has suggested that non**ambulatory**, home-bound seizure patients should receive supplements of vitamin D. Normally, 1–3 drops/day of Drisdol, an activated vitamin D preparation, prevents the deficit. An excess of vitamin D can lead to nausea, thirst, and neurological abnormalities.

Vitamins E and K   Vitamin E, or tocopherol, is contained in most foods. A deficiency of this vitamin is rare except in premature infants, where it leads to anemia (Oski & Barness, 1967). Supplements of vitamin E are now used in some preterm infants to decrease the risk of anemia and intraventricular hemorrhage.

Also unusual is a deficiency of vitamin K. This may occur in premature infants and in children with cystic fibrosis or severe developmental disabilities; it results in a

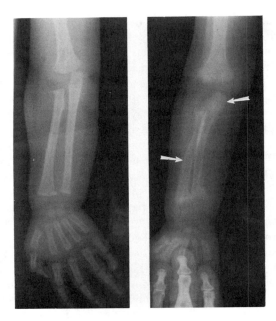

Figure 9.1.   X rays of arm in a normal child (left) and in a child with rickets (right). The upper arrow points to the widened, frayed part (metaphysis) of the bone. The lower arrow points to the decreased density of the bone shaft; both of these are typical findings in rickets.

blood clotting abnormality (American Academy of Pediatrics, 1971b; Suttie, 1969). Vitamin K is commonly found in vegetables, soybeans, and alfalfa.

Water Requirements

Water is second only to oxygen as an essential for life. The water content in infants (70%) is higher than that in adults (60%). It is replenished by the fluids we drink and is also provided in foods. Our requirements for water are related to caloric consumption and average about 1 milliliter of water per 1 calorie in persons of all ages. (Keep in mind that 1 milliliter is ⅟₃₀ of an ounce.) Thus, an infant needs to consume much larger amounts of water for his or her weight than an adult, because infants take in more calories. In young infants, the average intake of fluid should be about 90–150 milliliters/kilogram/day, or 1.5–2.5 ounces per pound of weight each day (American Academy of Pediatrics, 1979). In older infants and children, eating solid foods also provides water. Table 9.7 shows the liquid content of various foods.

In illnesses such as stomach flu or **gastroenteritis**, water is lost through vomiting and diarrhea. If it is not replaced, the individual may become dehydrated and require hospitalization and intravenous feedings of sugar, water, and minerals. This is a particular hazard for a child with multiple handicaps, because he or she becomes dehydrated more easily and may not be able to ask for a drink or obtain one alone very easily. Signs of dehydration include decreased and concentrated urinary

Table 9.7.   Liquid content of various foods

Food	Percentage of water
Strained fruits	80–85
Milk	87
Eggs	75
Meats	50–75
Fruits and vegetables	70–90
Breads	35
Cooked cereal	80–88

Source: Watt & Merrill (1963).

output, difficulty in forming tears and saliva, sunken eyes, and crinkled skin. These symptoms should prompt immediate medical attention.

Minerals

In addition to water, children and adults also need various minerals to ensure appropriate body functioning (Burgess, 1965). Some minerals are required in substantial amounts: calcium, magnesium, chloride, phosphorus, potassium, sodium, iodine, and iron (see Table 9.6). Other elements, such as fluorine, copper, zinc, and manganese, are needed in very small, or *trace*, amounts.

These diverse minerals perform different functions (Water and Electrolytes, 1975). For example, calcium, phosphorus, and magnesium are required for the formation of bone and teeth and for normal muscle contraction. A deficiency in these minerals leads to brittle bone structure, rickets, poor muscle tone, and poor growth (Hypomagnesia, 1971). For children with handicaps who have borderline nutrition, supplements of calcium carbonate (such as 1–3 tablets of TUMS a day) or calcium lactate syrup are useful. Calcium is commonly found in sardines, salmon, milk, cheese, and leafy green vegetables (Robinson & Lawler, 1977). Magnesium is contained in whole grains, nuts, beans, and leafy greens. Phosphorus is found in milk, milk products, and meats. Supplements of these two minerals are not necessary.

Potassium, chloride, and sodium maintain the body's fluid balance and are found in most foods. An imbalance of these minerals leads to muscle weakness, nausea, confusion, and seizures.

Iodine is a component of the thyroid hormone, thyroxine. An insufficiency leads to the development of **goiter** and hypothyroidism (Fierro-Benitez, Penafiel, De Groot, et al., 1969). Iodine is primarily found in shellfish, eggs, and dairy products, and is added to table salt.

Iron is an important constituent of hemoglobin, the pigment of the red blood cell. If a person does not take in enough iron, he or she becomes anemic. Children who eat insufficient amounts of liver, enriched cereals, legumes, or dried fruits are likely to develop iron deficiency anemia. This is especially true of children who are raised on a milk formula without iron supplement or without enriched cereals (Woodruff, 1977).

While a lack of one of the major minerals leads to certain known disorders, a deficiency in trace metals is rarely a cause of disease (Mertz, 1974; Underwood, 1977). Although recently it has been in vogue to link deficiencies in zinc and copper to all kinds of problems ranging from learning difficulties to mental retardation, no scientific evidence supports this thinking.

LEAD

One mineral that is harmful rather than helpful is lead. It may be present in paint on the walls of some homes. Combined with **pica** (the craving of some children for nonnutritive substances), lead poisoning has become a major health hazard in our inner cities.

Lead paint was outlawed for use in homes after World War II. However, older houses have many layers of paint, the oldest of which still contain lead. If these homes are not well maintained, flaking plaster provides a ready source of lead for the curious toddler. Minute amounts, less than 1 milligram, consumed repeatedly over months, will lead to lethargy, clumsiness, developmental regression, and anemia, all signs of lead intoxication (Lin-fu, 1973). If these symptoms are not recognized, the child may develop seizures, go into a coma, or even die. Once the symptoms of lead poisoning become apparent, it is likely that the child has suffered from brain damage; mental retardation and epilepsy often result.

The key to treatment of lead poisoning, therefore, is prevention or early treatment. Dr. Julian Chisolm (1973) at the Kennedy Institute for Handicapped Children, in Baltimore, was one of the first to recognize this. He set up outpatient clinics where inner city children between the susceptible ages of 1 and 5 years could be screened for increased levels of lead in their blood. Those children who have elevated lead levels are removed from their homes until the lead paint is stripped from the walls. The children are also treated both medically and behaviorally. Oral or intramuscular medications, such as **edetate calcium disodium (EDTA)** or **penicillamine**, are given. These drugs bind the lead in the body so that it can be excreted in the urine. Behavior modification is used to decrease the pica. Parents are instructed about the risk of lead poisoning and the danger areas in and around the home. The children continue to be followed in the outpatient clinics to make certain there is no recurrence of the poisoning.

Such a comprehensive approach has enabled great strides in the treatment and prevention of lead poisoning. However, these children may still suffer some degree of developmental delays, especially in language function (Lin-fu, 1973). The problem of lead poisoning will persist so long as there are dilapidated houses and inquisitive children whose fingers find paint chips.

TRADITIONAL DIETS: BREAST-FEEDING

In light of the variety of diets available and recommended, it is important to consider which ones are best nutritionally for children. For infants, breast milk is the best nourishment. It contains the correct ratio of carbohydrates to fats to protein, and it supplies needed calories and minerals. In addition, breast milk is more easily digestible than commercial formulas because of its lower protein and higher carbohydrate content (Fomon, 1974). It is also presterilized and provides the baby with immunity against certain infections. Finally, it is inexpensive and enhances maternal bonding. In underdeveloped countries, breast-feeding is often continued for 18 to 24 months (or until another baby is born). In these places, children develop severe malnutrition only after breast-feeding is terminated.

In the United States, 50% of women breast-feed during their baby's first weeks of life. However, fewer than 25% of women nurse after their children reach 5 months of age (Martinez & Nalezienski, 1981). Usually, women stop breast-feeding as a matter of convenience or because of other demands such as employment. For these infants, commercial formulas are an appropriate substitute for breast milk. They supply an adequate amount of calories, vitamins, minerals, proteins, fats, and carbohydrates. The average infant ingests about 3–5 ounces/kilogram/day of formula. Cereals and fruits are often added by 2 to 3 months of age, although they are not really needed until 6 to 9 months (Fomon, 1974) (Figure 9.2).

NONTRADITIONAL DIETS

In recent years, many nontraditional diets have become popular (Sinatra, 1984). Some of these, such as vegetarian and organic diets, provide adequate nutrition. Others, such as the megavitamin and macrobiotic diets, may actually harm a child.

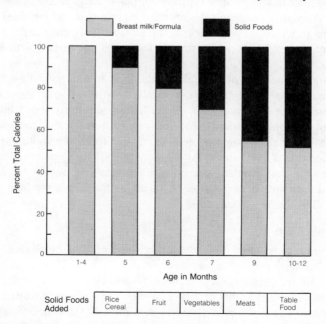

Figure 9.2. Suggested distribution of breast milk/formula and solid foods during first year of life. (*Source:* Ward, 1984.)

Vegetarian Diets

Vegetarian diets can be classified as lacto-ovo-vegetarian (vegetables plus dairy products and eggs) or vegan (plant foods only). People in many societies have practiced vegetarianism for centuries and have remained healthy, especially when they have supplemented their diet with milk or eggs. In fact, in many ways, the lacto-ovo-vegetarian diet is nutritionally similar to diets containing meats. In older children, vegan diets can be equally nourishing, as long as vegetarians select their foods carefully and make sure they receive sufficient calories, essential amino acids, and vitamins (Lappe, 1982; Register & Sonnenberg, 1973).

Yet, there are problems with a vegetarian diet for small children. If a nursing mother follows a vegan diet, her infant may develop deficiencies in calcium, vitamin D, vitamin B_{12}, and iron. The fat content of her milk also will be low. The child would have to receive supplements of vitamins and minerals. Also, for a toddler, vegetarian diets are so high in bulk that the child may be unable to eat a sufficient quantity of fruits and vegetables to receive adequate calories. An older child can eat legumes, wheat germ products, nuts, seeds, and dark green leafy vegetables to achieve an adequate caloric intake. However, even for this child, multivitamin/mineral supplements are necessary.

Organic Food Diets

Unlike vegetarian diets, natural or organic food diets are not restricted in their content. The main restriction here is in how the plants are grown or in how the animals are raised. To qualify as organic, plants must be grown in soil enriched with humus and compost in which no pesticides, herbicides, or inorganic fertilizers have been used. Animals must be reared on natural feeds and not treated with hormones or antibiotics.

Although proponents of these diets laud their results, no long-term study has shown the nutritional superiority of organically grown crops over those grown under standard conditions (Jukes, 1974). Nevertheless, concerns about hormones and additives are valid and, for some individuals, are sufficient reason to buy only organic foods. One important consideration is that these foods are more expensive than ordinary foods. In a 1982 survey by the New York City Department of Consumer Affairs, the foods in a standard marketlist of organically grown items purchased in a health food store often cost twice as much as those bought in a supermarket (Gourdine, Traiger, & Cohen, 1983).

Megavitamin Diets

In megavitamin diets, large doses of certain vitamins, usually 10 times or more the recommended daily allowance, are advocated.

The basis for megavitamin, or **orthomolecular**, therapy is the finding that certain patients with rare inborn errors of metabolism benefit from high doses of specific vitamins (see Chapter 8) (Scriver, 1973). Studies have found that some patients born with a defective enzyme require a much higher dose of a certain vitamin than normal to activate the enzyme. Others have expanded this finding to suggest that patients with disorders ranging from learning disabilities to mental retardation and childhood psychosis can successfully be treated with megavitamin therapy (Cott, 1972). Such usage is unsubstantiated (Arnold, Christopher, Heustis, et al., 1978). Furthermore, certain risks are inherent with ingesting large amounts of vitamins. For example, taking large doses of vitamin A can lead to nausea and increased intracranial pressure (Caffey, 1950). An excessive use of vitamin B_6 produces muscle weakness, and too much vitamin D results in hypercalcemia. Finally, an overdose of vitamin E can cause stomach pain and an increased risk of bleeding.

Macrobiotic Diets

While the ingestion of too many vitamins may be harmful, the use of a macrobiotic diet is definitely detrimental to growing children. The goals of such a diet are largely spiritual. One must follow 10 stages of dietary restriction beginning with the gradual elimination of animal products and leading to the elimination of fruits and vegetables. The highest-level diets allow only cereals; their caloric intake is very low. Strict adherence to such a diet may result in scurvy, rickets, anemia, hypocalcemia, malnutrition, and even death in infancy and childhood (Robson, Konlande, Larkin, et al., 1974).

SUMMARY

Considerable latitude exists in what parents can safely feed their children to ensure adequate nutrition. However, before embarking on any specialty diet, parents would be wise to consult a nutritionist or a physician. Some of the newer diets are dangerous for healthy children and may be devastating for a child with handicaps.

REFERENCES

American Academy of Pediatrics. Committee on Drugs and on Nutrition. (1971a). The use and abuse of vitamin A. *Pediatrics, 48,* 655–656.

American Academy of Pediatrics. Committee on Nutrition. (1971b). Vitamin K supplementation for infants receiving milk substitute infant formulas and for those with fat malabsorption. *Pediatrics, 48,* 483–487.

American Academy of Pediatrics. (1979). *Pediatric nutrition handbook.* Evanston, IL: American Academy of Pediatrics, Committee on Nutrition.

Arnold, L.E., Christopher, J., Heustis, R.D., et al. (1978). Megavitamins for minimal brain dysfunction. A placebo-controlled study. *Journal of the American Medical Association, 240,* 2642–2643.

Beeuwkes, A.M. (1948). Prevalence of scurvy among voyageurs to America, 1493–1600. *Journal of the American Dietetic Association, 24,* 300–303.

Bellinger, D.C., & Needleman, H.L. (1983). Lead and the relationship between maternal and child intelligence. *Journal of Pediatrics, 102,* 523–527.

Bowes, A.D.P., Church, C.F., Pennington, J.A.T., et al. (1984). *Bowes and Church's food values of portions commonly used* (14th ed.). Philadelphia: J.B. Lippincott Co.

Bray, G.A., Dahms, W.T., Swerdloff, R.S., et al. (1983). The Prader-Willi syndrome: A study of 40 patients and a review of the literature. *Medicine, 62,* 59–80.

Burgess, R.E. (1965). Fluids and electrolytes. *American Journal of Nursing, 65,* 90–94.

Caffey, J. (1950). Chronic poisoning due to excess of vitamin A. Description of clinical and roentgen manifestations in 7 infants and young children. *Pediatrics, 5,* 672–687.

Cochrane, W.A. (1965). Overnutrition in prenatal and neonatal life: A problem? *Canadian Medical Association Journal, 93,* 893–899.

Conners, C.K. (1980). *Food additives and hyperactive children*. New York: Plenum Press.

Cott, A. (1972). Megavitamins: The orthomolecular approach to behavioral disorders and learning disabilities. *Academic Therapy, 7,* 245–249.

Fierro-Benitez, R., Penafiel, W., De Groot, L.J., et al. (1969). Endemic goiter and endemic cretinism in the Andean region. *New England Journal of Medicine, 280,* 296–302.

Fomon, S.J. (1974). *Infant nutrition* (2nd ed.). Philadelphia: W.B. Saunders Co.

Fomon, S.J., Haschke, F., Ziegler, E.E., et al. (1982). Body composition of reference children from birth to age 10 years. *American Journal of Clinical Nutrition, 35,* 1169–1175.

Galler, J.R., Ramsey, F., & Solimano, G. (1984). The influence of early malnutrition on subsequent behavioral development. III. Learning disabilities as a sequel to malnutrition. *Pediatric Research, 18,* 309–313.

Galler, J.R., Ramsey, F., Solimano, G., et al. (1984). The influence of early malnutrition on subsequent behavioral development. IV. Soft neurologic signs. *Pediatric Research, 18,* 826–832.

Gourdine, S.P., Traiger, W.W., & Cohen, D.S. (1983). Health food stores investigation. *Journal of the American Dietetic Association, 83,* 285–290.

Hahn, T.J., Hendin, B.A., Scharp, C.R., et al. (1975). Serum 25-hydroxy-caliciferol levels and bone mass in children on chronic anticonvulsant therapy. *New England Journal of Medicine, 292,* 550–554.

Hamill, P.V.V., Drizd, T.A., Johnson, C.L., et al. (1977). NCHS growth curves for children, birth–18 years. In *Vital & Health Statistics,* Series 11, No. 165 (pp. 56–61). Hyattsville, MD: U.S. Department of Health, Education & Welfare, Public Health Service.

Harrison, H.E., & Harrison, H.C. (1979). *Disorders of calcium and phosphate metabolism in childhood and adolescence.* Philadelphia: W.B. Saunders Co.

Haussler, M.R. (1974). Vitamin D: Mode of action and biomedical applications. *Nutrition Reviews, 32,* 257–266.

Herbert, V., & Jacob, E. (1974). Destruction of vitamin B_{12} by ascorbic acid. *Journal of the American Medical Association, 230,* 241–242.

Hodges, R.E., Baker, E.M., Hood, J., et al. (1969). Experimental scurvy in man. *American Journal of Clinical Nutrition, 22,* 535–548.

Hurley, L.S. (1980). *Developmental nutrition.* Englewood Cliffs, NJ: Prentice-Hall.

Hypomagnesia in protein-calorie malnutrition. (1971). *Nutrition Reviews, 29,* 89–90.

Jukes, T.H. (1974). The organic food myth. *Journal of the American Medical Association, 230,* 276–277.

Karlberg, P., Engstrom, I., Lichtenstein, H., et al. (1968). The development of children in a Swedish urban community. a prospective longitudinal study. III. Physical growth during the first three years of life. *Acta Paediatrica Scandinavica, 187 (Suppl.),* 48–65.

Krick, J., & Van Duyn, M.A.S. (1984). The relationship between oral-motor involvement and growth: A pilot study in a pediatric population with cerebral palsy. *Journal of the American Dietetic Association, 84,* 555–559.

Lappe, F.M. (1982). *Diet for a small planet* (10th anniversary ed.). New York: Ballantine.

Lin-fu, J.S. (1973). Vulnerability of children to lead exposure and toxicity. *New England Journal of Medicine, 289,* 1229–1233.

Loomis, W.F. (1967). Skin-pigment regulation of vitamin-D biosynthesis in man. *Science, 157,* 501–506.

Maclean, W.C., & Graham, G. (1982). *Pediatric nutrition in clinical practice.* Menlo Park, CA: Addison-Wesley Publishing Co.

Martinez, G.A., & Nalezienski, J.P. (1981). 1980 update: The recent trend in breast-feeding. *Pediatrics, 67,* 260–263.

Mertz, W. (1974). Recommended dietary allowance up to date—trace minerals. *Journal of the American Dietetic Association, 64,* 163–167.

Miller, J.Z., Nance, W.E., Norton, J.A., et al. (1977). Therapeutic effect of vitamin C. A co-twin control study. *Journal of the American Medical Association, 237,* 248–251.

Oski, F.A., & Barness, L.A. (1967). Vitamin E deficiency: A previously unrecognized cause of hemolytic anemia in the premature infant. *Journal of Pediatrics, 70,* 211–220.

Pauling, L.C. (1976). *Vitamin C, the common cold & the flu.* San Francisco: W.H. Freeman & Co.

Pratt, E.L. (1984). Historical perspectives: Food, feeding, and fancies. *Journal of the American College of Nutrition, 3,* 115–121.

Register, U.D., & Sonnenberg, L.M. (1973). The vegetarian diet. Scientific and practical considerations. *Journal of the American Dietetic Association, 62,* 253–261.

Riley, D.J., Santiago, T.V., & Edelman, N.H. (1976). Complications of obesity—hypoventilation in childhood. *American Journal of Diseases of Children, 130,* 671–674.

Robinson, C.H., & Lawler, M.R. (1977). *Normal and therapeutic nutrition* (15th ed.). New York: Macmillan Co.

Robson, J.R., Konlande, J.E., Larkin, F.A., et al. (1974). Zen macrobiotic dietary problems in infancy. *Pediatrics, 53*, 326–329.

Scriver, C.R. (1973). Vitamin-responsive inborn errors of metabolism. *Metabolism, 22*, 1319–1344.

Shils, M.E., & Goodhart, R.S. (1980). *Modern nutrition in health and disease* (6th ed.). Philadelphia: Lea & Febiger.

Sinatra, F.R. (1984). Food faddism in pediatrics. *Journal of the American College of Nutrition, 3*, 169–175.

Smith, D.W. (1977). *Growth and its disorders: Basics and standards, approach and classifications, growth deficiency disorders, growth excess disorders, obesity.* Philadelphia: W.B. Saunders Co.

Stein, Z., & Susser, M. (1975). The Dutch famine, 1944–45, and the reproductive process. I. Effects or six indices at birth. *Pediatric Research, 9*, 70–76.

Suskind, R.M. (Ed.). (1981). *Textbook of pediatric nutrition.* New York: Raven Press.

Suttie, J.W. (1969). Control of clotting factor biosynthesis by vitamin K. *Federation Proceedings, 28*, 1696–1701.

Underwood, E.J. (1977). *Trace elements in human and animal nutrition* (4th ed.). New York: Academic Press.

U.S. National Research Council, Food and Nutrition Board. (1980). *Recommended dietary allowances.* Washington, D.C.: National Academy of Sciences.

Wait, B., Blair, R., & Roberts, L.J. (1969). Energy intake of well-nourished children and adolescents. *American Journal of Clinical Nutrition, 22*, 1383–1396.

Ward, L. (1984). *An infant feeding guide.* Baltimore: Johns Hopkins Medical Center, Department of Nutrition.

Water and electrolytes in malnutrition. (1975). *Nutrition Reviews, 33*, 74–76.

Watt, B.K., & Merrill, A.L. (1963). *Composition of foods—raw, processed, prepared* (rev. ed.). Washington, DC: U.S. Department of Agriculture, Agriculture Handbook No. 8.

Williams, R.R. (1961). *Toward the conquest of beriberi.* Cambridge, MA: Harvard University Press.

Winick, M. (Ed.). (1979). *Nutrition, pre- and postnatal development.* New York: Plenum Press.

Woodruff, C.W. (1977). Iron deficiency in infancy and childhood. *Pediatric Clinics of North America, 24*, 85–94.

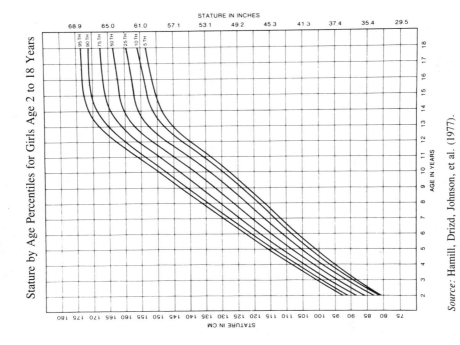

Stature by Age Percentiles for Girls Age 2 to 18 Years

Source: Hamill, Drizd, Johnson, et al. (1977).

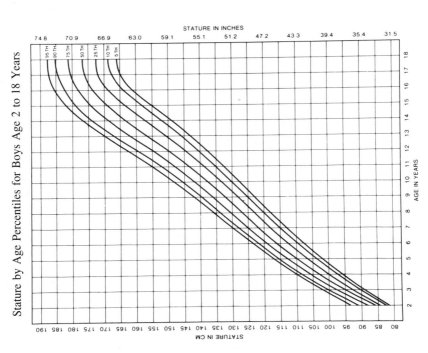

Stature by Age Percentiles for Boys Age 2 to 18 Years

Source: Hamill, Drizd, Johnson, et al. (1977).

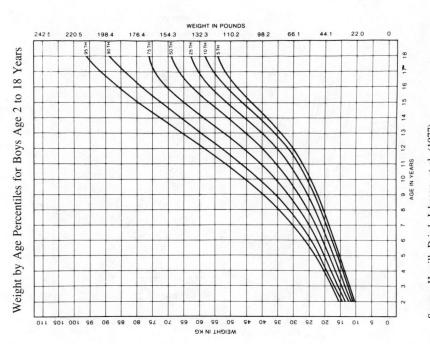

Weight by Age Percentiles for Girls Age 2 to 18 Years

Source: Hamill, Drizd, Johnson, et al. (1977).

Weight by Age Percentiles for Boys Age 2 to 18 Years

Source: Hamill, Drizd, Johnson, et al. (1977).

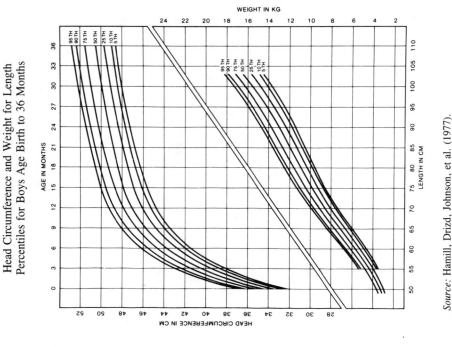

Head Circumference and Weight for Length Percentiles for Boys Age Birth to 36 Months

Source: Hamill, Drizd, Johnson, et al. (1977).

Head Circumference and Weight for Length Percentiles for Girls Age Birth to 36 Months

Source: Hamill, Drizd, Johnson, et al. (1977).

Chapter 10

Feeding the Child with Handicaps

Upon completion of this chapter, the reader will:
—understand the function and structure of the gastrointestinal tract
—be aware of the feeding problems of children with handicaps
—know some of the ways to treat these problems

Children with multiple handicaps face special problems in getting adequate nutrition. These children may have a decreased appetite, be unable to communicate their hunger, or be unable to obtain food on their own. In addition, they may have difficulty sucking, chewing, or swallowing. Problems with **gastroesophageal reflux** and constipation add further difficulties. In this chapter, the anatomy and function of the gastrointestinal tract are explained. Feeding and digestive problems are discussed along with possible ways to treat these problems.

THE GASTROINTESTINAL TRACT

For optimal nutrition to take place, the gastrointestinal tract must be able to complete the digestive process and perform its three major functions: the controlled movement of food from the mouth to the anus, the digestion of food, and the absorption of nutrients.

The complex acts of chewing and swallowing begin this process. Once food is chewed, it collects into a **bolus** or lump and passes to the back of the mouth. It is then reflexively sent into the pharynx and the **esophagus**. A small flap of tissue, called the **epiglottis**, covers the trachea during this process so that food will not be **aspirated** into the lungs (Figure 10.1). The food then passes down the esophagus and enters the stomach. A muscle **sphincter** at the junction of the esophagus and the stomach prevents the backward flow of food (reflux) once it has entered the stomach.

As soon as the stomach receives the food, it secretes acid to destroy infectious agents in the food, adds fluid, and churns the mixture up in a washing machine–like

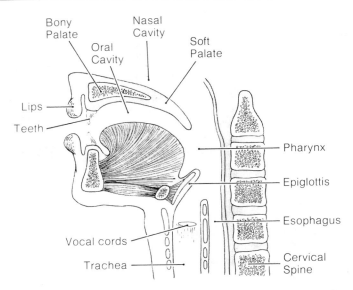

Figure 10.1. Anatomy of swallowing. Once food is taken, the lips close and the food is passed by the tongue to the pharynx. As the food drops down, the epiglottis falls over the tracheal opening, preventing aspiration into the lungs. The food passes easily down the esophagus into the stomach.

fashion. The stomach's contents then gradually flow into the **duodenum**, the upper part of the small intestine. (Incidentally, the intestines are referred to as small or large because of their diameter, not their length.) Normally, the duodenum (Figure 10.2) takes care of the most important part of the digestive and absorptive processes. Enzymes and other substances from the pancreas and bile ducts are released into the duodenum and aid in the breakdown of food particles into their major parts: proteins, fats, and carbohydrates. These compounds are further simplified into sugars, such as **lactose**, fatty acids, amino acids, and vitamins. The **ileum**, or lower small intestine, absorbs these digested nutrients. The water and electrolytes added in the stomach are recycled when they are reabsorbed by the ileum.

The leftovers, including the remaining water and electrolytes, then pass to the large intestine or colon (see Figure 10.2). In the adult, the colon receives about 50 ounces of fluid a day but discharges only about 3 to 6 ounces as stool. The rest of the fluid is normally reabsorbed. Movement through the colon is much slower than through the rest of the digestive tract and depends on the volume of nonabsorbable nutrients, often called **bulk** or **fiber**, that is contained in the food. While movement from the stomach to the end of the ileum may take only 30 to 90 minutes, passage through the colon may require 1 to 7 days. Rapid movement, which happens, for example, during a stomach flu, leads to diarrhea. Conversely, slower movement causes more water to be absorbed and results in hard stools and constipation. For proper movement to take place, an individual needs to be able to coordinate muscle activity, including control of the rectal sphincter muscles that facilitate voluntary defecation.

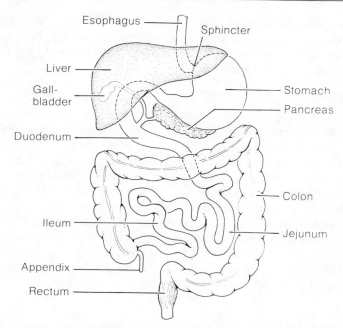

Figure 10.2. The digestive tract. Food enters the stomach through the esophageal sphincter, which prevents reflux (backward flow) of the stomach's contents. The partially digested food then passes through the three segments of the small intestine (duodenum, jejunum, and ileum). There, digestive juices from the pancreas and the gallbladder are added. The remaining water and electrolytes pass to the colon where water is removed. Voluntary stooling is controlled via the rectal sphincter muscle.

It is in the colon that bacteria alter nondigestible residues and form substances that give the stool its odor. The absence of this bacteria in an infant's colon accounts for the lack of smell in the stool during the first few months of life.

FEEDING PROBLEMS OF THE CHILD WITH HANDICAPS

For a child with handicaps, problems in eating and digestion range from inability to suck, chew, or feed him- or herself to problems in digestion and motility (movement) of the gastrointestinal system.

Sucking

In infancy, sucking is the only way to obtain nutrition. To suck, a child must be able to purse the lips and then rhythmically raise and lower the body of the tongue, creating a vacuum. Food can then be pulled into the mouth and swallowed.

For the child with handicaps, especially with cerebral palsy, a number of problems may interfere with sucking. These include abnormal muscle tone, lip and tongue **retraction**, involuntary movement, and nasal regurgitation. Abnormal body muscle tone may force the child into an arched, extended position, making feeding more difficult and increasing the likelihood of vomiting. When the lips are retracted or tightly drawn back, they are more difficult to purse to make a seal necessary for sucking. Similarly, retracting the tongue lowers it and hinders the creation of a vacuum. In nasal regurgitation caused by uncoordinated swallowing, food or liquid is ejected through the nose rather than down the pharynx.

Spoon-feeding

Normally, a child progresses from sucking to spoon-feeding around 4 months of age. At this point, the child begins to eat solid foods. Some children with handicaps, however, are unable to move to this next step. To spoon-feed, a child must be able to respond appropriately to the touch of a spoon to his or her lips. When abnormal muscle tone exists, this becomes difficult. Children with handicaps may have a tonic bite reflex that leads to a sudden closure of the jaw when the teeth or gums are lightly touched. If this happens, the bite does not release for some time. The spoon is stopped before it even delivers the food. An opposite problem is one in which the jaw does not close around the spoon. Then, the food merely slides out of the mouth. Similarly, a reflexive tongue thrust in a child with handicaps may actually push the food out of the mouth rather than down the throat. Lastly, the child may be hypersensitive to the touch of the spoon or food and even refuse to open his or her mouth.

Chewing

Once a child is able to be spoon-fed, the next developmental step is chewing. Usually this starts at around 6 months of age when the child is capable of moving the food from side to side and can keep it on the side of the mouth for chewing. Chewing then consists of a rhythmical bite-and-release pattern with a series of jaw openings and closings. Some children with handicaps will never have the skills needed to chew. Even those who have the potential may be delayed in chewing because of abnormalities in muscle tone, involuntary tongue movement, or the persistence of primitive reflexes such as the tonic bite reflex or the tongue thrust.

Swallowing

Swallowing has three phases: oral, pharyngeal, and esophageal. An individual must be able to form a bolus and coordinate the contraction of his or her muscles to move the food from the back of the tongue to the pharynx and then down the esophagus (see Figure 10.1). As mentioned earlier, the epiglottis must then fold over the opening of the trachea to prevent the food from being inhaled into the lungs. Poor coordination of these muscle contractions may interfere with adequate food intake or increase the risk of aspiration of food into the lungs, a problem that leads to recurrent pneumonia.

Gastroesophageal Reflux

Gagging, vomiting, and **rumination** (the regurgitation and rechewing of swallowed food) provide further problems for the child with developmental disabilities. Whether these problems are voluntary or involuntary, they interfere with adequate nutrition. One contributing factor is *gastroesophageal reflux*. Here the muscular part of the lower esophagus that normally prevents food from backing up from the stomach into the esophagus does not work properly. Food and stomach acid juices can then surge up from the stomach after a meal and cause vomiting or aspiration into the lungs. In addition, the escape of stomach acid can cause an inflammation of the esophagus that may make eating uncomfortable.

The Small Intestine

While problems of sucking and swallowing are common in children with handicaps, their digestive systems are usually able to absorb nutrients once they reach the small intestine. Occasionally, however, in handicapped as well as normal children, there may be malabsorption that interferes with adequate nutrition (Ament, 1972).

The most common malabsorptive disorder is lactose intolerance. Approximately 10%–20% of black and Jewish children have this problem (Bayless & Christopher, 1969). Symptoms include vomiting and diarrhea after swallowing milk products. The cause of the intolerance is the inherited deficiency of the enzyme **lactase**, which normally breaks down milk sugar (lactose) and allows its absorption. Unabsorbed lactose irritates parts of the gastrointestinal tract and causes vomiting and diarrhea (Stephenson & Latham, 1974). Now, an affected individual can take lactase in a capsule before ingesting any milk products, and thus can prevent or decrease the symptoms.

Another disorder associated with digestive problems is cystic fibrosis. In this case, pancreatic enzymes are not secreted; this interferes with the normal absorption of fats and vitamins and leads to diarrhea and malnutrition (Berry, Kellogg, Hunt, et al., 1975; Crozier, 1974). Children with cystic fibrosis also have severe lung disease.

Still another cause of malabsorption is **celiac disease** (Ruffin, Kurtz, & Borland, 1964). This involves an intolerance to cereal products due to a deficiency of an enzyme needed to break down the **gluten** contained in cereals. Malnutrition may result. With all three of these disorders, enzyme supplements or a diet restricted in the problem nutrient can improve the child's condition.

The Large Intestine

For the child with handicaps, the major problem with the function of the large intestine or colon is constipation. This is due to an inadequate fluid and fiber intake combined with uncoordinated muscle contractions and poor rectal sphincter control. The result is the retention of stool for prolonged periods of time. The longer the stool remains in the colon, the more water is absorbed, and the harder and more immobile the stool becomes. The end result is constipation (Benson, 1975).

HANDLING FEEDING PROBLEMS

Handling feeding problems in children with handicaps can be difficult and time consuming. Such problems may also hinder parent-child relationships. Following are some recommendations:

1. *Improve appetite.* If possible, parents should offer their child food he or she likes, especially when his or her appetite is poor. When doing this, parents must

remember to keep the child's overall diet balanced. Parents may also use preferred food as rewards for eating less favored but more nutritious foods. In some cases, the use of Periactin, an antihistamine drug, has been effective in stimulating appetite.

2. *Enhance sucking and chewing.* While it is impossible to hasten the neurological maturation of these responses, physical therapists, occupational therapists, and speech pathologists have developed ways of handling children with handicaps that enhance these actions.

The first step involves the appropriate positioning of the child when feeding. A child who lies in an extended position should be cradled in a flexed posture so that body parts needed for eating are lined up properly. Such positioning may allow the child to better suck from a bottle or chew solid foods. Next, manually pursing the child's lips and holding the jaw stable may help the child develop improved tongue and lip control. Another way to help develop such control in older children is to teach the child to drink from a straw. Both of these approaches diminish the effects of abnormal responses such as tongue thrusting and lip or tongue retraction. Thickening liquid formula with cereal may also help a child better handle liquids. Varying the texture of food and its ingredients may also stimulate the child's interest in eating. Chewing may be enhanced by placing food between the upper and lower back teeth; this forces the child to use his or her tongue and to move the jaw to remove the food.

3. *Decrease regurgitation.* Once food is swallowed, vomiting, gagging, and rumination may present further problems. A number of approaches including positioning, medications, surgery, and behavior modification may control these difficulties. The simplest method is positioning. The child should be fed in an upright position and then placed in a **prone** (face down) position after feeding (Orenstein, Whitington, & Orenstein, 1983). This allows the food to flow more readily through the stomach and decreases the risk of gastroesophageal reflux. Furthermore, medications such as propantheline (ProBanthine) and metoclopramide (Reglan) (Temple, Bradby, O'Connor, et al., 1983) tighten the esophageal sphincter muscle so that it remains closed once the food passes through. Again, the risk of reflux is reduced. Also, the drug, cimetidine (Tagamet) is sometimes used to decrease stomach acidity and to lower the risk of an inflammation of the esophagus.

One of the main concerns with gastroesophageal reflux is the risk of **aspiration pneumonia**. In a child who has had recurrent episodes of pneumonia despite the efforts just described, surgery may be necessary. The operation is called a **fundal plication** (Wilkinson, Dudgeon, & Sondheimer, 1981). In it, the surgeon tightens the muscle around the opening of the esophagus. This decreases reflux and allows for normal oral feeding.

Rumination, unlike reflux, is more behavioral than physiological in origin. The child chews and swallows the food part way, then regurgitates it and chews it again, like a cow chewing its cud. For these children, a behavior modification approach has met with some success. The child is positively reinforced for not gagging and vomiting and receives negative reinforcement for continuing to vomit and gag (Holvoet, 1982).

4. *Individualize dietary intake.* While the required ratio of fats to carbohydrates and proteins is the same for all children, the caloric requirements of children with handicaps are different from those of normal children. For instance, the requirements for children with handicaps are more appropriately calculated per unit of height than per unit of weight (Smith, 1976). Ambulatory children who have developmental disabilities and who have various types of motor dysfunction require about the same number of calories per unit of body height as those who do not have motor dysfunction. However, if the child is nonambulatory, then only about 75% of the normal caloric intake is required.

5. *Use alternative methods of feeding.* In some cases, sufficient oral feeding may become impossible because of an inadequate suck, a swallowing problem, or frequent bouts of aspiration pneumonia. For these children, nasogastric tube feedings or the placement of a **gastrostomy** tube is often required. With nasogastric tube feedings, a tube is passed through the nose into the esophagus and then into the stomach. Once it is inserted, a small amount of air is pushed into the tube before food is given. The parent listens for rumblings in the stomach. If no rumblings are heard, the tube may have lodged in the trachea instead of the esophagus. As soon as it is correctly placed, the tube can handle a liquid diet. One can either use commercially available formulas, such as Isocal, or blended feedings composed of a regular diet combined with milk.

The main problem with nasogastric tube feeding is that it can usually only be used for a few months at a time because the tube irritates the esophagus and can cause aspiration if it is incorrectly placed. Therefore, in children for whom adequate oral feeding becomes impossible, a gastrostomy tube is placed. A small hole is surgically made in the abdominal and stomach walls, and a tube is placed through the hole into the stomach. Feeding can then be done through the gastrostomy tube in a manner similar to nasogastric tube feeding. The placement of a gastrostomy tube does not interfere with normal oral feeding. Frequently, these children require both a gastrostomy and a fundal plication.

6. *Avoid constipation.* Constipation is a chronic problem for most children with developmental disabilities. Not only is it uncomfortable, but it may also decrease their appetite. While no cures for constipation are known, the following suggestions may be helpful. As much fluid as possible should be added to the diet. Bulky and high-fiber foods, such as whole-grain cereals, bran, and raw fruits and vegetables, should also be eaten to increase movement through the gastrointestinal tract. A commercially available fiber product, Unifiber, has also been helpful. Prune or apricot juice can be given to act as a mild laxative. Stool softeners, such as Colase, may be used regularly to help coat the stool and facilitate its movement through the intestines. Active or passive physical exercise is also important to aid the movement of the stool.

When laxatives or suppositories are necessary, milk of magnesia, Malt Supex, Senokot, Dulcolax, or glycerine suppositories are usually effective. Enemas may also help the problem of constipation, but their constant use may interfere with rectal sphincter control (Clayden, 1976). Therefore, it is wise to use enemas sparingly. Remember, it is not necessary for all children to have one stool a day; once every 3 days may suffice.

SUMMARY

Feeding a child with handicaps often requires the implementation of a number of creative approaches and the involvement of a variety of health care professionals. When effective, these methods enable the children to receive the necessary combination of nutrients and fluids to help them grow and remain healthy.

REFERENCES

Ament, M.E. (1972). Malabsorption syndromes in infancy and childhood. Part I. *Journal of Pediatrics, 81,* 685–697.

Bayless, T.M., & Christopher, N.L. (1969). Disaccharidase deficiency. *American Journal of Clinical Nutrition, 22,* 181–190.

Benson, J.A., Jr. (1975). Simple chronic constipation: Pathophysiology and management. *Postgraduate Medicine, 57,* 55–60.

Berry, H.K., Kellogg, F.W., Hunt, M.M., et al. (1975). Dietary supplement and nutrition in children with cystic fibrosis. *American Journal of Diseases of Children, 129,* 165–171.

Clayden, G.S. (1976). Constipation and soiling in childhood. *British Medical Journal, 1,* 515–517.

Crozier, D.N. (1974). Cystic fibrosis: A not-so-fatal disease. *Pediatric Clinics of North America, 21,* 935–950.

Culley, W.J., & Middleton, T.O. (1969). Caloric requirements of mentally retarded children with and without motor dysfunction. *Journal of Pediatrics, 75,* 380–384.

Holvoet, J.F. (1982). The etiology and management of rumination and psychogenic vomiting: A review. *Monographs of the American Association of Mental Deficiency, 5,* 29–77.

Morris, S.E. (1977). *Program guidelines for children with feeding problems.* Edison, NJ: Childcraft Education Corp.

Orenstein, S.R., Whitington, P.F., & Orenstein, D.M. (1983). The infant seat as treatment for gastroesophageal reflux. New England Journal of Medicine, 309, 760–763.

Ruffin, J.M., Kurtz, S.M., & Borland, J.L., Jr. (1964). Gluten-free diet for nontropical sprue. Immediate and prolonged effects. *Journal of the American Medical Association, 188,* 42–44.

Smith, M.A.H. (Ed.). (1976). *Guides for nutritional assessment of the mentally retarded and the developmentally disabled.* Memphis: University of Tennessee Center for the Health Sciences, Child Development Center.

Stephenson, L.S., & Latham, M.C. (1974). Lactose intolerance and milk consumption: The relation of tolerance to symptoms. *American Journal of Clinical Nutrition, 27,* 296–303.

Talbot, N.B., Kagan, J., & Eisenberg, L. (1971). *Behavioral science in pediatric medicine.* Philadelphia: W.B. Saunders Co.

Temple, J.G., Bradby, G.V., O'Connor, F.O., et al. (1983). Cimetidine and metoclopramide in oesophageal reflux disease. *British Medical Journal, 286,* 1863–1864.

U.S. Maternal and Child Health Service, Children's Bureau. (1970). *Feeding the child with a handicap.* Washington, DC: U.S. Government Printing Office, Publication No. 2091.

Wallace, H.M. (1972). Nutrition and handicapped children. *Journal of the American Dietetic Association, 61,* 127–133.

Wilkinson, J.D., Dudgeon, D.L., & Sondheimer, J.M. (1981). A comparison of medical and surgical treatment of gastroesophageal reflux in severely retarded children. *Journal of Pediatrics, 99,* 202–205.

Wilson, J.M. (1978). *Oral-motor function and dysfunction in children.* Chapel Hill: University of North Carolina, Department of Medical Allied Health Professionals, Division of Physical Therapy.

Chapter 11

Dental Care

Upon completion of this chapter, the reader will:
—understand the development and structure of the teeth
—recognize malformations such as cleft lip and palate and their effect on nutrition and speech
—be aware of the effects of thumb sucking, teeth grinding, mouth breathing, and tongue thrusting on oral health
—know how dental decay and periodontal disease occur and what prophylactic steps can be taken to prevent these problems
—understand what procedures are commonly used during routine dental checkups and dental surgery

Our teeth are important for the preparation of our food for swallowing and digestion. In children, the emergence of teeth also stimulates the growth of the jaw. Besides these functions, teeth help us produce certain sounds when we speak. Children with handicaps are at an increased risk for both dental malformations and dental disease. Thus, those who care for these children need to be careful to provide them with appropriate dental care.

In this chapter, teeth formation and the problems that may occur during this process are addressed. Various types of dental disorders are then discussed, followed by a consideration of the appropriate kinds of dental care.

THE FORMATION OF TEETH

Tooth buds first appear when the human embryo is only 6 weeks old. As the pregnancy progresses, the outer layer of these buds, made up of **epithelial** cells, forms the dental enamel. This enamel is deposited over the softer inner tissue or dentin (Nowak, 1976) (Figure 11.1). The dentin is gradually **calcified**; nerves, blood, and lymph vessels develop to form the pulp of the mature tooth. Ten primary or **deciduous** teeth are formed in what is to become the upper jaw (the **maxilla**) and 10 more in the lower jaw (the mandible). These primary teeth also keep the proper spacing in the dental arch that is needed for the later development of permanent teeth.

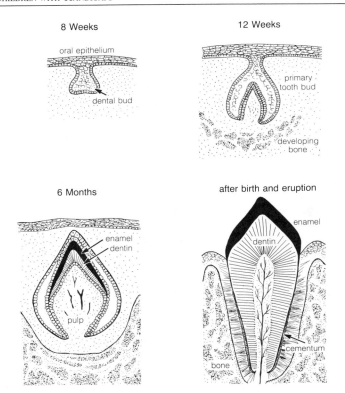

8 Weeks

oral epithelium

dental bud

12 Weeks

primary tooth bud

developing bone

6 Months

enamel
dentin

pulp

after birth and eruption

enamel

dentin

cementum

bone

Figure 11.1. Development of teeth. By the time the fetus is 8 weeks old, the dental (tooth) bud has formed and, by 12 weeks, it is beginning to assume a tooth-like shape. At 6 months gestation, the layers of the tooth—enamel, dentin, and pulp—are evident. After birth, when the child is about 16 months old, this primary cuspid, completely formed, erupts.

If there is a disturbance in the formation of dentin or enamel, or if foreign material is incorporated in this process, the texture, thickness, or color of the teeth can be affected.

By the third month of gestation, the permanent tooth buds have started to form under the primary teeth. After birth, these teeth begin to calcify. When a child is around 6 years of age, they start to grow and push up the roots of the primary teeth, causing the primary teeth to be shed. Thus, the primary teeth have a life cycle that begins with their formation in fetal life and ends with their shedding during childhood.

PROBLEMS AFFECTING THE DEVELOPMENT OF TEETH

In most children, the teeth's developmental process moves along smoothly. However, a number of problems may affect tooth development. Among these is the use of the antibiotic, tetracycline, by a woman when she is pregnant. If the tetracycline is taken between the fourth and the last month of pregnancy, the infant's teeth may have a brownish-yellow discoloration, and the enamel may be thinned (Josell & Abrams, 1982a). Not only is this discoloration unattractive, but thinned enamel also makes the teeth more susceptible to decay. If a child takes tetracycline between 4 months and 8 years of age, his or her permanent teeth may also be discolored. Thus, it is suggested that pregnant women and young children avoid taking tetracycline.

Besides tetracycline, other conditions can cause tooth discoloration. With congenital rubella, the virus causes pigment deposits in the dental enamel (Nowak, 1976). Similarly, in Rh incompatibility, bilirubin leads to the same problem (Stewart & Poole, 1982).

More serious are the dental malformations associated with various genetically inherited syndromes. Anodontia, or the absence of teeth, is found in **Ellis–van Creveld syndrome** and **Hallermann-Streiff syndrome** (D. Smith, 1982). Thin-enameled, abnormally shaped teeth are found in Down Syndrome and **mucopolysaccharide** disorders (D. Smith, 1982). These abnormalities affect eating patterns and increase the incidence of tooth decay and malocclusion of the jaw.

Finally, cleft lip and palate create a number of dental problems (Ranta & Rintala, 1982). These defects occur when fusion of the pharyngeal arches does not take place during fetal development (Figure 11.2). In about 1 out of 1,000 live-born infants, the cells that should grow together to form the lips and palate do not move in the proper direction. This creates a cleft, or opening. Such a defect may be an isolated one, unassociated with mental retardation or other handicaps, or it may be part of a more complex syndrome.

The resultant dental problems associated with cleft lip and palate include extra or missing teeth. The spacing of the teeth also may be abnormal. In addition, even with the surgical closure of the cleft at 1–2 months of age, long-term dental problems may exist.

Cleft palate can also affect speech and nutrition. The formation of various sounds in speech may be more difficult. Before it is repaired, the cleft interferes with the baby's ability to suck from a breast or bottle. The jaw may also grow abnormally, distorting the face. Lastly, though unrelated to dental problems, the child is at increased risk for middle ear infections (Rood & Stool, 1981).

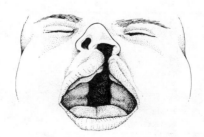

Figure 11.2.   Cleft lip and palate result from incomplete fusion of the pharyngeal arches.

THE EMERGENCE OF TEETH

A baby's first tooth, the lower, central incisor, appears around 6 months of age (Figure 11.3A). In rapid succession, the child sprouts another incisor, a cuspid or pointed tooth, and two molars on either side of his mouth, in the upper and lower jaws. By 18–30 months of age, the child has a total of 20 primary teeth. When the child is about 6 years old, the first of these teeth is shed and is replaced shortly by an adult central incisor (Table 11.1). Over the next 6–12 years, the rest of the primary teeth are shed and are eventually replaced by a total of 32 permanent teeth (Figure 11.3B) (Forrester, Wagner, & Fleming, 1981). Children with developmental delays also often have delays in the emergence of their teeth. Thus, this timetable may not hold true for them (Wessels, 1979).

DENTAL PROBLEMS

A number of factors affect our dental health. Certain behaviors, such as mouth breathing and finger sucking, may lead to dental difficulties in the future. Other problems include malocclusion, dental decay, **periodontal** disease, and dental injuries.

Problem Behaviors

At least four behaviors may adversely affect the teeth and the jaw. These are mouth breathing, tooth grinding, finger sucking, and tongue thrusting (Schneider & Peterson, 1982). Children with handicaps tend to exhibit these behaviors more often than normal children. For instance, mouth breathing is much more common in children with retardation, especially those with Down syndrome. Although breathing through the mouth is normal for infants, it often continues for longer periods of time in children with mental retardation. Over time, this can lead to an inflammation of the gums and periodontal disease.

Table 11.1. Timetable for emergence and shedding of teeth

	Age (months) at emergence		Age (years) at shedding	
	Lower	Upper	Lower	Upper
Central incisor	6	7½	6	7½
Lateral incisor	7	9	7	8
Cuspid	16	18	9½	11½
First molar	12	14	10	10½
Second molar	20	24	11	10½
Incisors	Range = ±2 mos.		Range = ±6 mos.	
Molars	Range = ±4 mos.			

Source: Massler, M., & Schour, I. (1958) *Atlas of the mouth*. Chicago: American Dental Association. Copyright by the American Dental Association; reprinted by permission.

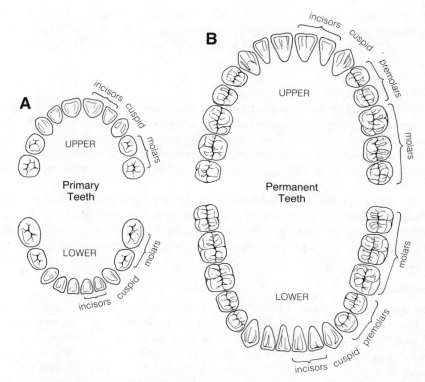

Figure 11.3. Primary and permanent teeth. A) There are 20 primary teeth: 4 incisors, 2 cuspids, and 4 molars on the top and on the bottom of the mouth. B) There are 32 permanent teeth: 4 incisors, 2 cuspids, 4 premolars, and 6 molars on the top and on the bottom.

Tooth grinding, or **bruxism**, is also more common in children with retardation; it occurs in over half of the children who have severe mental retardation. For these children, tooth grinding is a form of self-stimulatory behavior. Grinding of the molar teeth interferes with normal chewing.

For children with extrapyramidal cerebral palsy, tongue thrusting is often a problem. This not only hinders eating by pushing food out of the mouth, but it may also lead to malocclusion because the tongue pushes forward against the front teeth.

Finally, the most common troublesome behavior in both children with handicaps and normal children is finger sucking, usually thumb sucking. Approximately 45% of all 4-year-olds suck their fingers (Josell & Abrams, 1982a). The principal hazard with this behavior is malocclusion, caused by increased pressure against the front teeth.

Treating these problem behaviors is often difficult. For example, mouth breathing may result from a partial obstruction in the nasal passages. Until this obstruction is removed and corrected, the child will continue to breathe through the mouth. Similarly, tongue thrusting is an involuntary behavior; retainers or other mouth inserts are used to deal with this problem. Bruxism and thumb sucking are especially difficult behaviors to control. Some behavior modification techniques have met with a measure of success (Rosenstein, 1978), including rewarding the child for periods of time when he or she does not engage in the troublesome behavior (Azrin, Nunn, & Frantz-Renshaw, 1980).

Malocclusion

Malocclusion means the improper fitting together of the upper and lower teeth. It is common in the general population but occurs even more frequently in children with handicaps (R. Smith, 1982). Poor oral motor control and tongue thrusting, found in children with cerebral palsy, affects the normal alignment of the teeth. Facial abnormalities such as the flat face of the Down syndrome child also predispose a child to malocclusion.

Treatment of these irregularities falls under the domain of the **orthodontist**. Although the correction of this improper alignment of the teeth is often thought of as simply being cosmetic, the use of braces to separate and properly space the teeth also decreases the incidence of dental decay and gum disease by making routine oral hygiene easier.

Dental Decay

Dental decay (or caries), which causes cavities, mainly occurs in children and adolescents. Dental caries begins with plaque formation. Plaque is composed of bacteria, bacterial by-products, saliva, and food particles that combine to form a clear, sticky mass that clings to the teeth and gums (Rule, 1982). The bacteria in plaque feed off the food sugars, especially sucrose, that come in contact with the teeth. The baby who is put to sleep with a bottle of milk or juice or who sucks on a honey-coated pacifier will have a greater chance of dental caries because of the prolonged contact of the sugar with the teeth. The bacteria ferments the sugar; this then releases acids that can destroy the enamel and the dentin of the tooth. Over months or years, this process may gradually demolish the tooth. In addition, unremoved plaque calcifies as tartar (calculus) and can cause tenderness and swelling of the gums. Calculus can eventually destroy bony supports of the tooth and, thus, may loosen the tooth as well.

Periodontal Disease

As noted earlier, teeth become loose when the gums and bony supports of the teeth are damaged. This may be because of a buildup of plaque and diseases of the gum, or it may result from some sort of trauma. Gum disease is a much more common disorder in older adults, but it can also be a problem in children with handicaps. For example, a high incidence of gum disease has been found in institutionalized Down syndrome children. Mild gum inflammation, called gingivitis, results from an accumulation of plaque and exists in roughly 40% of normal children. This inflammation seems to reach a peak incidence in adolescence (Lesco & Brownstein, 1982). The best treatment of gingivitis is good dental care at home, including thorough daily brushing and flossing.

In children with handicaps, the most frequent occurrence of gum disease is in those who receive Dilantin to control seizures. Thirty-five percent of the individuals who receive this drug over a long period of time develop enlarged gums that are prone to infection, trauma, and bleeding (Figure 11.4) (Livingston & Livingston, 1969). Reducing the amount of Dilantin an individual must take usually causes the gums to shrink. If the gums become very enlarged, the dentist may have to trim them surgically.

Dental Injuries

Tooth fractures, also called avulsions, occur in approximately 25% of all children (Josell & Abrams, 1982b). These fractures usually result from an injury suffered in sports, fights, falls, or from thrown objects. A child with seizures is at greater risk of injury from falls than other children. The most commonly injured teeth are the maxillary incisors, or front teeth, especially in the first 2–3 years after their emergence and particularly when they are flared or protruded (buck teeth) (Ferguson & Ripa, 1979). The severity of the damage to the tooth correlates with the prognosis (Josell & Abrams, 1982b). A crown fracture involving only the enamel and dentin will probably heal so long as the pulp has not been traumatized. Even a tooth that has been completely knocked out can be reimplanted within an hour of the accident if the tooth has been kept moist. This is best done by placing the tooth in milk or salt water, but tap water or even saliva has worked. Also, the tooth should not be cleaned as this could remove tissue useful in reattachment (American Dental Association, 1982; Andreasen, 1981).

In any kind of tooth injury, one must be careful to protect against the child's inhaling the tooth or tooth fragments. The best treatment is prevention; children with severe seizures and those who play in contact sports should wear mouth guards for protection.

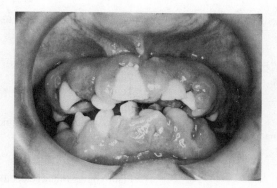

Figure 11.4. Enlarged, inflamed gums associated with chronic ingestion of Dilantin for control of seizures. (Photograph courtesy of Dr. Seth Canion, Kennedy Institute for Handicapped Children, Baltimore.)

DENTAL CARE AND TREATMENT

Dental care and treatment consist of **prophylactic** dental care in the home, routine dental checkups, and dental surgery. The special needs of the child with handicaps deserve particular attention.

Prophylactic Dental Care

Four forms of prophylactic dental care can significantly reduce the likelihood of caries and periodontal disease. These are 1) healthful eating habits, 2) tooth brushing and flossing, 3) fluoridation, and 4) regular professional dental care (Shelton & Ferretti, 1982). In terms of diet, if possible, children should eat sweets sparingly and only as part of a meal. In this way, other foods can dilute and neutralize the effects of the carbohydrates. Preferably, between-meal snacks should include fresh fibrous vegetables and nuts such as carrots and peanuts rather than candies and other sweets. Foods that are good to eat as snacks are listed in Table 11.2.

Besides a proper diet, toothbrushing and flossing are essential ingredients for healthy teeth and gums. Ideally, one should brush after every meal. Realistically, a thorough brushing and flossing once a day is probably sufficient. A small, soft, multibristle brush should be used and should be held at a 45° angle to the gums. Brushing is done in a circular motion for a few minutes. After brushing, one should use dental floss, a waxed or unwaxed nylon filament. This is gently pulled between the teeth. The floss removes foreign matter, stimulates the gums and, most importantly, breaks up the plaque that accumulates between the teeth.

Another component of dental care is fluoridation. Fluoride reacts with certain chemical compounds in tooth enamel to form a more acid-stable enamel that resists decay. It also affects bacterial growth and metabolism (Hamilton, 1977). Most water is now fluoridated, and many brands of toothpaste contain fluoride. Thus, in most cases, it is unnecessary to take fluoride tablets or vitamins that contain fluoride every day. Fluoridation has resulted in a halving of the incidence of dental cavities since the

Table 11.2. Foods that are good to use as snacks to maintain dental health

Raw vegetables	
Carrot sticks	Green pepper rings
Celery sticks	Lettuce wedges
Cauliflower bits	Radishes
Cucumber sticks	Tomatoes
Drinks	
Milk	Unsweetened vegetable juices
Sugar-free carbonated beverages	
Other snacks	
Nuts	Soda crackers
Popcorn	Plain yogurt (unsweetened)
Peanut butter (unsweetened)	Sugarless gum or candy
Cheese	

Source: American Dental Association, 1983; Forrester, Wagner, & Fleming, 1981.

1950s. The average number of cavities is now 5 per child between birth and adulthood (National Caries Program, 1981).

Dental Care for the Child with Handicaps

For the child with handicaps, the most common dental problem is an increased risk for developing dental caries (Johnson & Albertson, 1972). This occurs for a number of reasons. First, the child, especially one with cerebral palsy, may not be able to eat highly textured foods and may require carbohydrate supplements to maintain weight. Thus, the teeth do not receive as much natural cleansing with fiber and may be exposed to more sugars. In addition, the child may drink less water and may not use toothpaste in cleaning the teeth because he or she might inhale the toothpaste. Thus, the intake of fluoride may be insufficient to be an effective deterrent. Lastly, toothbrushing and flossing may be difficult. The child may not be able to perform the action alone and may need to rely entirely on the parent or caregiver. These difficulties, combined with a possible predisposition to caries because of thin enamel or other teeth malformations, increase the risk of tooth decay in the child with handicaps (American Dental Association, 1982).

Caregivers of these children may try a number of methods to decrease this risk. The first step is to improve toothbrushing and to increase the intake of fluoride. If necessary, once-a-day brushing before bedtime must suffice. Occupational therapists can adapt the handles of toothbrushes to help children who lack fine motor dexterity. Another option is the use of a washcloth, a piece of gauze, or a cotton-tipped applicator impregnated with a mild abrasive. Electric toothbrushes may also be used. When responsibility for toothbrushing falls to the parent or caregiver, appropriate positioning of the child must be considered (Johnson & Albertson, 1972). Toothpaste is not essential. However, the child may have to take fluoride tablets or drops, especially if he or she does not use toothpaste. Fluoride treatments at a dentist's office every 6 months help to restore needed minerals to the tooth enamel. The use of an oral irrigating device such as a Water Pik or similar tool may help to remove food, foreign bodies, and dental plaque. Finally, one can use a tablet or solution that contains a harmless dye that highlights plaque so that areas needing more attention can be identified.

Routine Dental Checkups

Besides practicing prophylactic dental care in the home, by age 2 or before all the primary teeth have erupted, children should begin to visit their dentist regularly for "preventive maintenance." Children with disabilities should visit a dentist within 6 months after their teeth begin to emerge. These visits generally involve a visual inspection of the teeth for signs of decay, gum inflammation, and the position of the teeth (Coll & Conlan, 1982). The teeth are cleaned using a high-speed brush to remove tartar; often, a fluoride treatment is given. The dentist or dental hygienist also probes for cavities. Periodically, an X ray is taken to look for hidden decay and for the progress of the secondary teeth. Children also receive instructions about brushing and flossing. In addition, some dentists are now using a new pit and fissure sealant procedure. In this technique, the biting surface of the molars, the teeth most susceptible to decay, is etched with a mild acid and coated with a plastic sealant. This covering provides added protection against cavities.

Despite the rather benign nature of the visit to the dentist, many children—and adults—express fear about going. Children may learn from their frightened parents that the dentist is someone to avoid. To decrease anxiety, it is helpful to explain before the visit what will happen. The child should be told that the dentist is someone who will help him or her, will count the teeth, clean them, and apply tooth nourishment—fluoride. Often dentists use music or cartoons to allay fears; some reward the children with small gifts after the visit. Once the pattern of a pleasant visit has been established, most of the children will trust the dentist, and future treatment becomes easier to administer.

Dental Surgery

The most common type of dental surgery is the filling of a cavity. To do this, the dentist begins by using a high speed drill to remove the decay. This creates a larger hole that is then filled, often with a silver amalgam compound. Normally, the procedure takes less than 10 minutes.

To make the procedure more comfortable, a local anesthetic, usually Xylocaine, is used to deaden temporarily the nerve of the tooth being repaired. After the surgery, the child's mouth will feel numb for about 2 hours, but he or she should feel no pain. If the child is anxious, the dentist may administer nitrous oxide ("laughing gas") to relax the child. Other useful drugs include Valium, scopolamine, and chloralhydrate. Valium is used as an antianxiety agent and chloralhydrate as a sedative. Scopolamine decreases the flow of saliva and, thus, makes the dental work easier to perform.

If the individual has a congenital heart defect, the dentist will probably also treat him or her with penicillin prior to surgery. This is done to prevent the rare occurrence of subacute bacterial **endocarditis** (SBE), an infection of the lining of the heart that may be induced by bacteria released during dental surgery (Holbrook, Willey, & Shaw, 1983).

SUMMARY

Oral health is important for adequate nutrition and speech. For a child with handicaps, the maintenance of healthy teeth is complicated because of malformations, mal-occlusions, diet, and medication. Dental trauma is a further complication, especially in individuals with seizures. These problems accentuate the importance of prophy-lactic dental care and routine dental checkups.

REFERENCES

Aasenden, R., & Pebbles, T.C. (1974). Effects of fluoride supplementation from birth on human deciduous and permanent teeth. *Archives of Oral Biology, 19,* 321–326.
American Academy of Pediatrics, Committee on Nutrition. (1979). Fluoride supplementation: Revised dosage schedule. *Pediatrics, 63,* 150–152.

American Dental Association. (1982). *Caring for the disabled child's dental health*. Chicago: American Dental Association, Bureau of Health Education and Audiovisual Services.

American Dental Association (1983). *Diet and dental health*. Chicago: American Dental Association, Bureau of Health Education and Audiovisual Services.

Andreasen, J.O. (1981). *Traumatic injuries of the teeth* (2nd ed.). Philadelphia: W.B. Saunders Co.

Azrin, N.H., Nunn, R.G., & Frantz-Renshaw, S. (1980). Habit reversal treatment of thumbsucking. *Behavior Research and Therapy, 18*, 395–399.

Braham, R.L., & Morris, M.E. (Eds.). (1980). *Textbook of pediatric dentistry*. Baltimore: Williams & Wilkins Co.

Carlos, J.P. (1982). The prevention of dental caries: Ten years later. *Journal of the American Dental Association, 104*, 193–197.

Coll, J.A., & Conlan, J.G. (1982). The pediatric dental office. *Pediatric Clinics of North America, 29*, 743–759.

Ferguson, F.S., & Ripa, L.W. (1979). Prevalence and type of traumatic injuries to the anterior teeth of preschool children. *Journal of Pedodontics, 4*, 3–8.

Forrester, D.J., Wagner, M.L, & Fleming, J. (Eds.). (1981). *Pediatric dental medicine*. Philadelphia: Lee & Febiger.

Hamilton, I.R. (1977). Effects of fluoride on enzymatic regulation of bacterial carbohydrate metabolism. *Caries Research, 11* (Suppl. 1), 262–291.

Hennon, D.K., Stookey, G.K., & Muhler, J.C. (1969). Prevalence and distribution of dental caries in preschool children. *Journal of the American Dental Association, 79*, 1405–1414.

Holbrook, W.P., Willey, R.F., & Shaw, T.R. (1983). Prophylaxis of infective endocarditis. *British Dental Journal, 154*, 36–39.

Johnson, R., & Albertson, D. (1972). Plaque control for handicapped children. *Journal of the American Dental Association, 84*, 824–828.

Josell, S.D., & Abrams, R.G. (Eds.). (1982a). Symposium on oral health. *Pediatric Clinics of North America, 29*, 429–771.

Josell, S.D., & Abrams, R.G. (1982b). Traumatic injuries to the dentition and its supporting structures. *Pediatric Clinics of North America, 29*, 717–741.

Lesco, B.A., & Brownstein, M.P. (1982). Recognition of periodontal disease in children. *Pediatric Clinics of North America, 29*, 457–474.

Livingston, S., & Livingston, H.L. (1969). Diphenylhydantoin gingival hyperplasia. *American Journal of Diseases of Children, 117*, 265–270.

Massler, M., & Schour, I. (1958). *Atlas of the mouth*. Chicago: American Dental Association.

National Caries Program, National Institute of Dental Research. (1981). *The prevalence of dental caries in United States children, 1979–1980: The national dental caries prevalence survey*. Bethesda, MD: U.S. Department of Health and Human Services, Public Health Service, National Institutes of Health, Publication No. 82-2245.

Nowak, A.J. (Ed.). (1976). *Dentistry for the handicapped patient*. St. Louis: C.V. Mosby Co.

Ranta, R., & Rintala, A. (1982). Tooth anomalies associated with congenital sinuses of the lower lip and cleft lip/palate. *Angle Orthodontist, 52*, 212–221.

Rood, S.R., & Stool, S.E. (1981). Current concepts of the etiology, diagnosis, and management of cleft palate related otopathologic diseases. *Otolaryngologic Clinics of North America, 14*, 865–884.

Rosenstein, S.N. (1978). *Dentistry in cerebral palsy and related handicapping conditions*. Springfield, IL: Charles C Thomas.

Rule, J.T. (1982). Recognition of dental caries. *Pediatric Clinics of North America, 29*, 439–456.

Sanger, R.G., & Casamassimo, P.S. (1983). The physically and mentally disabled patient. *Dental Clinics of North America, 27*, 363–385.

Schneider, P.E., & Peterson, J. (1982). Oral habits: Considerations in management. *Pediatric Clinics of North America, 29*, 523-546.

Shelton, P.G., & Ferretti, G.A. (1982). Maintaining oral health. *Pediatric Clinics of North America, 29*, 653–668.

Smith, D.W., with assistance of Jones, K.L. (1982). *Recognizable patterns of human malformation: Genetic, embryologic and clinical aspects* (3rd ed.). Philadelphia: W.B. Saunders Co.

Smith, R.J. (1982). Development of occlusion and malocclusion. *Pediatric Clinics of North America, 29*, 475–501.

Starks, D., Market, G., Miller, C.B., et al. (1985). Day to day dental care: A parents' guide. *Exceptional Parent, 15(4)*, 10–17.

Stewart, R.E., Barber, T.K., Troutman, K.C., et al. (1982). *Pediatric dentistry: Scientific foundations and clinical practice*. St. Louis: C.V. Mosby Co.

Stewart, R.E., & Poole, A.E. (1982). The orofacial structures and their association with congenital abnormalities. *Pediatric Clinics of North America, 29*, 547–584.

Sweeney, E.A. (1981). Pediatric dentistry. *Current Problems in Pediatrics, 11*, 1–51.

Wessels, K.E. (Ed.). (1979). *Dentistry and the handicapped patient*. Littleton, MA: PSG Publishing Co., Inc.

Chapter 12

The Brain and Nervous System
Our Computer

Upon completion of this chapter, the reader will:
—be able to trace the development of the central nervous system
—know the structure of the neuron, how it operates, and how messages are transmitted
—be aware of the areas of the brain and their function
—know the location and purpose of the basal ganglia
—understand the interaction between the cerebellum and the cerebrum
—comprehend the workings of the peripheral nervous system and how it aids in movement
—know the function of the autonomic nervous system
—be able to describe the flow of the cerebrospinal fluid in addition to knowing its origin and function
—know what hydrocephalus involves

The nervous system is the body's computer; it coordinates and directs our various bodily functions. Its major components are the **central nervous system** (CNS), consisting of the brain and spinal cord, the **peripheral nervous system,** and the **autonomic nervous system**. Each component controls some aspect of our behavior and affects our understanding of the world around us. For example, the brain is not only involved in perception and thought; it also initiates voluntary movement. The impairment of any part of this system makes us less able to adapt to our environment and can lead to disorders as varied as mental retardation, learning disabilities, cerebral palsy, and epilepsy. This chapter gives an overview of the structure and function of this intricate system.

DEVELOPMENT OF THE CENTRAL NERVOUS SYSTEM

The central nervous system begins to form during the third week after fertilization, when the embryo is merely 1.5 millimeters long (Carpenter & Sutin, 1983). Part of the ectodermal layer forms an elongated, shoe-shaped body called the *neural plate*. With further development, this plate expands and rises to become the *neural fold*, later taking the form of the *neural tube* (Figure 12.1). At this time, the central nervous system looks like a closed tubular structure with a tail and a head. The tail portion will become the spinal cord, and the broader head portion will form the brain. Lack of closure of the neural tube at this stage leads to the development of spina bifida or anencephaly.

By the third week of gestation, the head portion of this tubular structure has three distinct bulges that will eventually form the basic subdivisions of the brain: the *cerebral hemispheres,* the *cerebellum,* and the *brain stem* (Figure 12.2).

Within about 3 more weeks, these parts of the brain start to bend into their adult shape. The forebrain develops into the cerebral hemisphere, the midbrain into the brain stem, and the hindbrain into the cerebellum. When fully developed, the cerebral hemispheres rest on top of the brain stem, and the cerebellum lies behind it. The cerebellum is the last part of the central nervous system to be formed and is still immature at birth (see Figure 12.2).

When the fetus is 4 months old, the basic brain structures are all in place. Yet, internally, enormous changes are continuing to take place.

THE NERVE CELL

The *neuron,* or nerve cell, is the basic functional unit of the nervous system (Noback, 1981). Similar to other cells, the neuron has a cell body consisting of a nucleus and cytoplasm. Unlike other cells, it also has a long fiber—called an axon—extending from the cell body and many, shorter, jutting tendrils called *dendrites* (Figure 12.3).

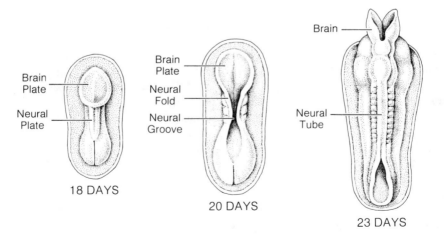

Figure 12.1.   Development of the central nervous system during the first month of life. This is a longitudinal view showing the gradual closure of the neural tube to form the spinal column and the rounding up of the head region to form the primitive brain.

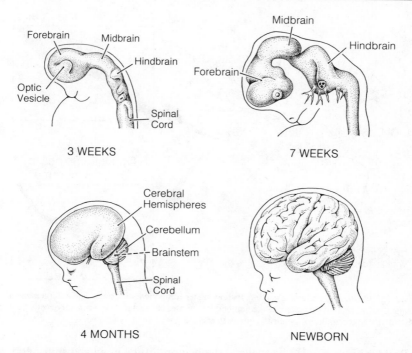

Figure 12.2. Development of the brain during fetal life. This is a side view illustrating the increasing complexity of the brain over time. The forebrain develops into the cerebral hemispheres, the midbrain into the brain stem, and the hindbrain into the cerebellum. Although all brain structures are formed by 4 months, the brain grows greatly in size and complexity during the final months of prenatal development.

Axons and dendrites have different functions. The axon carries impulses away from the nerve cell body, while the dendrites receive impulses from other neurons and carry them toward the cell body. Attached along the length of the dendrites are tiny projections, or spines, that increase the surface area of the dendrites and enable a more elaborate transmission of messages. It is interesting to note that children with Down syndrome have dendritic spines that are fewer in number and narrower than those of normal children (Purpura, 1974). The narrower the spine, the more difficult it is to communicate messages because the resistance to electrical current is increased (see Figure 12.3).

Arrangement of Nerve Cells in the Brain and Spinal Cord

While there is only one cell layer during early fetal life, nerve cells in the adult brain are arranged in six layers. As the brain expands in size, so do the number and complexity of the nerve cell layers. The nerve cell bodies migrate from the bottom layer toward the top layer (Figure 12.4). Incomplete migration of nerve cell bodies has been discovered in a number of types of severe mental retardation. Why such cells do not complete their migration is unknown.

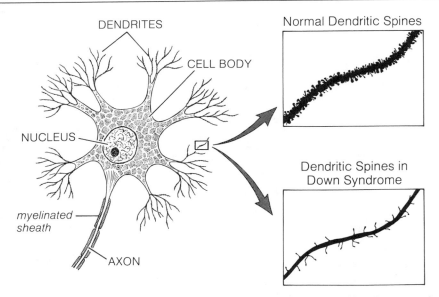

Figure 12.3. Idealized picture of a nerve cell showing its component elements. The enlargements show the minute dendritic spines that increase the number of synapses or junctures between nerve cells. Note the diminished size and number of dendritic spines in a child with Down syndrome.

Besides being divided into layers, the neurons of the brain and spinal cord are further separated into two distinct regions called the *gray* and the *white matter*. The gray matter contains the nerve cell bodies; it appears grayish in color. The white matter is made up of axons sheathed with a protective covering called *myelin*.

During fetal life, most of the axons have no myelin coating. After birth, the axons gradually develop this glistening sheath that aids in more rapid conduction of nerve impulses. The dendrites also change, increasing in number and expanding in complexity. During the first 2 years of life, the proliferation of the nerve fibers

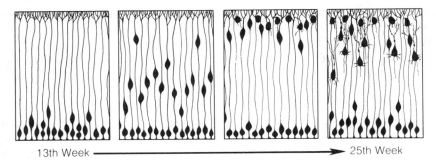

Figure 12.4. Growth of nerve cells in the cortex between 3 and 6 months gestation. The cell bodies climb toward the upper layers of the cortex and sprout dendrites. There is an increase both in the number of cells and in the complexity of their projections.

changes the appearance of the neural network from that of a barren seedling to an arboreal structure of great beauty and complexity.

Transmission of Messages

Impulses jump from one neuron to another across a juncture, or **synapse**. Here the terminal of the axon of one neuron almost touches either the dendrite or the cell body of another neuron (Figure 12.5). When a nerve cell generates an electrical impulse, that impulse can travel down the axon only as far as the edge of the axon, called the *presynaptic membrane* (see Figure 12.5). It cannot cross without a bridge. In this case, the bridge consists of a chemical called a **neurotransmitter**. Each neuron has a specific neurotransmitter. These substances include norepinephrine, acetylcholine, dopamine, serotonin, and GABA; they are contained in small pouches near the *presynaptic membrane*. Upon stimulation by an electrical impulse, the pockets open and release the neurochemical into the opening or *synaptic cleft*. The nerve impulse's electrical energy is first transformed into chemical energy and then back again to electrical energy at the receptor on the tip of the other neuron, called the *postsynaptic membrane* (Gilman & Winans, 1982). It can then continue on its way to the next synapse, eventually reaching its final destination.

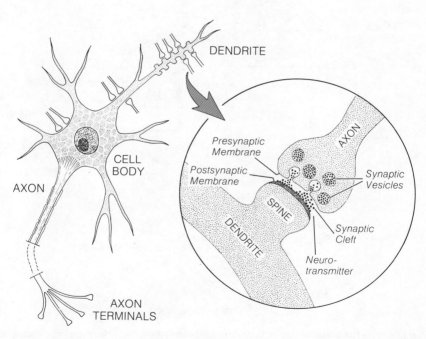

Figure 12.5.   Central nervous system synapse. The enlargement shows the abutting of an axon against a dendritic spine. The space separating the two is the synaptic cleft. Neurotransmitter bundles are released into the cleft from vesicles in the presynaptic membrane. These permit transmission of an impulse across the juncture.

THE CENTRAL NERVOUS SYSTEM: BRAIN AND SPINAL CORD

The central nervous system consists of the brain and the spinal cord. In an adult, the brain weighs about 3 pounds; it has four main components: the *cerebrum,* the *diencephalon,* the *brain stem,* and the *cerebellum.* The cerebrum is the largest of these parts.

The Cerebrum

The cerebrum contains two cerebral hemispheres joined together in the middle by the fibrous tissue of the **corpus callosum** and separated at the top (Figure 12.6A). Each hemisphere is functionally divided into four lobes. The *frontal lobe* occupies the front, or anterior, third of the hemisphere, and the *occipital lobe* takes up the back, or

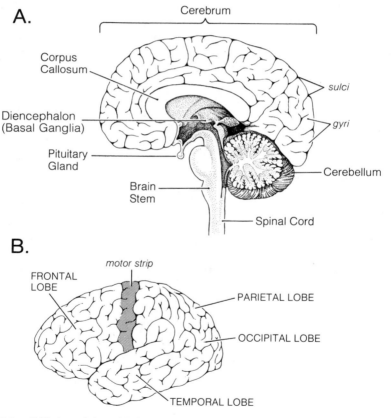

Figure 12.6. A) Horizontal view of the brain showing the component elements: cerebrum, diencephalon, cerebellum, brain stem, and spinal cord. B) Side view of the cortex. The cortex is divided into four lobes: frontal, parietal, temporal, and occipital. The motor strip, lying at the back of the frontal lobe, is highlighted. It initiates voluntary movement and is damaged in spastic cerebral palsy.

posterior, fourth of each hemisphere. The *parietal lobe* sits in the middle-upper part of the cerebrum, while the *temporal lobe* is in the lower-middle region (Figure 12.6B).

In the fetus, the cerebral surface appears smooth. As the complexity of the brain increases, indentations gradually appear. By late childhood, the surface of the cerebrum has become very convoluted with many furrows and humps called **sulci** and **gyri**. In an adult, a smooth, unconvoluted cerebrum, called **lissencephaly**, is associated with some forms of severe mental retardation and seizures.

The substance underlying the surface of the cerebral hemisphere is called the *cortex* and is composed mainly of nerve cell bodies, or gray matter. Below the gray matter lie the nerve fibers, or the white matter. The cerebral cortex initiates motion and thought and adds to the capability of the more reflexive and involuntary brain stem. Each cortical lobe takes care of particular activities and functions.

The Frontal Lobe   The frontal lobe is involved both in initiating voluntary muscle movement and in cognition. The motor strip of the frontal lobe, lying just in front of the parietal lobe, controls voluntary motor activity. The different areas of the body are represented topographically along this strip. The tongue and larynx, or voice box, are at the lowest point. They are followed in an upward sequence by the face, hand, arm, trunk, thigh, and foot (Figure 12.7). The tongue, larynx, and hand occupy a particularly large area along this strip because the motor activities involved in speech and fine motor dexterity are so complex and require elaborate control.

Thus, voluntary movement is begun with stimulation of a nerve impulse in this strip. This impulse passes down the pyramidal tract, which connects the cortex with the diencephalon, the brain stem, and the spinal cord. At the spinal cord, the impulse is passed across a synapse to a peripheral nerve that leads to some body part. The end result is muscle movement. This movement in turn sets off a sensory, or **afferent**, communication back to the cerebrum to complete the circuit.

If there is damage either to the motor cortex or to the pyramidal tract, **spasticity** results. Voluntary movement becomes difficult, and muscle tone is increased. Conversely, if the entire motor strip rather than a specific area is stimulated at one time, a massive, simultaneous contraction of all muscles, called a **tonic** seizure, occurs. This is what happens in a **grand mal** seizure.

Besides controlling voluntary movement, the frontal lobe also contains areas that are involved in abstract thinking. Years ago, some patients with severe **psychosis** or with antisocial behavior were treated by undergoing a prefrontal leukotomy, an operation in which part of the frontal lobe is cut. This diminished the aggressive outbursts, but the patients became messy, lost some of their initiative, were easily distracted, and had poor judgment (Benson, Stuss, Naeser, et al., 1981).

The Occipital Lobe   The occipital lobe is primarily concerned with vision. It is here that the visual stimuli terminate in what is called the visual-receptive area. Images are reconstructed and "seen" in this area. The image is processed further in another part of the occipital lobe and then is passed on to the temporal and parietal lobes. In the parietal lobe, the images are integrated with what has been heard and felt

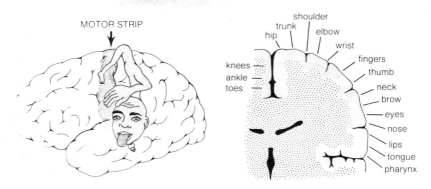

Figure 12.7.   The motor strip. The cartoon shows a representation of body parts at various points on the strip. Note that the areas of facial and hand muscles are very large. This is because of the intricate control necessary for speech and fine motor coordination. A cross-sectional view of the motor strip is shown at right.

so an intelligent interpretation can be made. Damage to the occipital region leads to "cortical blindness." Although the eyes can see, the occipital lobe does not receive the image. The person, therefore, is functionally blind.

The Parietal Lobe   Besides aiding in vision, the parietal lobe integrates other stimuli, making a whole impression from various inputs received from the different senses. Within this lobe are distinct areas for visual, auditory, touch, pain, smell, and temperature sensations. Few specific diseases have been associated with damage to this lobe. However, some researchers believe that the visual-perceptual problems experienced by children with learning disabilities are the result of abnormal functioning in this lobe (Hynd & Cohen, 1983). In addition, the difficulty a child with attention deficit disorder has in performing fine-motor tasks may result from changes in this area of the brain.

The Temporal Lobe   This area of the cerebrum is mainly involved in communication and sensation. It helps us form and understand language and stores visual and auditory experiences. When the temporal lobe malfunctions, a number of disorders may result. The two most common are **receptive aphasia** and partial complex or psychomotor seizures.

In receptive aphasia, which is basically an adult disorder, Wernicke's area of the temporal lobe (see Figure 17.1) is damaged by a tumor, stroke, or traumatic injury (Brown, 1972). The person cannot understand the words he or she hears (see Chapter 17).

As is true of receptive aphasia, the problem in a psychomotor seizure also rests in the temporal lobe (Gold, 1974). Before the seizure begins, the individual may experience a "dèjá vu," or flashback, phenomenon caused by stimulation of this area of the brain. The person may also see strange images, smell unpleasant odors, or hear bizarre sounds (see Chapter 22).

The Diencephalon

Resting beneath the cortex in the center of the brain is an area called the diencephalon (see Figure 12.6a). It contains the basal ganglia and related structures. In lower vertebrates, this area controls motor activity. In human beings, however, this primitive part of the brain modifies and alters the instructions from the motor cortex that call for voluntary movement.

Besides the basal ganglia, the **labyrinth** in the inner ear and the cerebellum also affect voluntary movement. Together, these three parts of the nervous system serve as a series of checks and balances on our motor activity and balance.

As with other parts of the brain, damage to the diencephalon leads to abnormalities in movement. The most common of these disorders is called *extrapyramidal cerebral palsy* (see Chapter 21). Other diseases involving this region are **Parkinson's disease**, **Huntington's disease**, and **torsion dystonia**.

The Brain Stem

The brain stem lies between the cerebral hemispheres and the spinal cord. It has three regions: the medulla, the pons, and the midbrain (Figure 12.8). These parts together contain 11 cranial nerves that control such diverse functions as breathing, swallowing, seeing, and hearing. These nerves also affect facial expression, eye and tongue

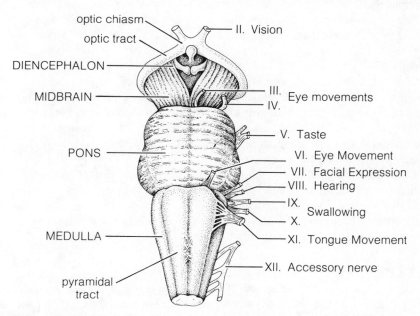

Figure 12.8. The brain stem. The three regions are shown: midbrain, pons, and medulla. The placement and function of 11 cranial nerves are illustrated. Note that the pyramidal tract runs from the cortex into the brain stem. The pyramidal fibers cross over in the medulla. Thus, the right hemisphere controls left-sided movement.

movement, and salivation. Besides these cranial nerves, the brain stem also contains sections of the pyramidal and extrapyramidal tracts as well as other nerve tracts that flow from the cortex to the spinal cord.

Children with cerebral palsy often have damage to the brain stem or to pathways that end in the brain stem. This explains why these children have a high incidence of sucking and swallowing problems, **strabismus**, excessive salivation, and speech disorders.

The Cerebellum

The last of the major parts of the brain, the cerebellum, hangs over the brain stem and rests just below the cerebral hemispheres (see Figure 12.6a). The cerebellum coordinates the action of the voluntary muscles and times their contractions so that movements are performed smoothly and accurately.

For us to move efficiently, the work of the cerebellum must be integrated with the work of the cerebral hemispheres and the basal ganglia. To illustrate, consider the following example. Uncle Harry and Aunt Jane are dancing at their 40th anniversary party, and Uncle Harry drank a bit too much and is unsteady. He steps on Aunt Jane's foot. His foot transmits a message to the cerebellum, advising it of the progress of his voluntary movement. Touch, auditory, and visual stimuli also send impulses to his tipsy cerebellum. Harry feels Jane's toes under his and hears her cry, "Ouch!" These messages are integrated and correlated. After evaluating the significance of all the messages, the cerebellum compensates for inaccuracies in motor movements and tells the motor cortex to correct any mistakes. Uncle Harry lifts his foot and smiles sheepishly. "My cerebellum is a little pickled," he might well say.

While voluntary movement can take place without the presence of the cerebellum, such movement is clumsy and disorganized. The walk of a person with abnormal cerebellar functioning is called **ataxic** and is most commonly seen in an inebriated person. Also, the hands of a person with cerebellar damage will tremble, his or her eyes will twitch (also called nystagmus), and he or she will overshoot the mark when reaching for an object.

In childhood, the most common cause of cerebellar dysfunction is drug intoxication (Holcomb, Lynn, Harvey, et al., 1972). For example, a child with a seizure disorder who receives too much Dilantin will weave while walking and have difficulty reaching precisely. This is because Dilantin has a direct effect on cerebellar function. When the drug level falls to normal, these problems disappear.

The Spinal Cord

Under the brain lies the spinal cord. It is a cylindrical structure that extends from the brain stem to the lower back. Surrounding both the brain and the spinal cord are three layers of covering called the **meninges** (Figure 12.9). The spinal cord is enlarged in the neck, or **cervical**, region and in the **lumbar**, or lower back area. These enlarged areas contain many **anterior horn cells**, cells that send messages to the peripheral nerve fibers that lead to the arms and legs.

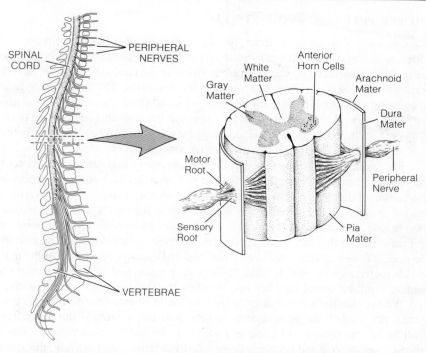

Figure 12.9. The spinal column. The spinal cord extends from the neck to the lower back. It is protected by the bony vertebrae that form the spinal column. The enlargement to the right shows a section of the cord taken from the upper back region. Note the meninges (the dura, arachnoid, and pia mater) surrounding the cord and the peripheral nerve on its way to a muscle. This nerve contains both motor and sensory components. The spinal cord, like the brain, has both gray and white matter. The gray matter consists of various nerve cells, most important of which are the anterior motor horn cells. These are destroyed in polio. The white matter contains nerve fibers wrapped in myelin that gives the cord its glistening appearance.

Primarily a conduit, the spinal cord transmits motor and sensory messages. However, if the spinal cord is damaged—for example, because of an injury or congenital malformation such as spina bifida—the messages from the brain to the peripheral nerves below the lesion or area of injury are short-circuited. The result may be the loss both of sensation and of movements in the affected limbs.

Damage to the spinal cord can also come from an infection. The polio virus, now virtually eradicated in the United States, led to paralysis in many children during the 1950s because it destroyed the anterior horn cells of the spinal cord. While the sensory pathways remained intact, the motor path was interrupted (Bell & McCormick, 1981). The child could feel touch and pain but could not move. Another infection affecting the spinal column is meningitis, caused by either a virus or bacteria. In meningitis, the infectious agent attacks the meninges, or coverings of the spinal cord and brain. Except in infants, the effects of meningitis are usually reversible. In **encephalitis**, a related viral infection, the infection invades the brain tissue itself; this is a much more dangerous type of infection (Bell & McCormick, 1981).

THE PERIPHERAL NERVOUS SYSTEM

For voluntary movement to occur, the nerve impulse that passes from the motor cortex to the anterior horn cells in the spinal cord must connect with a peripheral nerve. This nerve then takes the impulse from the spinal cord to the muscle. Actually, peripheral nerves have fibers that run in both directions. The motor, or **efferent**, fibers bring signals from the brain to the muscles and cause movement. The sensory, or **afferent**, fibers carry signals from the muscle to the brain that indicate the position of a joint and the tone of the muscle following the movement. The interaction between these two types of nerves allows us to move smoothly.

For normal muscle tone to occur, the proper relationship between the motor and the sensory fibers must exist. Even when at rest, muscles have some tone because of this constant interchange between the motor and sensory nerves. In other words, it is not the muscle itself but rather the activity of the nervous system that maintains muscle tone. For example, if a muscle is stimulated by moving a joint, a person will feel resistance to this movement, that is, an increase in muscle tone. The activity of the muscle at rest and the involuntary reaction that opposes the stretch of the muscle are characteristics of muscle tone. This tone is decreased when the motor fibers leading from the spinal cord are cut, or when the sensory fibers are abnormal.

When either the anterior horn cells or the motor fibers of the peripheral nervous system are injured, an individual may lose both the voluntary and the reflexive qualities of the muscle and become paralyzed. Beside the paralysis, the affected muscle loses its tone and becomes floppy, or **hypotonic**. After a while, the affected muscle and limb begin to shrink, or atrophy, from lack of use. This is what happens to a person who has polio or a severed spine.

If there is damage to either the pyramidal tract or the extrapyramidal tract, muscle tone is also affected. When the pyramidal tract is injured, the tone and reflexes actually increase. Muscle resistance is strong at the beginning of movement but then gives way in a sudden, clasped-knife fashion as more force is applied. Also, a quick stretch of a tendon will produce **clonus**, a sustained series of rhythmic jerks. The combination of these characteristics is called *spasticity* and is the hallmark of a kind of cerebral palsy aptly called *pyramidal* or *spastic cerebral palsy* (see Chapter 21) because it arises from an abnormality in the motor cortex or pyramidal tract.

The changes resulting from damage to the extrapyramidal tract are quite different. With damage to this system, voluntary movement is possible, but it may be exaggerated in a twisting, squirming pattern called **choreoathetosis**. In addition, rigidity rather than spasticity characterizes the changes in tone and is the hallmark of *extrapyramidal cerebral palsy* (see Chapter 21).

THE AUTONOMIC NERVOUS SYSTEM

The preceding discussion has focused on control of voluntary movement. There is also an entirely different nervous system that takes care of involuntary activities—the autonomic nervous system. This system controls the functioning of the cardiovascular, respiratory, digestive, endocrine, urinary, and reproductive systems. The tracts of this system start in either the diencephalon or the spinal cord and move on to the particular organ with which they are involved.

While the voluntary nervous system is concerned with individual muscle movements, the autonomic nervous system has an "all or none" effect. The best example of this is the "fight or flight" response (Figure 12.10). When a person is frightened, several physiological changes take place simultaneously. The pupils dilate, the hair stands on end, and the functioning of the digestive system is suspended so that blood can be diverted to more important areas such as the brain. Heart rate and blood pressure increase, and the bronchioles of the lung expand in size. All of these changes are controlled by the autonomic nervous system and prepare the individual to react to the emergency.

A more common function of the autonomic nervous system is the control of bowel and bladder function. In infants, this function is purely reflexive. When the bladder or bowel fills, the outlet muscles release and the child urinates or stools. Between the ages of 12 to 18 months, the child gradually gains control over these activities. The cerebral cortex sends fibers to the spinal cord and, from there, to the muscles of the bowel and bladder. These fibers inhibit the autonomic nervous system's reflexive response so that the action of urinating or stooling is reduced.

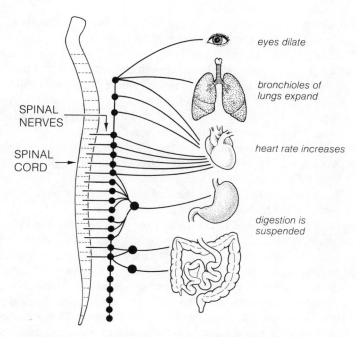

eyes dilate

bronchioles of lungs expand

SPINAL NERVES

heart rate increases

SPINAL CORD

digestion is suspended

Figure 12.10. Autonomic nervous system. These nerves control such involuntary motor activities as breathing, heart rate, and digestion. This system is involved in "fight or flight" reactions.

Thus, when an older child feels the need to urinate or to stool, he or she can tighten the necessary muscles until he or she reaches a bathroom. Damage to the pyramidal tract or the spinal cord causes a loss of this inhibition of the autonomic nervous system. This is why most children with cerebral palsy or severe mental retardation have great difficulty controlling bladder and bowel function.

THE CEREBROSPINAL FLUID

The cerebrospinal fluid is a clear, watery liquid that bathes the spinal cord and flows through the four ventricles, or cavities, within the brain (Figure 12.11). Totaling about 4 ounces in an adult, this fluid serves as a buffer for the central nervous system against sudden pressure changes and also helps provide this system with nutrition. Produced in a tangle of cells that hang down from the roof of the ventricles, called the **choroid plexus**, and absorbed on the surface of the brain, this fluid is constantly being recirculated.

After it is produced in the roof of the **lateral ventricles**, the cerebrospinal fluid flows through the third ventricle toward the fourth ventricle via a narrow passageway called the *aqueduct*. Openings in the roof of the fourth ventricle allow some of the cerebrospinal fluid to flow into the small space surrounding the brain. Much of the fluid, however, goes from the fourth ventricle down the meninges surrounding the spinal cord to the base of the spine.

If this flow is obstructed, it backs up in the ventricles and leads to increased intracranial pressure. This condition is called hydrocephalus (Figure 12.12) (Milhorat, 1972). In an infant, a significant increase in intracranial pressure is prevented because the brain can expand by pushing open the unfused bones of the skull. This results in an increase in the infant's head circumference. In an older child, however, the cranial bones are fused, and the brain has no room to expand. If untreated, this intracranial pressure will build up and cause the child to vomit, become lethargic, and go into a coma. Such a situation requires emergency treatment.

The causes of hydrocephalus are many. In some children, it is inherited. In others, it follows meningitis or an intraventricular hemorrhage. The infection or bleeding causes a blockage either of the openings on the surface of the brain or of the aqueduct. Both abnormalities hinder the flow of the cerebrospinal fluid. In some cases, the cause of the hydrocephalus is unknown.

Treatment of hydrocephalus involves either medication or the surgical placement of a bypass, called a *shunt*. Physicians have successfully used the drugs Lasix and Diamox to treat some children with developing hydrocephalus, especially after an intraventricular hemorrhage (Shinnar, Gammon, Bergman, et al., 1985). These drugs work by decreasing the production of cerebrospinal fluid by the choroid plexus. In most cases of hydrocephalus, however, treatment involves the surgical placement of a **ventriculo-peritoneal** (V-P) **shunt** (Vintzileos, Ingardia, & Nochimson, 1983). A plastic tube is inserted through a hole in the skull into one of the lateral ventricles. Another tube runs under the skin from the skull to the abdominal cavity. Extra tubing is left within the abdominal cavity and uncoils as the child grows. Just under the skin

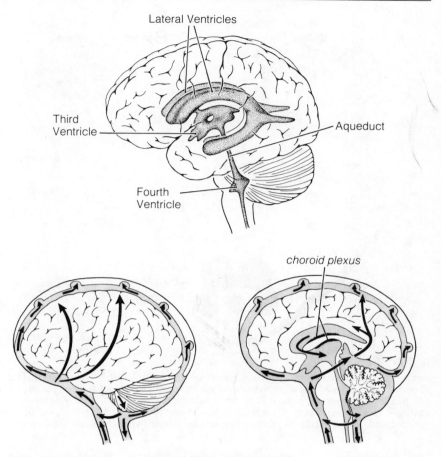

Figure 12.11. Ventricular system of the brain. The major parts of the ventricular system are shown above. The flow of cerebrospinal fluid is shown below. The fluid is produced by the choroid plexus in the roof of the lateral and third ventricles. Its primary route is through the aqueduct, into the fourth ventricle, and then into the spinal column, where it is absorbed. A secondary route is around the surface of the brain. A blockage, most commonly of the aqueduct, leads to hydrocephalus. (Lower illustrations redrawn with permission from Milhorat, T.H. [1972]. *Hydrocephalus and the cerebrospinal fluid*. Baltimore: Williams & Wilkins Co. Copyright © 1972, The Williams & Wilkins Co., Baltimore.)

on the skull, the two tubes are connected to a reservoir with a one-way valve (see Figure 12.12). This system allows the fluid to drain from the ventricles into the abdominal cavity, bypassing the block. In this way, intracranial pressure is decreased, and further enlargement of the head is prevented. Recently, a shunt was even placed in a fetus diagnosed prenatally as having hydrocephalus (Frigoletto, Birnholz, & Greene, 1982). Unfortunately, so far, this kind of prenatal treatment has met with a high incidence of failures and miscarriages.

While this treatment generally works well after a child is born, the shunt may become blocked later in life. If this happens, the intracranial pressure may suddenly

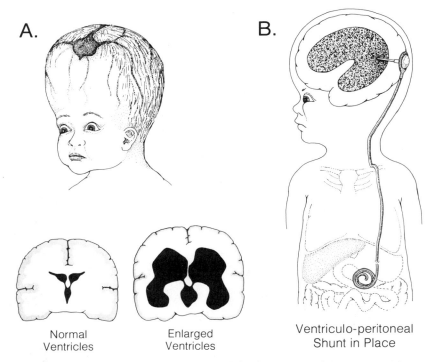

Normal Ventricles   Enlarged Ventricles   Ventriculo-peritoneal Shunt in Place

Figure 12.12.   Hydrocephalus. A) The head is enlarged, as is the "soft spot." A cross-section of the brain shows markedly enlarged lateral ventricles. B) A ventriculo-peritoneal shunt has been placed. A plastic tube is inserted into one of the lateral ventricles. Another tube runs under the skin from the skull to the abdominal cavity. Enough extra tubing is left in the abdomen to uncoil as the child grows. The block is bypassed, and cerebrospinal fluid can then flow directly from the ventricles to the abdominal cavity.

increase, causing lethargy and vomiting. Replacement of the malfunctioning shunt takes care of the problem, but it must be done immediately to avoid a dangerous buildup of pressure.

Children who have these ventriculo-peritoneal shunts can participate in all activities other than contact sports. Hydrocephalus is not necessarily associated with mental retardation or other disabilities, and many of these children grow up to lead normal lives (Prigatano, Zeiner, Pollay, et al., 1983).

SUMMARY

The nervous system has three major subunits: the central nervous system, the peripheral nervous system, and the autonomic nervous system. Within the central nervous system are the cerebrum, the diencephalon, the brain stem, the cerebellum, and the spinal cord. The messages from these components control the other two nervous systems.

Developmental disabilities result from damage to some portion of the nervous system. Disorders such as attention deficit disorder, learning disabilities, cerebral palsy, and epilepsy are discussed in later chapters.

REFERENCES

Bell, W.E., & McCormick, W.F. (1981). *Neurologic infections in children* (2nd ed.). Philadelphia: W.B. Saunders Co.

Benson, D.F., Stuss, D.T., Naeser, M.A., et al. (1981). The long-term effects of prefrontal leukotomy. *Archives of Neurology, 38,* 165–169.

Brown, J.W. (1972). *Aphasia, apraxia, and agnosia: Clinical and theoretical aspects.* Springfield, IL: Charles C Thomas.

Carpenter, M.B., & Sutin, J. (1983). *Human neuroanatomy* (8th ed.). Baltimore: Williams & Wilkins Co.

Clewell, W.H., Johnson, M.L., Meier, P.R., et al. (1982). A surgical approach to the treatment of fetal hydrocephalus. *New England Journal of Medicine, 306,* 1320–1325.

Frigoletto, F.D., Jr., Birnholz, J.C., & Greene, M.F. (1982). Antenatal treatment of hydrocephalus by ventriculoamniotic shunting. *Journal of the American Medical Association, 248,* 2496–2497.

Geschwind, N. (1979). Specializations of the human brain. *Scientific American, 241,* 180–199.

Gilman, S., & Winans, S. (Eds.). (1982). *Manter & Gatz's essentials of clinical neuroanatomy and neurophysiology* (6th ed.). Philadelphia: F.A. Davis.

Gold, A.P. (1974). Psychomotor epilepsy in childhood. *Pediatrics, 53,* 540–542.

Hayden, P.W., Shurtleff, D.B., & Stuntz, T.J. (1983). A longitudinal study of shunt function in 360 patients with hydrocephalus. *Developmental Medicine and Child Neurology, 25,* 334–337.

Holcomb, R., Lynn, R., Harvey, B., Jr., et al. (1972). Intoxication with 5.5 diphenylhydantoin (Dilantin): Clinical features, blood levels, urinary metabolites, and metabolic changes in a child. *Journal of Pediatrics, 80,* 627–632.

Hynd, G.W., & Cohen, M. (1983). *Dyslexia: Neuropsychological theory, research, and clinical differentiation.* New York: Grune & Stratton.

Illingworth, R.S. (1980). *The development of the infant and the young child: Normal and abnormal* (7th ed.). New York: Churchill Livingstone, Inc.

Milhorat, T.H. (1972). *Hydrocephalus and the cerebrospinal fluid.* Baltimore: Williams & Wilkins Co.

Noback, C.R. (1981). *The human nervous system: Basic principles of neurobiology* (3rd ed.). New York: McGraw-Hill Book Co.

Prigatano, G.P., Zeiner, H.K., Pollay, M., et al. (1983). Neuropsychological functioning in children with shunted uncomplicated hydrocephalus. *Child's Brain, 10,* 112–120.

Purpura, D.P. (1974). Dendritic spine "dysgenesis" and mental retardation. *Science, 186,* 1126–1128.

Shinnar, S., Gammon, K., Bergman, E.W., Jr., et al. (1985). Management of hydrocephalus in infancy: Use of acetazolamide and furosemide to avoid cerebrospinal fluid shunts. *Journal of Pediatrics, 107,* 31–37.

Vintzileos, A.M., Ingardia, C.J., & Nochimson, D.J. (1983). Congenital hydrocephalus: A review and protocol for perinatal management. *Obstetrics and Gynecology, 62,* 539–549.

Chapter 13

Bones and Muscles
Support and Movement

Upon completion of this chapter, the reader will:
—be able to explain the structure and development of bone
—know some of the most common bony deformities and their treatment
—recognize the various types of joints
—be aware of what happens when a person has arthritis
—know the function of tendons and ligaments
—understand how the musculoskeletal and nervous systems work together
—be able to identify some of the major diseases affecting movement

---

Although the nervous system initiates movement, without bones and muscles to respond to the signals, nothing would happen. We would be immobile. Our musculoskeletal system (composed of muscle and bone) assists movement through the interworkings of the bone, cartilage, ligaments, tendons, and muscles. This chapter explores how these various tissues function and examines what can go wrong.

BONE

Bone forms our skeleton, the internal structure of our body. Our bones range in size from the 0.5-inch **phalanges** of the finger to the roughly 18-inch femur, or thigh bone. Some of our bones, such as the skull, are flat; others, such as the femur, are tubular. Even though bones are hard and immobile, they are actively growing. Just as the body is dependent on the skeleton for support, so the skeletal system relies on the body for its maintenance and growth.

Structure and Development of Bone

The height of a child increases because of growth of the long, tubular bones. To understand how this works, it is helpful first to examine the structure of a bone. Consider the femur as an example. This bone consists of a shaft or *diaphysis,* a spongy, upper portion called a *metaphysis,* and a growth plate near the end of the

167

bone, called the *epiphysis* (Figure 13.1A). Surrounding the bone is a tough, fibrous, protective layer called the **periosteum**. Calcium crystals imbedded in a protein complex make up about one-third of a bone. It is this mineral-protein mixture that lends strength to the bone. The central core, the bone marrow, is where blood cells are formed. Weaving through the bone's structure are blood vessels that supply oxygen and nutrition necessary for growth.

Bone grows from the epiphysis. Here, cartilage cells are first laid down on top of the existing bone. The cartilage is soon invaded by bone-forming cells, or **osteoblasts**. These cells contain calcium and gradually transform the cartilage into bone. Both ends of the long bone then lengthen, and the child gets taller (Figure 13.1B).

As growth takes place, the bone undergoes different stresses, and it begins to remodel or change in shape. This increases its strength and stability. If bone were not capable of this reshaping, it would be more susceptible to fracture. While growth involves the osteoblast cells, this reshaping is performed by a different cell type, the **osteoclast**. The osteoblast adds calcium, and the osteoclast removes it from already formed bone and returns it to the blood stream. A part of the bone, therefore, is constantly disappearing, and new bone is being laid down in its place. The result is a sleeker, longer bone. On the average, a section of a child's bone lasts about a year and

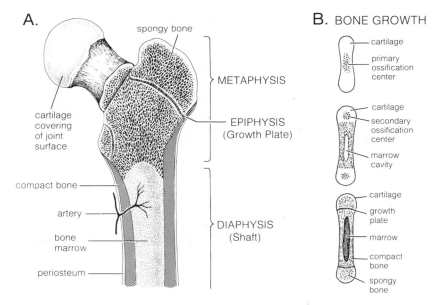

Figure 13.1.   A) The structure of a typical long bone, the femur. New bone grows from the epiphysis and the femur lengthens. The upper portion of the bone is the metaphysis, and the shaft is called the diaphysis. The bone marrow, which produces blood cells, lies in the center of the shaft. Surrounding the bone is a fibrous protective sheath, the periosteum. The bone facing the joint space is covered by flexible cartilage. B) The long bone starts off as a mass of cartilage in fetal life. Gradually the center is invaded by osteoblasts. These cells lay down minerals that form bone. The ossification centers spread and the bone enlarges and hardens. After birth, further bone growth occurs only from the epiphysis.

is then replaced by new bone. Thus, bone is a living organ that continually grows and reshapes to increase its effectiveness. In an adult, the reshaping continues even though growth has stopped. The average bone segment of an adult lasts about 7 years (Rosse & Clawsson, 1970).

Bony Deformities

Bony deformities may occur *in utero* or after birth. Two of the most common types are club foot and congenital dislocation of the hip.

In most cases, club foot, or *talipes equinovarus,* comes from a defect in fetal development of the foot (see Figure 4.6). The instep of the foot does not develop normally, and the foot turns in and appears shortened. This may affect one or both feet, with the result that the foot has a limited range of motion. Walking is also hindered. The deformity can be corrected either through casting or with **orthopedic** surgery.

While club foot is more common in boys, congenital dislocation of the hip occurs more frequently in girls. This condition seems to be associated with a delivery by breech position. A hereditary factor may also contribute to the defect. Whatever the cause, the result is a misshapen pelvis that has an abnormal **acetabulum**, or bony socket. Thus, the "ball"-shaped head of the femur does not fit properly into the shallow socket of the abnormal pelvis (Figure 13.2). Spreading back the hips when the child is an infant, using either a **Pavlik harness** or a **Frejka pillow**, will often avoid the need for corrective surgery.

Club foot and congenital hip dislocation represent isolated deformities. Other

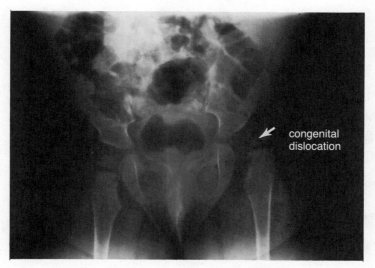

congenital dislocation

Figure 13.2.   Congenital dislocation of the left hip. The arrow indicates the point of dislocation. (X ray courtesy of Dr. Sandra Kramer, Department of Pediatric Radiology, The Johns Hopkins Hospital, Baltimore.)

bony disorders may involve the entire skeleton. One such example is achondroplasia, or short-limbed dwarfism. In a child with this disorder, the long bones are all short and stubby so he or she has shortened arms and legs (Figure 13.3). Since this disorder is inherited as an autosomal dominant trait, an affected parent will pass on the disorder to approximately half of the offspring.

Another example of a multiple bone deformity is **arthrogryposis**. In this disorder, usually because of fetal paralysis or an inadequate amount of amniotic fluid, the fetus remains in a fixed position for a prolonged period of time. This results in multiple **contractures** at the joints. Surgery and/or the repeated use of casts are usually needed to treat the deformities.

In addition to these problems, bony deformities may also develop after birth. For example, in cerebral palsy, the asymmetrical pull of various muscles may lead to a dislocation of the hip. In this case, splints do not suffice. Either a surgical procedure called an adductor tenotomy and obturator neurectomy (ATON), or a **varus osteotomy**, discussed in Chapter 21, is required to correct the problem. Besides the complication of a dislocated hip, an asymmetrical pull of spinal muscles on the vertebral column may cause scoliosis, or curvature of the spine (Figure 13.4).

Lastly, certain metabolic disorders can lead to the buildup of abnormal compounds in the bone. This causes the bony structure of the body to change. For example, over time, children with Hurler's syndrome (discussed in Chapter 8) develop a coarse facial appearance and short stubby limbs.

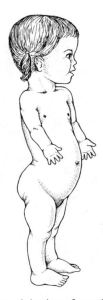

Figure 13.3.   Achondroplasia, an autosomal dominant form of short-limbed dwarfism.

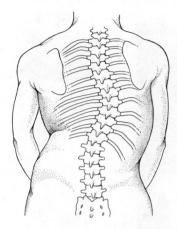

Figure 13.4. Scoliosis, or spinal curvature, caused in this case by asymmetrical muscle pull in a child with cerebral palsy.

Fractures

Any person may fracture, or break, a bone. A fracture occurs when force is brought to bear against the bone, sufficient to break the bone (Figure 13.5). Young children have a greater risk of fracture than adults because the diameter of their bones is smaller and cannot sustain as much force. The most common causes of fractures in children are household and automobile accidents, sports injuries, and child abuse.

Some children experience fractures, called *pathological fractures,* even when there does not seem to be force sufficient to break the bone. For example, such a child might suffer a broken leg merely by being lifted from a lying to a sitting position. Nonambulatory children with handicaps have frail bones and are frequent victims of these fractures. As discussed in Chapter 9, it may be important to add vitamin D and calcium supplements to the diets of these children. Fractures also may occur in children who have leukemia or other tumors that invade the bone marrow and weaken the internal structure of the bone. Children with rickets who have not formed normal calcium deposits are common victims of pathological fractures. In addition, an inherited disorder called *osteogenesis imperfecta* is associated with brittle bones that fracture easily. These children may suffer multiple fractures during their delivery. As they grow up, they may have as many as 20 to 30 fractures of various bones (McKusick, 1972).

For proper healing, fractures must have a cast put around them, usually for 6 to 8 weeks. Casts are made of plaster in a fashion similar to papier mâché. The cast serves to stabilize the bone fragments and hold them together after they have been manually realigned. This allows the bone to heal in the normal position. Healing takes place by a process called **callus** formation (see Figure 13.5). The callus starts off as a blood clot, the result of bleeding from tiny blood vessels inside the bone. Within a few weeks, osteoblasts invade the clot and gradually lay down new bone. By 6 to 8 weeks

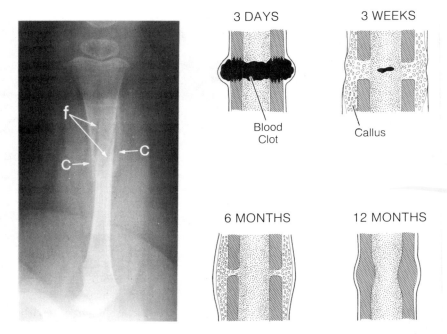

3 DAYS

Blood Clot

3 WEEKS

Callus

6 MONTHS

12 MONTHS

Figure 13.5.   Bone fracture. The X ray shows the fracture lines (f). This was taken 3 weeks after the accident, and callus formation can be seen (C). The mechanism of healing is outlined to the right. Initially, there is bleeding from bone capillaries damaged in the accident. Soon this blood clot is invaded by osteoblasts that lay down extensive bony tissue forming a callus. By 6 months, the bones are almost fused, but the bony structure is still enlarged. At 12 months, fusion is complete and the bone is strong and looks fairly normal. Further reshaping over time will make all signs of fracture disappear.

following the fracture, weight can be exerted on the bone, and it can usually function again. However, the remodeling process continues after that time. Eventually, the bulging callus disappears. Within 6 to 12 months, a normal appearing bone is seen on X ray (Rosse & Clawsson, 1970).

Unfortunately, in children with multiple handicaps, this healing process does not proceed so smoothly or so rapidly. While the healing time for normal children is 6–8 weeks, 8–12 weeks may be required for a fracture to heal in a child with handicaps. Remodeling also takes longer because these children are often non-ambulatory and do not have as many reshaping forces at work. Thus, for these children, the fractured bone may remain enlarged and callused.

JOINTS

A joint is defined as the union of two or more bones. It is made up of the epiphyses and cartilage of the two connecting bones, the small, lubricated space called the *joint cavity,* and the ligaments and muscles that bind the bones together and make the joint stable (Figure 13.6).

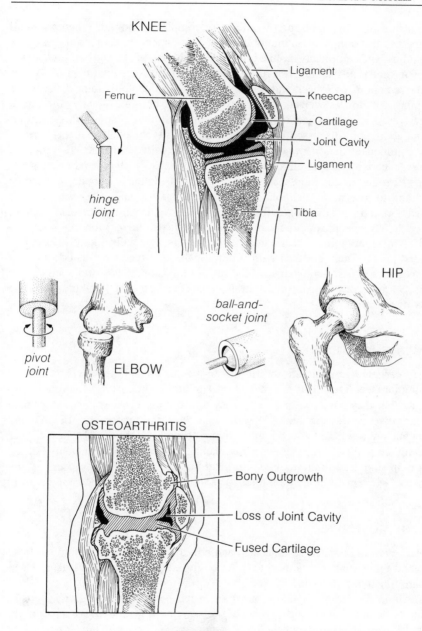

KNEE

Ligament

Kneecap

Cartilage

Joint Cavity

Ligament

Femur

hinge
joint

Tibia

pivot
joint

ELBOW

ball-and-
socket joint

HIP

OSTEOARTHRITIS

Bony Outgrowth

Loss of Joint Cavity

Fused Cartilage

Figure 13.6.   Joints. A normal knee joint is shown above as compared to an arthritic knee joint below. Normally there is a lubricated joint cavity separating the femur and tibia bones. Muscles cross the joint attached to the ligaments. In the diseased joint, the cavity has disappeared, and there is fusion of the opposing bones. This severely limits movement. The different types of joints are also illustrated: hinge (knee), pivot (elbow), and ball-and-socket (hip).

Joints may be immobile, partly mobile, or completely mobile. Where the skull bones meet is an example of an immobile joint. The fingers are composed of slightly mobile joints, and completely mobile joints include hinge, pivot, and ball-and-socket joints. The knee is an example of a hinge joint that can flex (see Figure 13.6). At this joint, movement of 145° back and forth is possible. In the elbow joint, a pivot and hinge joint, rotation as well as hinge movement can be done. Lastly, the hip, a ball-and-socket joint, can accomplish movement in all three planes—flexion, rotation, and abduction (discussed later in the section on types of movement).

A common affliction of joints is arthritis. Actually, arthritis is a group of disorders, each with its own characteristics and problems. In all cases, however, the cartilage surrounding the joint space is damaged, causing the joint space to become smaller and to lose its lubrication. The bones hit against each other and become inflamed. Sometimes, the bones fuse. The result is pain and a decrease in joint mobility. In older people and in handicapped individuals, the most common form of arthritis is **osteoarthritis** (see Figure 13.6). This is especially likely to occur in dislocated joints. Thus, children with cerebral palsy and recurring dislocations not only experience a loss of movement at the various joints but may suffer from painful arthritis. Surgery correcting the dislocation includes repairing the joint, thus reducing the risk of arthritis.

LIGAMENTS AND TENDONS

As noted earlier, ligaments are the fibrous tissues that attach one bone to another across a joint (see Figure 13.6). Tendons are similar in composition and function to ligaments, but they have looser fibers. They attach a muscle to a bone rather than connecting two bones (Figure 13.7). Both ligaments and tendons are flexible and resilient and are essential to keep joints moving properly. Unlike bone, these tissues have a limited ability to regenerate. Thus, damage to tendons or ligaments (all too common in athletes) often requires surgical repair. Even then, success is not guaranteed. Movement in the joint after such an injury may be limited and painful.

TYPES OF MOVEMENT

Before discussing how nerves, muscles, and bones work together, it is important to understand the various terms used to describe different kinds of movement. These terms are illustrated in Figure 13.8.

Flexion refers to the bending of a part of the body at a joint. *Extension,* the opposite of flexion, means to straighten out. *Abduction* is the moving of a part of the body away from the midline of the body, while *adduction* is movement toward the midline. The midline or middle segment of the body is also called the *median plane*. The outer parts of the body are the *lateral sections*. To illustrate, the umbilicus is in the median plane while the breasts are in the lateral sections of the body. *Anterior* refers to the top of a flat surface, whereas *posterior* is the rear or under part. Thus, the

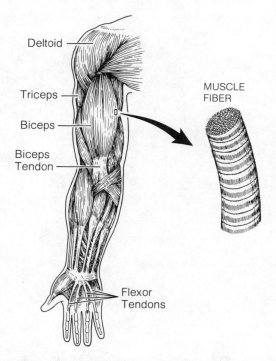

Figure 13.7.   Muscles. The major muscles in the arm. Note that the biceps and triceps are antagonists. The enlargement shows a muscle fiber, which is the unit of muscle tissue.

chest is anterior while the back is posterior. The word *superior* means up or above; *inferior* means below. The head is superior, and the feet are inferior to the shoulders.

When you lie on your back, you are in a *supine position*. You are *prone* when you lie on your stomach. A foot is *inverted* when the sole faces inward and *everted* when the sole turns outward. A *varus* position exists when the toes point toward each other making an A shape. When the heels are together and the toes apart, forming a V, the foot is in a *valgus* position.

MUSCLES AND THE NEUROMUSCULAR JUNCTION

Movement of a muscle across a joint is the result of a signal that begins in the brain, passes through the spinal cord, and ends in the peripheral nerve. Since the sole function of the muscle is to contract, its structure is very different from other body organs. The cell of a muscle is called the *muscle fiber* (see Figure 13.7). This fiber's chief components are two proteins, **actin** and **myosin**, that form highly organized subunits within the muscle fibers. It is these subunits that are stimulated by a nerve impulse to contract.

Such stimulation occurs at the neuromuscular junction, where the peripheral nerve reaches the muscle fiber. At this point, the nerve and muscle are separated by a

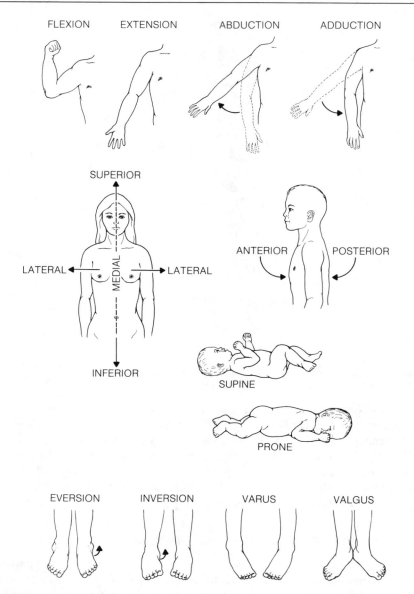

FLEXION   EXTENSION   ABDUCTION   ADDUCTION

SUPERIOR

LATERAL ◄───── MEDIAL ─────► LATERAL

ANTERIOR   POSTERIOR

INFERIOR

SUPINE

PRONE

EVERSION   INVERSION   VARUS   VALGUS

Figure 13.8.   Various types of movements and postures.

synaptic cleft (discussed in Chapter 12). The electrical impulse from the brain jumps this gap when it is converted into chemical energy by a neurotransmitter that is released into the cleft. The message then moves on to the muscle fiber. When the neurotransmitter bridges the gap, it stimulates the muscle to contract, and movement takes place.

Smooth movement happens so long as all the muscle groups around the joint act in concert. Each muscle group has *agonists* and *antagonists*. Antagonists are muscles that oppose the movement of the agonists, the primary muscles—for example, when the arm is flexed, the biceps (the agonist muscle) contract, and the triceps (the antagonist muscle) relax. If both muscle groups contracted, a painful muscle spasm or "charley horse" would develop. So, when the brain tells the arm to move, it actually sends out not one but a series of messages that tell some muscles to contract and others to relax.

NEUROMUSCULAR DISEASES

Neuromuscular diseases affect movement because of damage to either the anterior horn cells of the spinal cord, the peripheral nerves, the neuromuscular junction, or the muscle itself. Other disorders, such as cerebral palsy and torsion dystonia, also affect movement, but their defect is centered in the brain rather than in the musculoskeletal system.

Diseases of the Anterior Horn Cells

When an impulse leaves the brain to signal movement, it passes along the spinal cord to a point near the particular joint to be moved. Here it reaches an anterior horn cell (see Figure 12.9), which, in turn, passes the impulse to the peripheral nerve.

The two diseases most commonly associated with damage to the anterior horn cells are polio and **Werdnig-Hoffmann disease** (Emery & Holloway, 1982; Pearn, 1982). The polio virus selectively destroys the anterior horn cells and creates a gap between the central nervous system and the peripheral nerves. Paralysis takes place below the part of the spinal column that has been damaged by the infection. Polio is no longer a significant health problem in the United States, since the polio vaccine was first introduced in 1955 by Dr. Jonas Salk. Later, Dr. Albert Sabin developed an oral vaccine. Now, the immunizations that infants receive include three doses of oral polio vaccine in addition to their series of diphtheria, whooping cough (pertussis), and tetanus (DPT) shots.

Werdnig-Hoffmann disease also attacks the anterior horn cells. This is an autosomal recessive inherited disorder of unknown origin. Affected children are inactive *in utero* and very floppy after birth. Life expectancy is decreased, and a microscopic examination of the spinal cord reveals a severe deficiency of anterior horn cells. No treatment is available; these children often suffer from recurrent respiratory infections.

Disease of the Peripheral Nerves

Guillain-Barré syndrome is an example of an illness affecting the peripheral nerves. Its incidence is rare, approximately 1/100,000 (Bell & McCormick, 1981; Kaplan, Schonberger, Hurwitz, et al., 1983). Also called *acute polyneuropathy*, this disease causes paralysis similar to that seen in polio. It generally occurs after an upper respiratory infection and involves both sides of the body, starting in the lower extremities and moving upward for about 1 to 2 weeks. The upper extremities and diaphragm may also be affected, and breathing may be impaired. Thus, a person with this syndrome may need artificial ventilation to help him breathe. However, unlike polio, nerve damage may not be permanent in Guillain-Barré syndrome. Victims may recover over a period of months as the nerve fibers grow back together and function normally (Eisen & Humphreys, 1974).

Guillain-Barré syndrome is caused by an **autoimmune** response to a viral infection. The body identifies the infected nerve roots as foreign bodies and begins to damage them. No specific therapy exists. The physician simply tries to ride out the infection by supporting respiration and providing adequate nutrition during the acute illness. During the recovery phase, physical therapy is needed. As is true of polio, Guillain-Barré syndrome is not usually associated with brain damage or mental retardation.

Disease of the Neuromuscular Junction

Another disease involving the body's immune response is *myasthenia gravis*. This inherited disorder affects the neuromuscular junction. It occurs most frequently in young women, but children also occasionally suffer from this disease (Havard & Scadding, 1983; Rodriguez, Gomez, Howard, et al., 1983).

Muscle weakness is the main characteristic of myasthenia. Initially it affects the eyelids, making them droopy. Then it progresses to involve other muscle groups. A person with myasthenia gravis usually feels strong in the morning and increasingly weakens as the day goes on.

This disease results from antibodies blocking the receptors for acetylcholine, a neurotransmitter (Engel, Lindstrom, Lambert, et al., 1977). Consequently, when the nerve impulse moves down the peripheral nerve to the neuromuscular junction, it goes no further. Acetylcholine cannot be released into the synaptic opening, and muscle movement is either weak or does not happen at all.

Treatment involves increasing the level of acetylcholine in the synaptic cleft (Lisak, 1983). A medication called *neostigmine* prevents the breakdown of the acetylcholine so that more of the chemical is available to aid in the transmission of the nerve impulse. Strength improves within minutes of taking this drug. With proper treatment, individuals with myasthenia can lead quite normal lives.

Diseases of the Muscle Itself

Diseases of the muscle itself will obviously affect movement. The best known of these disorders is muscular dystrophy, the cause of which is unknown. The most common form of this disease is called *Duchenne's muscular dystrophy*.

Inherited as a sex-linked disorder (see Chapter 2), Duchenne's affects males and has an incidence of about 2/10,000 (Dubowitz, 1978; Dubowitz & Heckmatt, 1980). Parents are usually unaware of any problem until after the child starts walking. Then the child's walk resembles that of a duck, and he has difficulty climbing steps or getting up from a lying down position. Over a period of time, ranging from months to years, the child becomes weaker and less mobile, eventually ending up in a wheelchair. Pain, especially in the legs, is common, and the calf muscles become overdeveloped but weak. Children with Duchenne's also often have respiratory problems and mild mental retardation.

Diagnosing muscular dystrophy depends on finding an elevated level of **creatine phosphokinase (CPK)** in the blood. This enzyme is released by dying muscle cells. A muscle biopsy may show that the muscle fibers are in disarray and contain fatty tissue. Besides causing flaccid weakness in the voluntary muscles, this disease also damages the involuntary muscles of the heart and diaphragm. Because of this, children with muscular dystrophy often do not live to adulthood (Gilroy, Cahalan, Berman, et al., 1963).

Unfortunately, no effective treatment for muscular dystrophy exists. At one point, it seemed that the use of **steroids** held some promise, but this has not proved to be the case (Walton, 1981). Now treatment mainly focuses on helping to ensure mobility for as long as possible using braces, splints, and wheelchairs (Siegel, 1981).

MOVEMENT DISORDERS

Besides the already mentioned neuromuscular diseases, a number of other disorders affect movement. Their origins, however, are not in the musculoskeletal system. The most important of these is cerebral palsy, which is discussed at length in Chapter 21. Another example is torsion dystonia, or dystonia musculorum deformans.

As with muscular dystrophy, dystonia starts in childhood. Usually the first symptom is a turning in of one foot while walking. As time goes on, this unnatural position becomes more pronounced and is accentuated by movement (Wachtel, Batshaw, Eldridge, et al., 1982). Intermittent muscle spasms occur; they often disappear during sleep. Dystonia is typically associated with normal or superior intelligence (Marsden & Harrison, 1974; Wachtel, Batshaw, Eldridge, et al., 1982).

The underlying problem in this genetically inherited disorder seems to involve the basal ganglia of the brain. Some neurochemical imbalance may exist and may cause the unusual movements characteristic of dystonia.

Normally, treatment focuses on restoring the neurochemical balance in the basal ganglia. Two approaches have been used. The more conservative therapeutic approach is to use medications that increase the neurochemical levels in the brain. These drugs, such as L-dopa and Artane, are commonly used to treat Parkinson's disease, another movement disorder, in adults. But, they have also been helpful in treating dystonia in children. This kind of treatment has fewer side effects than surgery.

Neurosurgery is the more radical approach. A small needle is inserted through the skull bone into the **ventrolateral** nucleus of the **thalamus** (a part of the basal ganglia). An electrical current is run through the needle to destroy a small area of the nucleus. If successful, this operation, called a **thalamotomy**, may improve the dystonia. Unfortunately, improvement occurs in less than half of the cases. Furthermore, certain speech areas are located near the site of the operation, and 10%–20% of the children who undergo this surgery lose their ability to speak after the operation (Cooper, 1969).

SUMMARY

The musculoskeletal system both supports our physical structure and helps us carry out normal movement. Abnormalities of the bone lead to deformities such as club foot or short-limbed dwarfism, or diseases such as arthritis. Muscle diseases cause weakness and floppy tone, while peripheral nerve and anterior horn cell diseases result in paralysis. Because many of these diseases are difficult to treat, it is consoling to note that their incidence is rare. Fewer than 1% of all children suffer from these disorders.

REFERENCES

Bell, W.E., & McCormick, W.F. (1981). *Neurologic infections in children* (2nd ed.). Philadelphia: W.B. Saunders Co.

Bleck, E.E. (1979). *Orthopedic management of cerebral palsy*. Philadelphia: W.B. Saunders Co.

Cooper, I.S. (1969). *Involuntary movement disorders*. New York: Harper & Row.

Dubowitz, V. (1978). *Muscle disorders in childhood*. Philadelphia: W.B. Saunders.

Dubowitz, V., & Heckmatt, J. (1980). Management of muscular dystrophy. Pharmacological and physical aspects. *British Medical Bulletin, 36*, 139–144.

Eisen, A., & Humphreys, P. (1974). The Guillain-Barré syndrome. A clinical and electrodiagnostic study of 25 cases. *Archives of Neurology, 30*, 438–443.

Emery, A.E., & Holloway, S. (1982). Familial motor neuron disease. *Advances in Neurology, 36*, 139–147.

Engel, A.G., Lindstrom, J.M., Lambert, E.H., et al. (1977). Ultrastructural localization of the acetylcholine receptor in myasthenia gravis and in its experimental autoimmune model. *Neurology, 27*, 307–315.

Gilroy, J., Cahalan, J.L., Berman, R., et al. (1963). Cardiac and pulmonary complications in Duchenne's progressive muscular dystrophy. *Circulation, 27*, 484–493.

Havard, C.W., & Scadding, C.K. (1983). Myasthenia gravis. Pathogenesis and current concepts in management. *Drugs, 26*, 174–184.

Kaplan, J.E., Schonberger, L.B., Hurwitz, E.S., et al. (1983). Guillain-Barré syndrome in the United States, 1978–1981: Additional observations from the national surveillance system. *Neurology, 33*, 633–637.

Lisak, R.P. (1983). Myasthenia gravis: Mechanisms and management. *Hospital Practice, 18*, 101–109.

McKusick, V. (1972). *Heritable disorders of connective tissues* (4th ed.). St. Louis: C.V. Mosby Co.

Marsden, C.D., & Harrison, M.J.G. (1974). Idiopathic torsion dystonia (dystonia musculorum deformans): A review of forty-two patients. *Brain, 97*, 793–810.

Pearn, J.H. (1982). Infantile motor neuron diseases. *Advances in Neurology, 36*, 121–130.

Prosser, E.J., Murphy, E.G., & Thompson, M.W. (1969). Intelligence and the gene for Duchenne muscular dystrophy. *Archives of Disease in Childhood, 44*, 221–230.

Rodriguez, M., Gomez, M.R., Howard, F.M., Jr., et al. (1983). Myasthenia gravis in children: Long term followup. *Annals in Neurology, 13*, 504–510.

Rosse, C., & Clawsson, D.K. (1970). *Introduction to the musculoskeletal system*. New York: Harper & Row.

Siegel, I.M. (1981). Muscular dystrophy: Multidisciplinary approach to management. *Postgraduate Medicine, 69*, 124–128, 131–133.

Wachtel, R.C., Batshaw, M.L., Eldridge, R., et al. (1982). Torsion dystonia. *Johns Hopkins Medical Journal, 151*, 355–361.

Walton, J.N. (1981). *Disorders of voluntary muscle* (4th ed.). New York: Churchill Livingstone, Inc.

Chapter 14

Normal and Abnormal Development
Mental Retardation

with Bruce K. Shapiro

Upon completion of this chapter, the reader will:
—know the developmental milestones children attain
—be acquainted with Piaget's theory of intellectual development
—understand the definition and implications of the term *mental retardation*
—know the advantages and disadvantages of the principal intelligence tests used with children
—recognize the various approaches to the treatment of mental retardation
—be aware of the different levels of functioning and independence that individuals with mental retardation can achieve

---

At birth, a newborn responds primarily in an involuntary, or reflexive, way to his or her environment. Over the next 2 years, however, a combination of brain growth and learning experiences will enable the child to move from complete dependence on parents to active participation in the world. The child will learn to run, to talk, and to think creatively. This development occurs in a sequential, step-by-step fashion. Yet, some of the steps are steeper than others, and some children cannot manage all the steps. This chapter discusses the principles of normal development and developmental delay. It also defines the different forms of mental retardation and reviews some of the approaches to the treatment of mental retardation.

THE DEVELOPMENTAL SEQUENCE

The sequence of development has a number of characteristics. First, development is an ongoing process that begins with embryogenesis and continues throughout a

Bruce K. Shapiro, M.D., is a Developmental Pediatrician at The Kennedy Institute for Handicapped Children and Associate Professor of Pediatrics at The Johns Hopkins University School of Medicine, Baltimore, Maryland.

person's life. Second, this process is closely linked to the maturation of the central nervous system. Consequently, the most rapid intellectual development takes place when the brain is growing rapidly, during the first few years of life (Illingworth, 1983). Third, development progresses from head to foot, or in a cephalocaudal fashion. A child first gains head control, then sits, then crawls, and finally walks.

When discussing development, four major types of skills are usually considered: *gross motor, fine motor, language,* and *social-adaptive* (Gesell & Ilg, 1949). Language, the best predictor of future intellectual functioning, consists of expressive and receptive skills. Receptive language involves understanding what is said, while expressive language entails communicating with others by talking or by using other communicative tools (see Chapter 17).

The case of Michael, the child born of a normal pregnancy, as discussed in Chapter 6, is used here to illustrate the sequence of developmental milestones children pass as they grow from birth to 2 years of age (Table 14.1).

Gross Motor Development

As is true of all children, Michael's activity during the first 3 months of life was highly reflexive. In newborns, primitive reflexes are the primary means of responding to the world. As they grow, infants gradually integrate these primitive reflexes with voluntary movement. During early infancy, when Michael's mother, Karen, stroked the side of his lips, he rooted, or turned, toward her. When she placed her breast at his lips, he began to suck vigorously. If Michael turned his head to the right, his right arm and leg stretched out involuntarily while his left arm and leg flexed. Michael usually held his hands in a clenched position and, when pried open, his fingers automatically grasped Karen's fingers.

Yet, fairly quickly, he began to gain some control over his movements. For example, when pulled to a sitting position, he managed to hold his head up for a few seconds before it fell to rest on his chest. Also, when placed face down, Michael turned his head to one side or the other as if to breathe more comfortably.

As Michael grew, his actions became more purposeful. This development corresponded with the rapid growth and **myelination**, or sheathing, of the nerves in the central nervous system. This myelination allowed more rapid communication between the brain and the body. Thus, Michael was able to roll over from stomach to back at 5 months of age. To perform this action, his brain had to integrate certain primitive reflexes (Capute, Palmer, Shapiro, et al., 1984). If Michael were brain damaged, the primitive reflexes would have persisted and interfered with rolling over. Such persistence is a clue to the existence of cerebral palsy (see Chapter 21).

Continuing to develop on schedule, Michael next progressed to sitting up without support at 7 months of age. To accomplish this, he had to undergo a series of developmental steps. Initially, Michael had been unable to sit because he could not maintain his balance. A primitive reflex, called the tonic labyrinthine response, interfered by making Michael retract his shoulders and extend his arms whenever he lifted his head. He would then fall over. At 5 months of age, this reflex decreased in intensity, and Michael could sit up with support. The next step was to develop

Table 14.1. Development in the first 2 years of life (approximate ages of skill attainment)

Month	Gross motor	Fine motor	Social-adaptive	Language
1	Partial head control Primitive reflexes predominate	Clenched fists	Fixates objects and follows 90°	Alerts to sound Small sounds
2	Good head control Lifts chin in prone		Follows 180° Smiles responsively	
3	Lifts chest off bed Primitive reflexes less prominent	Hands held open Reaches toward objects Pulls at clothing	Follows 360° Recognizes mother	Coos
4	Swimming movements	Hands come to midline	Shakes rattle Anticipates food Belly laugh	Laughs aloud Produces different sounds for different needs
5	Rolls over stomach to back Holds head erect		Frolics when played with	Orients toward sound Gives a "raspberry"
6	Anterior propping response	Transfers objects Holds bottle Palmar grasp	Looks after lost toy Mirror play	Babbles Recognizes friendly and angry voices
7	Bounces when standing Sits without support	Feeds self cookie	Drinks from cup	Imitates noise Responds to name
8	Lateral propping responses	Rings bell Radial raking grasp	Separation anxiety begins Tries to gain attention	Nonspecific "Mama" Understands "no"
9	Crawls		Mouths objects	Recognizes familiar words

(continued)

183

Table 14.1. *(continued)*

Month	Gross motor	Fine motor	Social-adaptive	Language
10	Stands with support	Plays with bell Claps	Waves "bye-bye" Pat-a-cake	Specific "Da-da, Ma-ma"
11	Cruises around objects	Pincer grasp		Follows gesture command
12	Makes first steps	Throws objects Puts objects in containers	Aids in dressing Turns papers Takes turns	2–3 specific words
15	Climbs up stairs	Marks with pencil	Indicates when wet Spoon-feeds Builds tower with blocks Gives kisses Imitates chores	Low jargon Follows 1-step commands 4–6 words 1–body parts
18	Runs stiffly Handedness is determined Jumps	Constructive play with toys Scribbles Imitates lines Places objects in formboard	Places formboard Turns pages Parallel play Takes off shoes Does puzzles	High jargon Body parts Follows 2-step commands Points to one picture in book 10 words
24	Walks up and down steps	Imitates vertical lines Draws circle with pencil	Puts on and takes off shoes Plays alongside other children Negativistic Uses fork Indicates toileting needs	Uses "I" Four body parts Can form 3-word sentences Says "yes" and "no"

propping responses where his hands would reach out to help him balance himself whenever he began to topple over as he sat. Once this was perfected, he could sit with confidence.

Not satisfied with his sedentary existence, Michael next began the evolution of walking. At 7 months, he could stand when held, bearing weight on his feet. Then, at 9 months, he began to crawl, alternating both feet. He was able to pull himself up to a standing position at 10 months and started to walk around objects or cruise at 11 months. At last, at 13 months, Michael took his first independent steps. Five months later, he was running and, by 2 years of age, he could jump and walk up steps (Bloom, 1980; Caplan, 1978).

Fine Motor Development

Michael's fine motor development paralleled his gross motor development. During the first 2 or 3 months, he could do very little with his hands because they were usually held in a clenched position. Once they opened, at 3 months, Michael started to reach toward his colorful mobile and pull at his clothing. In the fourth month, he would clasp his hands together and then put them in his mouth, often chortling when he did this.

By 6 months of age, Michael could transfer objects from one hand to the other (Knobloch & Pasamanick, 1975; Yale University Clinic, Gesell, & Halverson, 1940). At this age, he was slightly more independent; he could feed himself a cookie and hold a bottle. Over the next few months, he started to explore his environment actively, reaching out to anything in sight and examining it. For example, if placed near a bell, Michael would grab it and ring it until one of his parents successfully substituted a quieter instrument. When he could crawl, at 9 months, he explored all the nooks and crannies of his house. At 12 months, his pincer grasp (using his thumb and forefinger) was refined and enabled him to pick up small objects. These objects usually ended up in his mouth, whether they were edible or not. When he reached 18 months of age, he could scribble with a pencil, creating many abstract works of art.

Communication Skills

As a newborn, Michael mainly communicated his needs by crying. After only a few weeks, he began to explore the world with his eyes. If Karen were lucky, she could hold his attention for a few seconds. He responded to a loud noise by stopping his movement for an instant and then returned to his seemingly random movements. When Michael was 2 months old, he rewarded his father's attention with a smile.

As time went on, Michael quickly developed more and more communication skills. He cooed in the third month and knew how to give a "raspberry" in the fourth. A month later, Michael started to turn his head toward a conversation as if to take part in it. In the sixth month, he started making babbling sounds. Four weeks later, he tried to imitate the sounds his parents made. He then responded to his name with a smile and a turn of the head. By the time Michael was 8 months old, he understood the command "no," although understanding it did not ensure his following it for very long. He began saying "mama" to everything and everyone in sight. At 11 months,

Michael spoke a few specific words (ma, bye) and could follow a simple command if it were accompanied by a gesture.

Unlike the development of motor skills that were simply refined during the second year of life, Michael's language skills exploded between 12 and 24 months. At 15 months, he had a 5–10 word vocabulary and used jargon or double-talked all the time. He also closed the door and sat down when commanded without a gesture as a guide (Knobloch & Pasamanick, 1975). When he was 18 months old, Michael could point to different parts of his body when asked to name them. He spoke unintelligible monologues, interspersing real words with jargon. He could name some pictures in a book, follow two-step commands such as "take the bell and put it on the table," and referred to himself as "I." Soon, he began to put together three-word phrases such as "I am hungry" or "I go outside." He was well on his way to having good communication skills.

Social-Adaptive Skills

Besides gaining motor and communication skills, Michael developed the ability to relate to the important people in his world and to differentiate some of his emotional responses. By the time he was 2 months old, Michael started to distinguish Karen from other people, giving her his best smile. During the fourth month, he began to laugh heartily and would reach for his bottle when it was brought into sight.

Michael's social interactions also became more sophisticated. Before he was a year old, he could play "peek-a-boo" and "pat-a-cake," wave "bye-bye," and throw a ball. During the second year, Michael started to help push his arms through a shirt and to take off most of his clothes. He also began to play alongside other children, not yet wanting to share with them at this age (Illingworth, 1983). When he was separated from his parents, he became upset (Bloom, 1980). By age 2, he became quite independent, feeding himself with a spoon and fork. As with his communication skills, his social skills had become much more refined.

PIAGET'S THEORY OF INTELLECTUAL DEVELOPMENT

The example of Michael illustrates that development involves a series of steps, which eventually enable a person to reason and solve problems. It is the inability to march up all of the steps that defines mental retardation. The problem in mental retardation is not so much that a mildly retarded child will only attain a mental age of 10 years instead of, for example, 16 years, but that certain abilities to understand information will be beyond the grasp of that child. This lifelong limitation restricts the individual's ability to adapt to his or her world.

To explain normal and abnormal intellectual development, Jean Piaget divided the process into four stages: 1) *the sensorimotor period,* which lasts from birth to approximately 18 months, 2) the *preoperational stage,* which lasts from 2 to 7 years of age, 3) *the stage of concrete operations,* which extends from ages 7 to 12 years, and 4) *the period of formal operations,* after 12 years of age (Cowan, 1978; Gruber & Voneche, 1977; Maier, 1978). Each stage is characterized by definite levels of achievement and abilities. The progression through these stages moves sequentially, with an adding on of abilities at each stage. Although some theorists have objected to Piaget's classifications because they give the impression that development neatly proceeds in defined steps, such delineations provide a framework to help us understand both the sequence of intellectual development and the limitations at the various levels of mental retardation.

The Sensorimotor Stage

During the sensorimotor stage, very primitive forms of intelligence are evident. Even before a child is able to use language well, he or she exhibits some complex behavior. The child begins to coordinate activities to reach certain goals, for example, to pull a string to reach a brightly colored ring attached to it. In addition, the child gradually becomes more interested in the world and less absorbed in him- or herself. In exploring the environment, the child, through experimentation, finds ways of acting and relating to achieve a goal. For example, an 18-month-old girl may want to reach for something out of her grasp. To do this, she will find a chair or stool and climb on it to reach the desired object. She is beginning to find her own solutions to concrete problems. However, she still cannot generalize what she learns to new situations. Most "discoveries" are made through trial and error. A child with severe retardation usually does not progress beyond this stage.

The Preoperational Stage

The preoperational stage is characterized by the use of meaningful language. In the first stage, the child deals with objects that surround him or her and are visible. With the use of language, beginning around age 2 years, the child can use symbols to represent objects that are not present. For example, at this age, a child may pretend a mud pie is a chocolate bar and may also pretend to eat it. A child at age 3 can make up a story and may reconstruct the recent past and project into the very near future.

Even with the use of language and the ability to think in more abstract terms, however, the preoperational stage of development remains a relatively primitive stage of intelligence. Although the child is beginning to be able to classify and group objects, he or she is not yet proficient at it. Also, while the child can distinguish between certain quantities—for example, big versus little—he or she is not yet able to perform what is called the operation of conservation. A 4-year-old boy, for example, believes that when water is poured from a tall, thin glass into a wide-mouthed, shorter glass, there is less water. He is taken in by the appearance of more water. The ability to understand that quantity cannot be judged by appearance alone, that is, the operation of conservation, is refined during the stage of concrete operations. A child with moderate retardation rarely progresses beyond this second stage.

The Stage of Concrete Operations

During the stage of concrete operations, a child becomes better able to order and classify objects and to see a relationship between different items. For example, a 9-year-old can speak of one object as being wider than another and shorter than something else. A child at this point can also arrange objects according to size or weight and can divide something into its parts. Children in this stage of development are able to solve some mathematical problems and to read well. They are also able to generalize learning to new situations and to begin to appreciate another person's point of view. However, these children still have difficulty dealing with hypothetical problems. In addition, although children in this stage are better able to understand the concept of past and future, this understanding is somewhat limited. Individuals with mild retardation usually remain at this level of development.

The Stage of Formal Operations

Piaget's final stage of intellectual development, that of formal operations, proceeds from age 12 throughout one's life. During this stage, children are able to project themselves into the future and to think about long-term goals. They also develop a sensitivity to the feelings of others and become, at the same time, increasingly more self-conscious. A notable characteristic is the development of an ability to reason using hypotheses. A classic example is Cyril Burt's test (Burt, 1959): If Edith is fairer than Susan and darker than Lilly, who is the darkest of all three? To solve this problem, a child must be able to form a system that includes all possible combinations of each element. As another example, a child may be asked to determine how many combinations can be formed with three colors. Once again, the child must be able to figure out all the possible combinations of the three colors to arrive at an answer. This ability is developed during the stage of formal operations. The use of higher mathematics is also possible. In other words, development of formal thought involves an ability to isolate a problem, to review it systematically, and to figure out all possible solutions to that problem.

Thus, Piaget's perspective on intellectual development involves the addition of more complex and abstract abilities with each stage. The child progresses from one stage to another. A person who is unable to progress through all the stages is limited in his or her ability to adapt as an adult. This person would have mental retardation.

MENTAL RETARDATION

The term *mental retardation* evokes different images in different people's minds. It is important for society in general to agree on a definition of mental retardation, to be aware of the degrees of retardation, and to be knowledgeable in how mental retardation is diagnosed. In addition, for parents and health care professionals, it is essential to understand the treatment approaches to mental retardation and to consider the long-term implications of mental retardation for the individual who is affected (Frankenberger, 1984).

Definition of Mental Retardation

To be classified as having mental retardation, a person must: 1) have intellectual functioning that is more than two standard deviations below the norm, 2) become mentally retarded as a result of an injury, disease, or problem that existed before age

18, and 3) be impaired in his or her ability to adapt to the environment (American Psychiatric Association, 1980).

The first part of the definition involves a statistical interpretation of intellectual functioning and of what is perceived as normal. Consider the average, or mean, intellectual functioning in a population to be the apex of a bell-shaped curve. Two standard deviations on either side of the mean encompass 95% of a population sample and define the range of normal (Figure 14.1). Since the average intelligence quotient, or IQ score, is 100, and the standard deviation of most IQ tests is 15 points, a score above 70 would fall within the normal range. A person scoring below 70 (two standard deviations below the mean) would be considered to have mental retardation (American Psychiatric Association, 1980). In addition, when one looks at Figure 14.1, one sees a second, smaller curve within the range of mental retardation, marking off a subgroup. This subgroup is the population that has mental retardation because of organic causes—for example, birth injuries, inborn errors of metabolism, and infections. The existence of this subgroup means that the incidence of severe mental retardation is higher than is predicted by the normal distribution curve.

The second part of the definition, concerning age of onset, is best illustrated by the following example: If a 3-year-old boy were in a car accident and suffered brain damage, he would be considered to have mental retardation, because the injury occurred during his developmental years. On the other hand, if his father sustained the same injury, he would have organic brain damage, not mental retardation, since he was no longer in his developmental years.

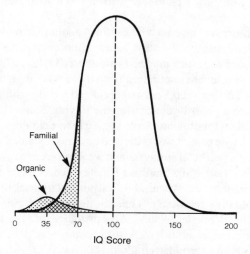

Figure 14.1. Bimodal distribution of intelligence. The mean IQ is 100. An IQ score of less than 70, or two standard deviations below the mean, indicates mental retardation. The second, smaller curve takes into account those individuals who have mental retardation because of birth trauma, infection, inborn errors, or other "organic" causes. This explains why more individuals have severe mental retardation than are predicted by the "familial" curve alone. (From Zigler, E. [1967, January]. Familial retardation: A continuing dilemma. *Science, 155*, 292–298, Figure 1; reprinted by permission. Copyright © 1967 by the American Association for the Advancement of Science.)

Finally, persons with mental retardation not only have limitations in their intellectual abilities but also are impaired in their ability to function in society. This impairment may range from mild to severe.

By definition, therefore, approximately 2.5% of our population has mental retardation, and another 2.5% has superior intelligence (see Figure 14.1). In the United States, this means roughly 5.5 million people have mental retardation. Over 85% of these people have IQ scores between two and three standard deviations below the mean and are called mildly or educably mentally retarded. Each lower stage of mental retardation refers to an additional 15 points, or one standard deviation, below the mean. Thus, mild retardation ranges from 55 to 69 in IQ score. Moderate retardation is from 40 to 54, severe retardation is 25 to 39, and profound retardation is less than 25.

Psychological Testing

To obtain a person's IQ score, certain tests, standardized for various age groups, are used. The most commonly used tests for children are the Bayley Scales of Infant Development, the Stanford-Binet Intelligence Scale, and the Wechsler intelligence tests for children (Goldman, Stein, & Guerry, 1983; Weaver, 1984; Wodrich, 1984).

The Bayley Scales are used to test the mental age of children who are from 2 months to 2½ years of age. It tests fine motor, gross motor, and language skills, along with visual problem solving. A single mental age (MA) and a developmental quotient (DQ) (similar to an IQ score) are calculated from the results. This test is well standardized and, by the time a child is 2 years old, is a good predictor of the child's future intellectual functioning.

With infants, however, one must be cautious about placing too much emphasis on this test's results because, for very young children, the test is dependent on nonlanguage items, and its results may be misleading (Bayley, 1958). It is possible to distinguish infants with severe retardation from those who are normal, but it is very difficult to draw the line between a normal child and a child with mild retardation or between a normal and a superior child using the Bayley Scales (Illingworth, 1971).

The Stanford-Binet Intelligence Scale is used to test children from 2 years of age through adulthood. In the past, it was criticized because it yielded a single mental age rather than providing a profile of strengths and weaknesses as do the Wechsler scales. However, the 1986 edition of the Stanford-Binet remedies these problems by giving scores in four different areas: verbal abilities, abstract/visual thinking, short-term memory, and quantitative reasoning. Thus, in its present form, this test is clearly competitive with the Wechsler scales. An advantage of this test is its superior evaluation of mathematical abilities. A disadvantage is it takes a long time to administer, up to 3 hours for older children.

Traditionally, the Wechsler Intelligence Scale for Children–Revised (WISC–R) has been the preferred test for children over 4½ years old. It contains a number of subtests in the areas of verbal and performance skills. These tests contain a number of subtests in the areas of verbal and performance skills. This allows the examiner to determine a series of IQ scores in different areas and, therefore, to obtain a more accurate picture of the strengths and weaknesses in the child's abilities. For example, a child with attention deficit disorder may have a wide scattering of scores over the various subtests, with normal scores in some verbal areas coupled with below-normal scores in some performance areas. A child with retardation, on the other hand, will seldom have any scores within the normal range.

Besides the various IQ tests, other tests are used to assess social-adaptive ability. Two such commonly used tests are the Vineland Social Maturity Scale and the American Association on Mental Deficiency Adaptive Behavior Scales (ABS) (Wodrich, 1984). The Vineland is older and is more frequently used. It tests such behavioral items as self-help behaviors (eating and dressing), interaction and cooperation with others, judgment, and self-control. The ABS has two parts. The first part, similar in content to the Vineland, assesses the child's level of self-sufficiency, independent functioning, and socialization. The second part is concerned with items that relate to emotional adjustment (Wodrich, 1984).

Clues to Developmental Delay

Often, parents are aware early in their child's life that he or she may not be developing like other children. This is true even when parents have not had any training in development, because they are able to compare that child to other children of the same age. However, in some mildly affected children, the delay may not become evident until school age.

To illustrate, consider the story of David, the child of Marie whom we mentioned in Chapter 6. David was born by cesarean section as a result of an abruptio placenta, a complication that led to brain damage. Marie noticed many of the signs in David's development that were indicative of developmental delay. (In the following paragraphs, the normal ages for these developmental milestones are indicated in parentheses after the age at which David achieved them.)

Marie noticed that David, as a tiny infant, showed little interest in his environment and was not very alert. He would sit in an infant seat for hours without complaint. Although Marie tried to breast-feed him, his suck was weak, and he frequently regurgitated his formula. He was floppy, and he had poor head control. His cry was high-pitched, and he was difficult to comfort. In gross motor development, David could hold his head up at 4 months (1 month), roll over at 8 months (5 months), and sit up at 14 months (7 months). He pulled himself to a standing position at 20 months (9 months).

In social and fine motor development, David also lagged behind the norm. David smiled at 4 months (2 months) and, generally, was not very responsive to his parents' attention. He transferred objects at 12 months (6 months). He did not start babbling until 13 months (6 months) and said "mama" at 20 months (10 months).

David's parents, concerned about their child's progress, consulted their pediatrician, who suspected that David had mental retardation when David was only 6 months of age. When given a Bayley Scale at 24 months, David's mental age was found to be 11 months, and he received a DQ (developmental quotient) of 52. Shortly after the testing, he began attending a preschool program for children with developmental disabilities.

When David was 6 years old, he was retested on the Stanford-Binet Intelligence Scale and achieved a mental age of 2 years 8 months, IQ of 45. He now attends a class for children with moderate retardation. The early diagnosis and treatment of David may help him better reach his potential and function more independently when he grows up.

David's case illustrates a number of points. First, David was a high-risk newborn who was followed closely for signs of developmental delay. Second, David's development did not follow a normal pattern, making the diagnosis of mental retardation more likely. Third, David's rate of development in motor, language, and social adaptive skills stayed about half the normal rate throughout infancy and into childhood. Because of this, David fell further and further behind his peers.

Keeping David's case in mind, one can readily see that it is important for parents and others who deal with children like David to have realistic expectations of their abilities. This is a difficult line to walk, since it is equally important not to expect too little of them. The best way to handle these children is for parents and professionals to have frequent discussions so that all are dealing with the child in a similar way and are consistent in their expectations.

Treatment of Mental Retardation[1]

Unfortunately, mental retardation has no cure. Despite this reality, some individuals have attempted to use various medications and diets to raise the IQ scores in children with mental retardation, especially in those with Down syndrome. One such example is a study done in 1981 by Dr. R.F. Harrell who used megavitamin therapy and mineral supplements to treat a group of individuals with mental retardation. She found a significant increase in IQ scores after the treatment. However, subsequent studies, using controlled conditions, could not replicate her results (Smith, Spiker, Peterson, et al., 1984).

Despite the failure of this and similar efforts, therapeutic approaches do exist that are beneficial to children with mental retardation (Batshaw & Shapiro, 1984). The most useful consists of a multidisciplinary effort to maximize the child's abilities and potential. Therapy is directed at a number of aspects of the child's life— education, social and recreational activities, behavior problems, and associated deficits (Colozzi & Pollow, 1984). Genetic and supportive counseling is also offered to the parents and siblings (see Chapters 3 and 24).

Early diagnosis is a prerequisite for effective treatment. This helps to ease the parents' anxiety and to allow for realistic goal setting and greater acceptance of the child. Children with moderate-severe retardation, like David, demonstrate developmental delays at a very young age, making the diagnosis clearer. However, many

---

[1]Portions of the information in this section on treatment of mental retardation have been taken from: Batshaw, M.L., & Shapiro, B. (1984). Mental retardation. In S.S. Gelles & B.M. Kagan (Eds.), *Current pediatric therapy* (11th ed.). Philadelphia: W.B. Saunders Co.; reprinted by permission.

children with mild retardation will not have significant developmental delays during the first years of their lives. For them, problems may not show up until they reach school age. Premature children, children who are small for gestational age, and infants who have had difficulties as newborns should be watched closely, as they are at greater risk for mental retardation than other children.

Once the diagnosis is made, the child should be referred to an interdisciplinary team at a public school, a state diagnostic and evaluation (D&E) center, or a university affiliated facility (UAF). There, a thorough evaluation is made by a group of professionals. Evaluation should include an examination by a developmental pediatrician, a clinical psychologist, and a social worker. The child may also need to be seen by a special education teacher, speech therapist, audiologist, and a behavioral psychologist.

A treatment plan is then developed (Menolascino, Neman, & Stark, 1983). The educational component of this plan should be based on the child's developmental level and his or her future goals for independence (Johnson & Werner, 1975). For instance, the child with mild retardation needs to gain basic academic and vocational skills, while the child with moderate retardation needs "survival" skills that can be used in a sheltered environment. At least yearly, the overall treatment plan should be reviewed to determine if it continues to meet the child's needs.

Besides education, the team needs to address the social and recreational aspects of the child's life. In general, children with mental retardation do better in individual or small-group activities than in team sports. Activities that utilize gross motor skills rather than fine motor coordination are most appropriate. Examples of these activities include track and field, swimming, and hiking. The Special Olympics provides many children with a framework for such activities. If the child has physical disabilities, certain precautions may need to be taken. For example, children with Down syndrome may need to be checked for abnormalities in the upper neck vertebrae before participating in certain sports.

To facilitate the child's socialization, behavior problems must be addressed. In assessing a retarded child's behavior, one must consider whether the behavior is appropriate for the child's mental age, while keeping his or her chronological age in mind. Although most children with retardation do not have behavioral problems, these problems do occur with greater frequency in such children than in normal children. The causes are complex and result from the interaction of a variety of factors, including inappropriate expectations of the child, organic problems, and family difficulties. Environmental change, such as a more appropriate classroom setting, may improve the problem behaviors. Family members can learn more about what to expect from their child, considering his or her developmental level. With certain problem behaviors, however, behavior modification and/or the use of medication may be necessary.

The theory behind behavior modification is explained in greater detail in Chapter 19. The technique involves the reinforcement of behaviors that are appropriate and the discouragement of inappropriate behaviors. In children with retardation, this approach is often used to encourage compliance with instructions and to treat self-stimulatory or self-injurious behavior (SIB). Such behavior, which includes head-banging, eye-gouging, scratching, and biting, occurs most frequently in children with severe retardation and may be life-threatening.

To discourage these behaviors, modification techniques such as extinction, timing-out, aversive conditioning, overcorrection, and/or differential reinforcement of other behaviors are used. In extinction, the relationship between a behavior and a subsequent reward is broken. For instance, if the behavior resulted in parental attention, such attention would be withdrawn. This must be used very carefully because the behavior may increase before later stopping. Timing-out involves removing the child from social contacts, usually in a separate room, after the occurrence of the problem behavior. Aversive conditioning links the behavior with a noxious response such as a water mist spray. Overcorrection, a mild punishment procedure, requires the child to exaggerate the correction of the behavior. One example would be to forcibly hold a boy's hand at his side for one minute following his gouging himself. Overcorrection and other approaches are often combined with teaching a child a new skill that is physically incompatible with the injurious behavior. For instance, one cannot hit oneself while stringing beads. Generally, behavior modification techniques are fairly successful in controlling these troublesome behaviors.

Although it is not necessary in most cases, some children may also need to receive medication to facilitate learning or to help suppress certain behaviors. Certainly, drugs must not be used as a substitute for effective, appropriate programming for these youngsters. The drugs that are most commonly used to control problem behaviors in children with mental retardation fall into three groups: **phenothiazines**, **butyrophenones**, and **amphetamines** (Platt, Campbell, Green, et al., 1984; Zimmerman & Heistad, 1982). Phenothiazines include chlorpromazine (Thorazine), thioridazine (Mellaril), and trifluoperazine (Stelazine). These drugs are sedatives and are used to lower levels of motor activity, anxiety, combativeness, and hyperactivity. However, they also decrease attention span. The usual dose in childhood for Thorazine or Mellaril is 25–200 milligrams/day, but this dosage must be individualized. Common side effects include excessive appetite and drowsiness. Uncommon toxic effects include abnormal liver function, skin eruptions, and increased occurrence of seizures. After prolonged treatment, usually over 5 years, an individual may develop a disorder called *tardive dyskinesia*. This disorder is characterized by marked physical restlessness, and the symptoms may be permanent (Burke, 1984). Haloperidol (Haldol), a butyrophenone, has similar therapeutic and toxic effects. Its usual dose is 1–5 milligrams/day.

Recent research has suggested that self-injurious behavior results from an alteration in the receptors for **endorphins**, the body's own opiates or "pleasure producers." If so, the child may engage in self-injurious behavior to stimulate him- or herself. If this is true, drugs such as naloxone and naltrexone, which block endorphin receptors, may help to treat this type of behavior.

Another category of drugs, amphetamines, which include methylphenidate (Ritalin) and dextroamphetamine (Dexedrine), is effective for the short-term control of hyperactivity and attention problems in children with normal IQs. However, they are less effective in controlling these problems in children with mental retardation. Yet, because these stimulants have fewer and less severe side effects than pheno-thiazines, they are still worth trying.

Preferably, trials of medication should be made. During this time, the teacher should keep a record of attention, behavior, and extent of hyperactivity. Each year, the child should be taken off the medication to evaluate the need for continued treatment.

Besides evaluating the educational, behavioral, and medication needs, the team must also assess the child for any associated deficits (Batshaw & Shapiro, 1984). Children with mental retardation also may have cerebral palsy, visual deficits, seizure disorders, speech disorders, autism, and other disorders of language, behavior, and perception. The severity and frequency of these disorders tend to be proportional to the degree of mental retardation. Failure to adequately assess and treat these problems may result in unsuccessful **habilitation** and may heighten behavior problems.

Finally, although the extent of mental retardation does not change appreciably over time, it is important periodically to review the assessment of the child. As the child grows, the parents need more information, goals must be reassessed, and programming may need changing. A review should include information about health status, family functioning, and the child's functioning, both at home and at school. Annual reviews are necessary throughout the school years.

Implications of Mental Retardation

A recurring question is whether it is useful or harmful to label a person as mentally retarded. A corollary is, to whom is it useful? We believe the answer to these questions depends on whether or not the designation is used to aid the individual. If such a designation enables a child to qualify for special educational programs or other assistance, then it makes sense to use the label. If the labeling results in the stigmatizing of a child or an avoidance of caring for that child's special needs, then it should not be used.

What implications does the label of mental retardation have for the individual? Most individuals with retardation fall into the range of mild mental retardation; many of them are able to gain economic and social independence with the equivalent of up to a fourth-grade education. Eighty percent of these people find work, mainly in unskilled or semiskilled jobs. More than 80% marry, usually to a spouse who has normal intelligence. As adults, they have a mental age ranging between 8 and 11 years of age, compared to an adult with normal intelligence who has a mental age of about 16 years (Illingworth, 1983).

Persons who have moderate retardation (approximately 10% of the retarded population) have more difficulty adapting to the outside world than those with mild retardation. For these individuals, the goal of education is to enhance self-help skills so they are better able to function in a vocational environment. While they cannot live independently, they can care for themselves under supervision and perform repetitive unskilled tasks. Few marry. Years ago, most of these people were institutionalized.

Now it is clear that virtually all of these individuals can function in a caring home environment or in small, community-based group homes. Throughout adulthood, these individuals need educational and work programs in a setting that can offer support services. As adults, their mental age ranges from 5 to 7 years.

For persons with severe and profound mental retardation (about 5% of the mentally retarded population), the ability to learn and care for themselves is very limited. Many of these individuals, besides having mental retardation, have other handicaps including seizures, cerebral palsy, hearing, or visual impairments. They are able to learn basic self-help skills but have extreme difficulty learning any academic skills. In the past, many of these individuals were institutionalized. Now, however, most live at home. Also, while their abilities are quite limited, activity centers exist in which they can use the abilities they have. The mental age in adulthood for persons with severe retardation is under 5 years, and for persons with profound retardation, it is under 3.

SUMMARY

Development is a step-by-step process that is intimately related to the maturation of the central nervous system. With mental retardation, development is altered so that adaptive and intellectual skills are impaired. Causes of mental retardation range from newborn trauma to infectious disease and from chromosomal abnormalities to inborn errors of metabolism. In more than 60% of the cases, the cause of mental retardation is unclear.

Most persons with mental retardation are mildly retarded and are able to achieve economic and social independence. The early identification of a developmental delay is important to ensure appropriate treatment and to enable the child to develop and use all of his or her capabilities.

REFERENCES

American Psychiatric Association. (1980). *Diagnostic and statistical manual of mental disorders (DSM III)* (3rd ed.). Washington, DC: American Psychiatric Association.
Batshaw, M.L., & Shapiro, B. (1984). Mental retardation. In S.S. Gelles & B.M. Kagan (Eds.), *Current pediatric therapy* (11th ed.). Philadelphia: W.B. Saunders Co.
Bayley, N. (1958). Value and limitations of infant testing. *Children, 5,* 129–133.
Berkler, M.S. (Ed.). (1978). *Current trends for the developmentally disabled.* Baltimore: University Park Press.
Bloom, M. (1980). *Life span development: Bases for preventive and interventive helping.* New York: Macmillan Co.
Burke, R.E. (1984). Tardive dyskinesia: Current clinical issues. *Neurology, 34,* 1348–1353.
Burt, C. (1959). General ability & special aptitudes. *Educational Research, 1,* 3–16.
Caplan, F. (Ed.). (1978). *The first twelve months of life.* New York: Bantam Books.
Capute, A.J., Palmer, F.B., Shapiro, B.K., et al. (1984). Primitive reflex profile: A quantitation of primitive reflexes in infancy. *Developmental Medicine and Child Neurology, 26,* 375–383.
Coburn, S.P., Schaltenbrand, W.E., Mahuren, J.D., et al. (1983). Effect of megavitamin treatment on mental performance and plasma vitamin B_6 concentrations in mentally retarded young adults. *American Journal of Clinical Nutrition, 38,* 352–355.

Colozzi, G.A., & Pollow, R.S. (1984). Teaching independent walking to mentally retarded children in a public school. *Education and Training of the Mentally Retarded, 19,* 97–101.
Cowan, P.A. (1978). *Piaget with feeling: Cognitive, social, and emotional dimensions.* New York: Holt, Rinehart, & Winston.
Fraiberg, S.H. (1959). *The magic years.* New York: Charles Scribner's Sons.
Frankenberger, W. (1984). A survey of state guidelines for identification of mental retardation. *Mental Retardation, 22,* 17–20.
Futterman, A.D., & Arndt, S. (1983). The construct and predictive validity of adaptive behavior. *American Journal of Mental Deficiency, 87,* 546–550.
Gesell, A.L., & Ilg, F.L. (1949). *Child development: An introduction to the study of human growth.* New York: Harper & Row.
Goldman, J., Stein, C.L., & Guerry, S. (1983). *Psychological methods of child assessment.* New York: Brunner/Mazel.
Grossman, H.J. (Ed.). (1983). *Classification in mental retardation.* Washington, DC: American Association on Mental Deficiency.
Gruber, H.E., & Voneche, J.J. (Eds.). (1977). *The essential Piaget.* New York: Basic Books.
Harrell, R.F., Capp, R.H., Davis, D.R., et al. (1981). Can nutritional supplements help mentally retarded children? An exploratory study. *Proceedings of the National Academy of Sciences, 78,* 574–578.
Illingworth, R.S. (1971). The predictive value of developmental assessment in infancy. *Developmental Medicine and Child Neurology, 13,* 721–725.
Illingworth, R.S. (1983). *The development of the infant and young child: Normal and abnormal* (8th ed.). New York: Churchill Livingstone, Inc.
Jablow, M.M. (1982). *Cara: Growing with a retarded child.* Philadelphia: Temple University Press.
Johnson, V.M., & Werner, R.A. (1975). *A step-by-step learning guide for retarded infants and children.* Syracuse, NY: Syracuse University Press.
Johnson, V.M., & Werner, R.A. (1977). *A step-by-step learning guide for older retarded children.* Syracuse, NY: Syracuse University Press.
Knobloch, H., & Pasamanick, B. (1975). *Gesell and Amatruda's developmental diagnosis: The evaluation and management of normal and abnormal neuropsychologic development in infancy and early childhood.* New York: Harper & Row.
Maier, H. (1978). *Three theories of child development* (3rd ed.). New York: Harper & Row.
Matson, J.L. (1984). Psychotherapy with persons who are mentally retarded. *Mental Retardation, 22,* 170–175.
Menolascino, F.J., Neman, R., & Stark, J.A. (Eds.). (1983). *Curative aspects of mental retardation: Biomedical and behavioral advances.* Baltimore: Paul H. Brookes Publishing Co.
Pader, O.F. (1981). *A guide and handbook for parents of mentally retarded children.* Springfield, IL: Charles C Thomas.
Platt, J.E., Campbell, M., Green, W.H., et al. (1984). Cognitive effects of lithium carbonate and haloperidol in treatment-resistant aggressive children. *Archives of General Psychiatry, 41,* 657–662.
Scheerenberger, R.C. (1983). *A history of mental retardation.* Baltimore: Paul H. Brookes Publishing Co.
Scheiner, A.P., & Abroms, I.F. (1980). *The practical management of the developmentally disabled child.* St. Louis: C.V. Mosby Co.
Singh, N.N. (1981). Current trends in the treatment of self-injurious behavior. *Advances in Pediatrics, 28,* 377–440.
Slater, B.R., & Thomas, J.M. (1983). *Psychodiagnostic evaluation of children: A casebook approach.* New York: Teachers College Press.
Smith, G.F., Spiker, D., Peterson, C.P., et al. (1984). Use of megadoses of vitamins with minerals in Down syndrome. *Journal of Pediatrics, 105,* 228–234.
Sprague, R.L., Kalachnik, J.E., Breuning, S.E., et al. (1984). The dyskinesia identification system—Coldwater (DIS-Co): A tardive dyskinesia rating scale for the developmentally disabled. *Psychopharmacology Bulletin, 20,* 328–338.
Thain, W.S., Casto, G., & Peterson, A. (1980). *Normal and handicapped children: A growth development primer for parents and professionals.* Littleton, MA: PSG Publishing Co., Inc.
Weaver, S.J. (Ed.). (1984). *Testing children: A reference guide for effective clinical and psychoeducational assessments.* Kansas City: Test Corporation of America.
Wodrich, D.L. (1984). *Children's psychological testing: A guide for nonpsychologists.* Baltimore: Paul H. Brookes Publishing Co.

Yale University Clinic of Child Development, Gesell, A.L., & Halverson, H.M. (1940). *The first five years of life: A guide to the study of the pre-school child.* New York: Harper & Row.

Zigler, E. (1967, January). Familial retardation: A continuing dilemma. *Science, 155,* 292–298.

Zimmerman, R.L., & Heistad, G.T. (1982). Studies of the long term efficacy of antipsychotic drugs in controlling the behavior of institutionalized retardates. *Journal of the American Academy of Child Psychiatry, 21,* 136–143.

Chapter 15

Vision

Upon completion of this chapter, the reader will:
—be able to describe the anatomy of the eye
—know the function of the major parts of the eye and some common problems
  associated with them
—be aware of some of the tests used to determine visual acuity
—understand how a child develops visual skills
—know the definition and some of the causes of blindness in children
—recognize some of the ways in which a blind child's development differs from
  a sighted child's and some approaches for treating a blind child

---

Vision may be the most important sense for interpreting the world around us. When
sight is impaired, it can have a detrimental effect on a child's physical, neurological,
and emotional development. Even as an isolated disability, blindness causes delays in
walking and talking, and creates a dependence on others. However, if visual loss is
identified early, various methods of treatment may improve the prognosis.

This chapter explores the embryonic development of the eye along with its
structure and function. It also examines diseases of the eye and common visual
problems of the child with handicaps. Finally, the development of visual skills and
the effect of blindness on a child's development are discussed.

STRUCTURE OF THE EYE

Reflected rays of light from an object strike the eye and are **refracted** at the surfaces
of the **cornea** and the **lens**. This refraction yields a focused image on the *retina*. The
image is then transmitted to the occipital lobe of the brain where it is interpreted. A
problem anywhere along this pathway causes some degree of visual loss.

In many ways, the structure of the eye is very similar to the inner workings of a
camera (Figure 15.1). The case of the eyeball is a thick, white fibrous covering called
the **sclera**. The shutter is the **iris**, the colored speckled area that opens and closes
according to light conditions. The **pupil** is the aperture in the center of the iris. The
cornea covers and protects the iris and is also the first and most important refracting

199

surface of the eye, focusing light toward the **macula** or **fovea centralis** in the center of the retina. The lens, the second refracting surface, transmits and further deflects the light rays. And the retina is the photographic film, a light-sensitive surface that records the image in an upside-down, back-to-front format.

The region between the cornea and the iris is called the *anterior chamber* and contains a watery fluid, the **aqueous humor**. Between the lens and the retina is a space filled with a translucent jelly-like substance, called the **vitreous humor**. These fluids maintain the shape of the eye.

The eye itself sits in a bony socket of the skull. The *extraocular muscles*, small fibers that turn the eyeball, and the *optic nerve*, which sends images from the eye to the brain, also lie in this space. A series of layers protect the surface of the eyeball. First, a thin, transparent layer called the **conjunctiva** covers the sclera and contains tiny blood vessels that give a "bloodshot" appearance to the eye when inflamed. Next, the *eyelids* intermittently sweep across the eye, wetting the cornea and washing dust and other foreign bodies from the eye. The *eyelashes* protect the eye from airborn debris. Tears are released from the **lacrimal** glands at the outer edge of the eye and are collected in the *tear ducts* in the inner corner of the eye.

DEVELOPMENT OF THE EYE

In the fetus, the eyes appear at 4 weeks gestational age as two spherical bulbs at the side of the head (Figure 15.2). These bulbs indent by 5 weeks to form the *optic cups*. The three cell layers in these cups then develop into the various parts of the eye. The ectoderm forms part of the lens and cornea. The **neuroectoderm** produces the retina and inner eye muscles, while the mesoderm forms the optic nerve, blood vessels and muscles of the eyeball, and the eyelids. By 7 weeks gestational age, when the embryo is only 1 inch long, the eyes have already assumed their basic form.

As fetal growth continues, the eyes gradually move from the side of the head to the center of the face. Malformations during the first trimester may lead to many defects—for example, anophthalmia, a lack of eyes, and microphthalmia, or small eyes. They may also prevent the complete fusion of the retina or the iris, a condition called a *coloboma* (Langman & Sadler, 1985). One syndrome resulting from such malformations is the **CHARGE association** (Pagon, Graham, Zonana, et al., 1981). Characteristics of this syndrome include coloboma (C), congenital heart disease (H), **atresia** of nasal passage (A), retarded growth (R), genital abnormalities (G), ear anomalies and/or deafness (E). Abnormalities occurring later in fetal life may lead to ocular **hypertelorism** or widely spaced eyes. Finally, viruses such as rubella (see Chapter 4) can invade the eye and cause **chorioretinitis** (an inflammation of the retina and **choroid**), **cataracts**, or **glaucoma**. Each of these conditions may produce severe visual loss.

FUNCTION AND DISEASES OF THE EYE

In this section, the functions of the cornea, lens, retina, optic nerves, and eye muscles are discussed along with some of the common disorders that affect them.

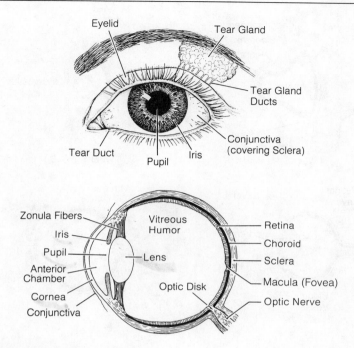

Figure 15.1. Anatomy of the eye.

The Cornea

The cornea helps to focus an image on the most light-sensitive part of the retina, the fovea centralis. This is accomplished in the following manner. When a person looks at a tree, his eyes see a series of parallel rays of light that leave the tree and reach the surface of the cornea. If these rays continued unfocused, they would each project to a different part of the retina, and the image would be blurred. However, as the parallel rays hit the **convex** surface of the cornea, they are turned or refracted. If everything works properly, the rays focus on the fovea, and a sharp image is transmitted to the brain (Figure 15.3).

For this to happen correctly, the eyeball must be the right size, and the cornea and lens must have the proper form. If the eye is too long or the refractive surfaces of the eye (cornea and lens) are too strong, the focused image (where all lines converge) is in front of the retina, and the picture is blurred (see Figure 15.3). This is called *myopia,* or nearsightedness. When the eye is too short or the cornea and lens are too weak, the image is formed behind the retina, also producing a blurred image (see Figure 15.3). In this instance, the person has *hypermetropia,* or farsightedness. The other common refractive problem is *astigmatism* (see Figure 15.3). Astigmatism occurs when the surface of the cornea has an irregular or barrel shape rather than a spherical one. Because of this change in shape, different sections of the cornea have different focal points, and the image is blurred. Both hypermetropia and astigmatism are common in infants and young children.

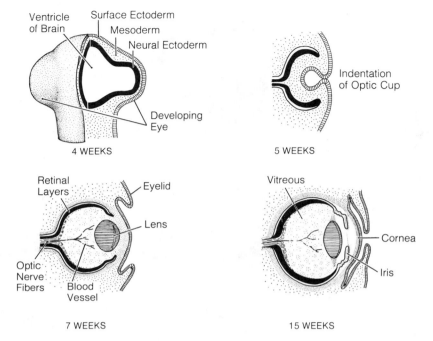

Figure 15.2. Embryonic development of the eye.

When any of these problems exists, people may have to wear either glasses or contact lenses. Myopic people wear **concave** lenses to move the focal point farther back, whereas the farsighted person wears convex lenses to move the focal point closer (see Figure 15.3). To correct astigmatism, a cylindrical lens is used that reduces the effect of the misshapen cornea (see Figure 15.3). For those with an astigmatism, a beneficial side effect of aging is that the cornea flattens, making astigmatism less apparent (Harley, 1983).

Glaucoma In the anterior chamber behind the cornea, the pressure is kept normal by the drainage of fluid through a passageway called Schlemm's canal (Figure 15.4). If this canal is blocked, the intraocular pressure rises and causes glaucoma. Signs of glaucoma include a large hazy cornea and excessive tearing. The individual experiences eye pain and discomfort in bright light. Diagnosis is made by measuring the intraocular pressure using a **tonometer**. If glaucoma is found, a surgical procedure, called a **goniotomy**, is performed to open up a passageway. If not treated, glaucoma usually causes blindness in the affected eye.

Although glaucoma is primarily an adult disease, a number of conditions in childhood are associated with it. These include certain metabolic disorders such as homocystinuria, some infections, chromosomal abnormalities, and other malformation syndromes. Glaucoma accounts for about 5% of blindness in children (Chew & Morin, 1983).

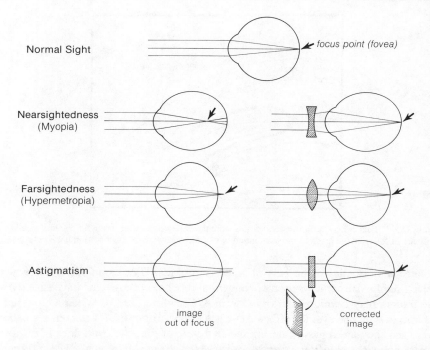

Figure 15.3.   Refractive errors. If the eyeball is too long, images are focused in front of the retina (myopia). A concave lens deflects the rays, correcting the problem. If the eyeball is too short, the image focuses behind the retina and is again blurred (hypermetropia). A convex lens corrects this. In astigmatism, the eyeball is the correct size, but the cornea is misshapen. A cylindrical lens is required to compensate.

The Lens

The lens, the second refracting surface of the eye, can change its shape to accommodate changes in the distance of an object from the eye. The lens rests suspended by **zonular** fibers behind the iris and in front of the vitreous humor (see Figure 15.1). It is convex on both sides and translucent. When light comes from a distant object, the rays are close together and well focused. Because little refraction is needed, the zonular fibers tighten and pull the lens so that it minimally refracts the rays of light (Figure 15.5). To see a nearby object where the rays are dispersed, the zonular fibers relax to allow the lens to become globular in shape with greater refractive power. The rays are sharply focused on the fovea. As a person ages, the lens becomes less flexible and less able to accommodate, a condition called **presbyopia**. The individual's vision becomes blurred. Wearing bifocals helps correct the problem because they heighten the refraction of light from close objects but do not do so for distant objects.

Cataracts   The major disease affecting the lens is the cataract, which may become dense enough to be seen as a white mass behind the opening of the pupil. Although this disorder is much more common in adults, it accounts for about 15% of blindness in children and occurs in about 1 in 250 births (Calhoun, 1983). It may be an

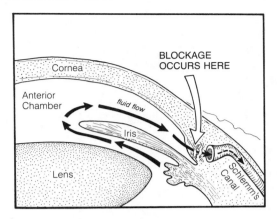

Figure 15.4. Glaucoma. Fluid normally drains from the anterior chamber through Schlemm's canal. A blockage in this passage leads to the accumulation of fluid and pressure, a condition called glaucoma.

isolated abnormality or be part of a larger problem. For example, children with galactosemia, Turner's syndrome, congenital rubella, or those who have suffered an eye trauma may develop cataracts (Merin & Crawford, 1972). When a child has a cataract in only one eye, the affected eye has a poor prognosis. If cataracts are in both eyes, and they are removed during the first year of life, the child does not usually experience a loss of vision, or **amblyopia** (Beller, Hoyt, Marg, et al., 1981). When a cataract is surgically removed, the lens of the eye is also removed. Without the refraction of the lens, the image in the eye is not focused. To compensate for the missing lens, the child wears contact lenses or glasses.

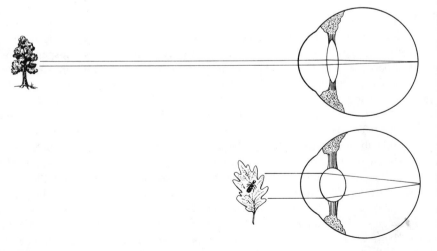

Figure 15.5. Accommodation. The lens changes shape to focus on a near or far object. The lens becomes thin and less refractive for distant objects, but rounded and more refractive for near vision.

The Retina

The retina is the light-sensitive "film" of the eye. Visual images are focused on it and then projected to the brain. Two layers, the sclera and the choroid, surround the retina and support, protect, and nourish it. Within the retina are two types of sensory cells, the *rods* and the *cones*. Both types of cells respond to light by undergoing a chemical reaction. Also, both contain a pigment called *retinol,* which is stored in the body as vitamin A. Retinol is bound to another molecule called **opsin** (Newell, 1978). The amount of retinol is the same in both rods and cones, but the type of opsin differs.

For detailed vision such as reading, seeing distant objects, and color vision, cones are needed. Each cone is sensitive to one of three distinct colors: red, green, or blue (Figure 15.6). The light from a colored object causes a different response from each type of cone and leads to a patchwork pattern that is interpreted in the brain as shades of color and shape. Cones are most numerous in the macula, the portion of the retina that contains the area of clearest vision, the fovea centralis.

In all other areas of the retina, the rods predominate. Rods distinguish light from dark and are necessary for night vision (see Figure 15.6). Unlike human beings, some animals have only rods or only cones. For instance, bats, which have only rods, fly at night. Squirrels only have cones and hunt in daylight.

A number of disorders involve abnormalities in the rods or cones (Eller & Brown, 1983). Some are birth defects such as color blindness, a sex-linked disorder that affects about 8% of men (see Chapter 2). In this disorder, one of the three types of cones is either abnormal or missing at birth (Harley, 1983). With this disorder, a person may be unable to discriminate red from green or blue from yellow or may confuse shades of red, green, and yellow.

Other diseases damage the cones or rods once they have already formed. For example, a dietary deficiency of vitamin A depletes the supply of retinol and initially

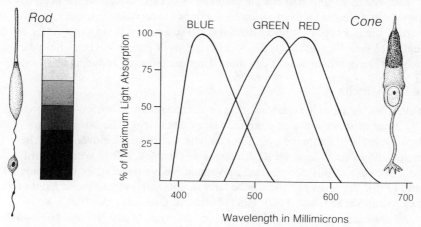

Figure 15.6. Rods permit black and white vision and allow us to see at night. Cones are needed for color vision. There are three types of cones, each of which is sensitive to one of three spectra of color: red, blue, or green. The absence of or damage to one type of cone leads to color blindness.

impairs night vision. If untreated, such a deficiency leads to blindness. It is the most frequent cause of vision loss in African children (Pirie, 1983). Another disorder, **retinitis pigmentosa**, which consists of a group of inherited diseases, gradually destroys the rods. Initially, it causes night blindness and then generalized visual impairment (Bloome & Garcia, 1981). Trauma that results in a hemorrhage in the retina may also produce visual loss in the affected eye (Von Barsewisch, 1979). Finally, degenerative nervous system disorders such as Tay-Sachs disease are associated with a deposit of toxic material in the choroid and retina, causing blindness.

The Optic Nerve

Deep within the retina, the rods and cones are connected to the cells of the optic nerve via bipolar neurons. Over a million of these nerve cells join together to form the second cranial nerve, the optic nerve. The part of the eye where this junction occurs is called the *optic disc*, or the blind spot of the eye (see Figure 15.1). If you cover one eye, stare straight ahead, and move one finger across the field of vision of your other eye, the finger will disappear at one point. This corresponds to the optic disc on the retina. Because this place contains nerve fibers but neither rods nor cones, no vision occurs.

One optic nerve emerges from behind each eyeball. A portion of the fibers of each crosses over at a point called the *optic chiasm* (Figure 15.7). This point rests within the skull, just before the nerves enter the brain. The nerve tract continues around the cerebral hemisphere to the occipital lobes (see Figure 15.7). There the image seen by the retina is perceived and coordinated with the sounds transmitted from the ear to form a complete message that is then interpreted (Hubel & Wiesel, 1979).

Damage to various parts of the pathway or to certain parts of the occipital lobe brings about different kinds of vision loss. For instance, damage to the right occipital lobe or to the right optic pathway itself will make a person blind to objects in the left visual field (see Figure 15.7). By identifying what part of a visual field a person cannot see, an ophthalmologist can often determine where the damage has occurred.

The Eye Muscles

Six eye muscles direct the eye toward an object and maintain binocular vision (Figure 15.8). Four of these rest along the four sides of the eye. The other two are placed obliquely and help rotate the eye. The complex, coordinated movement of these eye muscles allows us to look in all directions of our visual field without turning our heads. The loss of this coordinated movement leads to squint, or strabismus (Harcourt, 1976). The eyes can usually be held in good alignment by one month of age (Fox, Aslin, Shea, et al., 1980; Held, Birch, & Gwiazda, 1980).

Strabismus Abnormal alignment of the eyes occurs in about 3%–4% of children (Nelson, 1984). Two forms of strabismus, or squint, exist: *esotropia* and *exotropia*. When a child has esotropia, he is cross-eyed; the eyes turn in. If he has exotropia, he is wall-eyed, and the eyes turn out (see Figure 15.8). Esotropia is more

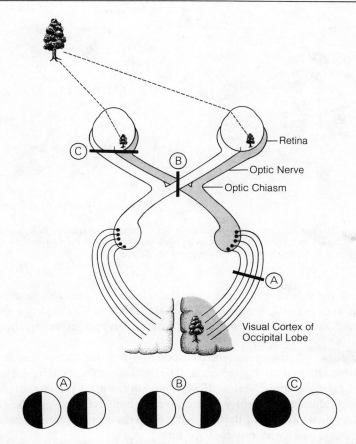

Figure 15.7. The visual pathway. An abnormality at various points along the route (upper figure) will lead to different patterns of visual loss (lower figure). These are illustrated: A) abnormality at the cortical pathway; B) damage to the optic chiasm; C) retinal damage.

common. The improper alignment may be present in one or both eyes, and it may be apparent all the time or only intermittently, such as when the child tires. Intermittent esotropia is unlikely to cause visual problems, whereas uncorrected, ongoing esotropia results in dimmed vision, or amblyopia (see next section). In addition, children with congenital esotropia are more likely to develop visual problems than those who develop it later in childhood.

Strabismus may result from an abnormality in the eye muscles or in the nerve supplying these muscles or from brain damage. In some children, farsightedness may be the reason for the esotropia. By wearing glasses to correct the farsightedness, the child's esotropia is also corrected (Jampolsky, Parks, & Robb, 1977).

In cerebral palsy, brain damage may alter the brain's signals to the eye muscles and cause strabismus (Scheiman, 1984). Here, glasses are not usually sufficient. The child may need to wear a patch over the good eye so that he or she uses and, therefore,

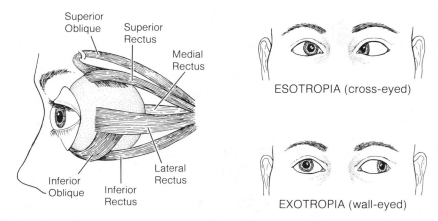

Figure 15.8. The eye muscles. Six muscles move the eyeball. A weakness in these muscles causes strabismus, or squint. In esotropia, the eye turns in, while in exotropia, the eye turns out. Strabismus can affect one or both eyes. Left esotropia and exotropia are illustrated.

strengthens, the weak eye. Corrective eye muscle surgery may also be necessary to realign the eyes (Kraft & Scott, 1984; Paakkala, 1982). It is extremely important to identify and treat strabismus early to prevent amblyopia in the weak eye (von Noorden, 1983).

Amblyopia Amblyopia involves a decrease in visual acuity, usually in one eye, for which there is no organic cause. The incidence of amblyopia is 1%–3%, in the school-age population (Nelson, 1984). Normally, when a person sees, the image of an object falls simultaneously on the fovea in each eye. The impulses carrying these images then travel along the optic pathway to the occipital cortex where the two images are fused into a **stereoscopic** picture.

Infants start fusing objects by 4 months of age (Held, Birch, & Gwiazda, 1980). From then on, if one eye points in one direction and the other in a different direction, two different images will fall on the foveas, and the occipital cortex will perceive two separate pictures. If this persists, the brain will start to suppress one of these images to avoid "double vision." If this suppression continues for a long period of time, the brain will eventually disregard the images received from the squinting eye (Ing, 1981). This leads to amblyopia in the weakened eye.

DEVELOPMENT OF VISUAL SKILLS

As with the acquisition of language and other skills, vision also has developmental milestones (Greenwald, 1983). A newborn can distinguish colors, focus on a human face, and follow the movement of the face 90° across his visual field (Miranda, Hack, Fantz, et al., 1977). By 1 month of age, a child can follow an object horizontally 180°, and by 2 months he or she can follow the same object vertically. At this age, a child can also imitate a smile. At 3 months, he or she can reach for and grab an object anywhere in the visual field. Visual acuity may be as good as 20/200 at birth, 20/40 at 6 months, and 20/20 (the standard for normal vision) by 1 year (Harley, 1983).

Because the infant normally has a number of visual skills, it is not difficult to identify a totally blind child. Determining a partial visual loss in infancy is more difficult. Furthermore, there is the possibility of mistakenly identifying a child with mental retardation as having a severe visual loss. Such a child may be delayed in the development of visual skills; however, this child's other developmental skills will be equally delayed. Tests of vision should help to discriminate the blind child from the child with mental retardation.

VISION TESTS

Different tests are used to evaluate visual acuity at various ages (Atkinson & Braddick, 1983). In infants, the most the clinician can do is identify children with significant visual impairment or detect differences between the two eyes (Lennerstrand, Andersson, & Axelsson, 1983). Three approaches have been used to assess visual acuity in infants: 1) checking the **opticokinetic** response, 2) measuring visual evoked responses(VERs), and 3) forced preferential looking (Dobson & Teller, 1978; Mohindra, Jacobson, Zwann, et al., 1983).

The opticokinetic response is determined by twirling a black and white striped cylinder in front of the baby (London, 1982). Similar to the effect of watching a picket fence from a passing car, the child's eyes should jiggle as they rapidly focus first on one stripe and then on another. If the child's eyes do not move, he or she may have a serious vision problem. However, it may also mean that the infant is simply not focusing on the stripes. Thus, this test is not a very accurate measure.

Another approach is measuring what are called visual evoked responses (Tyler, 1982). This technique ascertains the electrical reaction of the occipital cortex to a visual stimulus. In this test, electrodes are attached to the back of the child's head, and a light is flashed. Within a split second, the electrode that rests on the occipital lobe should record an electical impulse. If this does not happen, the abnormality in vision lies somewhere between the eye and the occipital cortex (Harley, 1983). However, here again, the child may simply not be focusing on the flashing signal, so this also is not a very accurate measurement (Hoyt, 1984).

Finally, forced preferential looking (Figure 15.9) involves alternating the position and size of a round striped board placed in a wall in front of the child (Lennerstrand, Andersson, & Axelsson, 1983). This test requires two examiners. One examiner changes the grids while the second observes the infant's eye movements. Because infants prefer to look at a pattern instead of a blank wall, they tend to focus on the grid. The child's visual acuity is then determined by varying the size of the grid.

For older children, the simplest approach to visual screening is to ask the child what he or she sees. In school-age children, this involves the use of the Snellen eye charts, which contain letters or numbers of various sizes (Figure 15.10). This card is placed 20 feet away from the person who covers one eye and reads from the largest

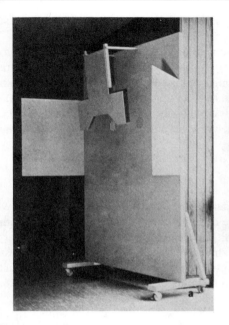
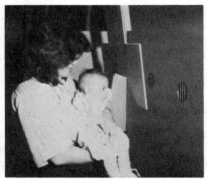

Figure 15.9. Forced preferential looking test. The infant is placed in front of a wall that has openings in which boards with patterns of various sizes are placed. The infant is expected to focus on the stripes. (From Fulton, A., Hansen, R., & Manning, K. [1981]. *Survey of Ophthalmology, 25,* 325–332; reprinted by permission. Copyright © 1981 by *Survey of Ophthalmology.*)

letter down to the smallest line he or she can distinguish. If a person can only read down to the 20/40 line, he or she is assumed to have a mild visual deficiency. This means that the smallest letter he or she can identify can be seen by a person with normal vision from 40 feet away. A person with a severe visual deficiency cannot read the 20/100 line.

Since a Snellen eye chart can only be used for children old enough to know the letters of the alphabet, a modification of this chart is used for preschool children (Hall, Pugh, & Hall, 1983). This is called the tumbling "E" chart (see Figure 15.10). Instead of having various letters, the chart contains only the letter "E" placed in different positions. The child is asked to point in the direction of the "legs" of the letter. Generally, this chart is useful for children between 3 and 6 years of age. A variation is a card with different-sized pictures of animals, toys, or other familiar objects.

If a visual deficiency is found, it most often is caused by a refractive error. When a significant refractive error is discovered, glasses or contact lenses are prescribed. Children older than 18 months who have vision problems should wear glasses. If the visual loss is solely a refractive error, the glasses or contact lenses usually correct the vision to 20/20. To determine the amount of refraction needed, an ophthalmologist or **optometrist** uses a **retinoscope** and tries various combinations of lenses to establish

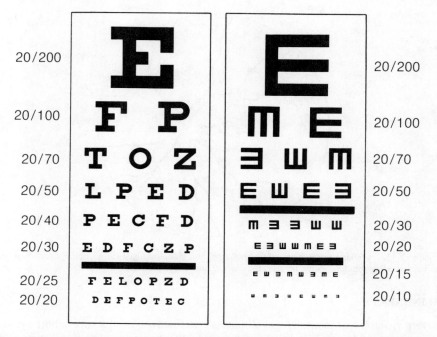

Figure 15.10. A Snellen eye chart and a tumbling "E" chart. A person reads down the chart as far as he or she can. The smallest line that the person can read is the one that indicates visual acuity. The "E" chart operates on the same principle and is used primarily for preschoolers.

what the prescription should be. The refractive power of the lens is measured in **diopters**. Therefore, a prescription for glasses or contact lenses indicates the number of diopters required in each lens.

A thorough eye examination also involves other tests. An ophthalmologist uses a slit lamp to examine the front part of the eye and an **ophthalmoscope** to examine the back portion. The slit lamp, a machine that produces a high-intensity band of light, is used to look for damage to the cornea and the lens. The ophthalmoscope, a device consisting of a series of magnifying lenses and a light source, is used to examine the retina, optic nerve, and retinal blood vessels (Figure 15.11). With it, an ophthalmologist can detect shrinkage or swelling of the optic nerve and damage to the retina or its blood supply. Finally, the tonometer is used to measure pressure in the eyeball to rule out glaucoma.

In a blind child, these tests may still not locate the source of the problem. For such a child, the electroretinogram (ERG) or the earlier-mentioned visual evoked response may prove helpful. The ERG measures electrical impulses generated by the retina when light stimulates it. If no electrical current is produced by the retina after a light is flashed, the retina is probably damaged. If the ERG is normal, but the visual evoked response is abnormal, it may indicate that damage exists somewhere along the pathway from the retina to the brain.

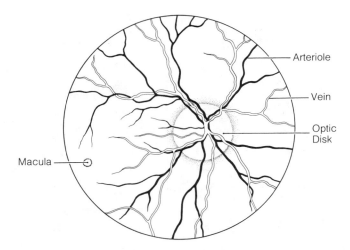

Figure 15.11.   Looking through an ophthalmoscope, an ophthalmologist can examine a portion of the retina, including the optic nerve or disc, the macula, and blood vessels.

BLINDNESS

Severe visual impairment or legal blindness is defined as visual acuity in both eyes of less than 20/200 or a visual field of less than 20° despite the best correction with glasses. A partially sighted person is one who has visual acuity ranging from 20/70 to 20/200 with correction (Smith & Keen, 1979). The overall incidence of blindness in children is 0.4/1,000; 46% of these children were born blind, and an additional 38% lost their sight before 1 year of age. Among blind children, approximately 25% are totally blind, 25% have some light perception, and the remaining 50% have enough vision to read enlarged type (National Society for the Prevention of Blindness, 1966). The most common sites of the visual impairment are the retina (35%), the optic nerve or pathways to the brain (22%), the lens (17%), and the eyeball (16%) (Jan, Freeman, & Scott, 1977).

When the cornea, lens, retina, and eyeball all appear normal but the child has severe visual impairment, this is called cortical blindness (Ackroyd, 1984). In such a child, visual evoked response testing elicits a markedly decreased response or none at all, while the electroetinogram is normal. This finding suggests that the abnormality rests either in the occipital lobe of the brain or in the pathway leading from the eye to the brain. Often, this type of blindness occurs after a head trauma or brain infection and may improve over time (Ronen, Nawratzki, & Yanko, 1983).

Causes of Blindness

In childhood, the causes of blindness are many and varied. The most common congenital causes are prenatal viral infections and eye malformations. Other causes of blindness include retinopathy of prematurity (ROP), trauma, infections, and tumors (Fraser & Friedmann, 1967; Jan, Freeman, & Scott, 1977). Blindness is far more prevalent in developing countries where nutritional disorders, such as vitamin A deficiency, and infections, such as **trachoma**, measles, tuberculosis, and chicken-pox, are common. Public health efforts, the use of silver nitrate at birth to prevent infections in infants' eyes, and immunization programs are gradually making an inroad into this tragic situation.

Retinopathy of Prematurity   Because retinopathy of prematurity is one of the most frequent causes of blindness after birth, it is discussed at length here. ROP occurs almost exclusively in premature infants who have received oxygen to treat respiratory distress syndrome (Alberman, Benson, & Evans, 1982). Now, it occurs in about 2%–4% of all premature babies who weigh less than 1.5 kilograms (roughly 3 pounds) at birth (Phelps, 1981). Between 1940 and 1953, the connection between oxygen and ROP was unknown, and many children were treated with 100% oxygen during the first weeks of life. In 1953, the correlation between high oxygen use and blindness was discovered, and preventive steps were begun (Ashton, Ward, & Serpell, 1953).

The development of ROP involves damage to the rapidly growing blood vessels in the infant's retina. High concentrations of oxygen destroy this network of delicate blood vessels (Figure 15.12). When the child is returned to breathing room air, the blood vessels grow back in a wildly disorganized fashion, with new capillaries growing into the vitreous humor (Silverman, 1980). The formation of fibers and scar tissue accompanies this new growth. The scar tissue begins to contract and gradually pulls the retina away from the choroid. Eventually, the retina may detach, and the child loses vision in that eye (Tasman, 1984).

Since 1954, much lower concentrations of oxygen, about 30%–45%, have been given to treat respiratory distress syndrome (Silverman, 1980). Also, an ophthal-mologist checks the retina of the premature infant periodically during the hos-pitalization. If new vessels are evident, surgical procedures as well as the use of lasers may prevent the retinal detachment. Because of these changes, the incidence of blindness caused by ROP has decreased.

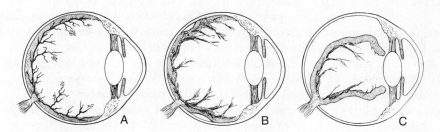

Figure 15.12.   Retinopathy of prematurity (ROP). An infant with respiratory distress syndrome is removed from oxygen therapy and returned to breathing room air. A) The blood vessels, destroyed by the oxygen, grow back in a haphazard fashion. Fibers and scar tissue also begin to form. B) As the scar tissue begins to contract, it pulls the retina away from the choroid. C) Eventually, the retina is totally detached, and the child becomes blind. Because of the danger of ROP, the concentration of oxygen given to premature infants must be closely monitored and the infant's eyes checked regularly during such treatment.

Other postnatal causes of blindness are less common (Harley, 1983). Infections such as meningitis can cause damage to the visual pathway into the brain. Trauma from car accidents or gunshot wounds may lead to hemorrhaging and may damage the retina. Tumors may impinge on the optic nerve or chiasm or arise from and obliterate the retina. One example of the latter is **retinoblastoma**, which may occur in one or both eyes. It is inherited and has an incidence of 1 in 17,000 (Harley, 1983; Shields & Augsburger, 1981). Removal of the affected eye, **chemotherapy**, **radiotherapy**, or **laser therapy** are used to treat the tumor.

Development of the Blind Child

As noted earlier, blindness may be an isolated disability or part of a multiply handicapping condition. For example, blindness caused by ROP is often an isolated finding, while blindness caused by congenital rubella is associated with congenital heart disease, hearing loss, cerebral palsy, and mental retardation.

Considering the infant who has blindness as an isolated handicap, several clues may point to a loss of vision. The parent of a blind infant may notice abnormalities in the movement of the child's eyes. The eyes will have random, jerky, uncoordinated movements called nystagmus; they neither focus on an object nor follow it. Strabismus is often present. Also, if a light is shone in the eyes, the pupils do not constrict. When a threatening gesture is made, the infant does not blink or cry.

Even with normal intelligence, a child who is blind from birth or early childhood is delayed developmentally (Teplin, 1983). Muscle tone is floppy, partly because its maintenance depends on visual perception (Jan, Freeman, & Scott, 1977; Teplin, 1983). Because of this, gross motor skills are delayed. The child may not sit until after 8 months and usually does not crawl at all (Figure 15.13). He may not take steps until 2 to 2½ years of age (Olson, 1983; Sonksen, Levitt, & Kitsinger, 1984).

Since we learn to speak by imitating mouth movements as well as by listening to sounds, language development is also delayed in blind children (Daugherty & Moran, 1982; Pring, 1984). The blind child must learn to speak using auditory means alone. This is a slow, painstaking process. Speech and language are usually normal by school age, but speech is accompanied by less body and facial expression.

In addition to the developmental delays, the blind child may exhibit unusual behavior. Self-stimulation involving rocking, eye gouging, light gazing, and head banging is common in blind children, even in those with normal intelligence (Eichel, 1978). This behavior can be controlled by using behavior modification techniques (Belcher, Conetta, Cole, et al., 1982) and tends to decrease by 4 years of age in children with normal intelligence (Schnittjer & Hirshoren, 1981). It usually persists, however, in blind children with mental retardation or hearing impairment.

Since the Bayley Scales of Infant Development and other infant developmental scales are based primarily on performance of visual skills, they are not very useful for evaluating blind children. Thus, IQ testing for these children is difficult before they reach 2½ years of age. After that, the verbal subtests of the Stanford-Binet and the Wechsler Intelligence Scale for Children are often used. These subtests may give an accurate picture of the child's intelligence and help in educational planning (Parmelee &

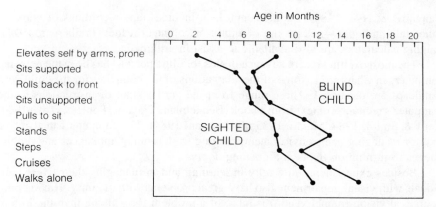

Figure 15.13. Chart of age or attainment of motor skills in sighted and blind children. The motor development of the blind child is delayed. (Adapted from Fraiberg, S. [1977]. *Insights from the blind*. New York: Basic Books. Copyright © 1977 by Selma Fraiberg. Used by permission of Basic Books, Inc., Publishers.)

Liverman, 1977). There is evidence that blind children have more difficulty with abstract concepts than sighted children, but they do well with numerical concepts. Another interesting finding is that blind children do dream, but they do not see images in their dreams unless they became blind after 7 years of age.

Caring for the Blind Child

The primary ways for the blind child to explore his or her world are through touch and sound. Therefore, parents should use textured objects placed within or just outside the child's reach, and they should encourage the child to explore the environment without fear (Vander Kolk, 1981). The child should be encouraged to lie on the stomach rather than on the back, to strengthen the neck and trunk muscles. He or she should also be urged to walk despite the risks of scrapes and bruises. In addition, it is important for parents to talk to their child, even during infancy, explaining and describing the world to him or her. They should try not to be discouraged by slow gross motor development (Fraiberg, 1971) and not to overprotect the child (Kastein, Spaulding, & Scharf, 1980). Touching and physical affection are also important as the child cannot respond to "body language."

By the time the blind child reaches school age, the extent of the visual loss is usually clear. If the child has partial vision, he or she can learn to read large-type books and be totally independent. If the child can see someone's fingers 12 inches away, he or she can get around a room without assistance, but reading will be difficult. If the child can only distinguish light and dark or has no visual perception at all, he or she will need braille, talking books, computers, and tutors.

Braille is a written language formed as a series of raised dots on a page and read from left to right. A good braille reader can read about one-quarter as fast as an average sighted reader (Karavatos, Kaprinis, & Tzavaras, 1984; Wood, 1981). A machine, an opticon, is quite useful because it converts typed text to braille (Cooper,

Gaitenby, & Nye, 1984). Supplemental help includes tape recordings of books—called talking books—and the use of a tutor or volunteer reader (Freiberger, 1974). Talking calculators are also available to assist in arithmetic.

The most exciting recent advance in aids for blind persons has been the personal computer. In Chapter 21, some of the adaptations of the computer for the child with handicaps are discussed. These range from the verbal input of instructions to the computer's recitation of text from a book (Beukelman, Traynor, Poblete, et al., 1984; Kelly & Smith, 1984; Maino, 1985; Zuckerman, 1984). The computer can also be a tool for managing one's environment, ranging from running appliances and dialing phones to turning on lights and opening doors.

Besides experiencing difficulty in learning and in managing their lives, individuals with visual impairment also have great problems with mobility. Having poor peripheral vision (tunnel vision) is more of a problem for walking than the loss of central vision, while the reverse is true for reading. However, any residual vision is better than none. Also, individuals who have acquired blindness generally have an easier time than those with congenital blindness because they have a better understanding of how the world looks. The use of aids for walking is in dispute. Some professionals advocate the use of seeing eye dogs. Others prefer the use of canes or a sonar-guided obstacle device. Most professionals believe that a child should use whatever works best for him or her to attain the greatest degree of independence.

Educational Services for Blind Persons

For a child with visual impairment, the educational placement depends both on the extent of visual loss and the presence of any other handicapping conditions. It is important to start an infant stimulation program when the child is about 6 months old. Usually, this involves a home-based program where the teacher visits and works with the child once a week. By 2 years of age, the child is usually ready for a special preschool program.

Those with a partial visual loss can often be mainstreamed into a regular school classroom with the use of visual aids and resource help. Technical and vocational training is generally incorporated into the high school curriculum. The bright child with visual impairment should be encouraged to go on to college and to seek a professional career. Most colleges now accept and make accommodations for students with visual impairments.

Children who are blind usually do best in a self-contained class. These children need to learn braille. In addition, they may require other aids such as computers, talking calculators, and opticons. The outcome for these children may be very positive, depending on the child's intelligence and the absence of other handicapping conditions.

The Multiply Handicapped Blind Child

When blindness is part of a multihandicapping condition, the prognosis becomes much worse (Warburg, 1983). The incidence of blindness in the population with multiple handicaps is more than 200 times that found in the normal population (Warburg, Frederiksen, & Rattleff, 1979). One-third of partially sighted and two-thirds of blind children have other disabilities including mental retardation (24%), hearing impairments (10%), seizure disorders (8%), congenital heart disease (7%), and cerebral palsy (6%) (Jan, Freeman, & Scott, 1977). Mental retardation limits the adaptability of the person. Learning is slower, and eventual independence is more limited. In one study, approximately 70% of blind children with mental retardation were severely-profoundly retarded. Cerebral palsy, which interferes with mobility and the sense of touch, was found in 61% of these children, seizure disorders in 70%, and hearing loss in 14%. Combined with blindness, hearing loss creates isolation from one's surroundings (Curtis & Donlon, 1984). Sixty-five percent of the children had two or more handicapping conditions besides blindness (Warburg, Frederiksen, & Rattleff, 1979).

In Warburg, Frederiksen, and Rattleff's study (1979), the most common causes of blindness in these children with multiple handicaps were malformations of the central nervous system (35%), prenatal and postnatal infections (13%), genetic disorders (17%), and prematurity (12%). The most frequent causes of visual impairments were optic atrophy (39%), cortical blindness (20%), retinal abnormalities (15%), cataracts (7%), and malformations of the eye (6%).

Treatment in these cases must address all the handicapping conditions and must use all the senses and abilities that remain. A multidisciplinary approach involving a wide range of health care professionals is essential for the treatment of these children.

The Story of Beth, a Blind Child

In 1953, Beth was born prematurely at 32 weeks gestation and weighed 2½ pounds. Because she had a severe case of respiratory distress syndrome, she received high levels of oxygen for many weeks. When she was discharged at 2 months of age, her parents were delighted with her progress. She was alert, active, and fed eagerly.

Since the doctors had warned Beth's parents that her development might lag because of her prematurity, they were not initially concerned when she neither seemed to focus her eyes nor smile. They did become concerned, however, when, at 3 months of age, she still showed no interest in brightly colored mobiles and would not smile socially. Beth's pediatrician also became concerned. She had just read an article about a newly discovered condition, retrolental fibroplasia (now called retinopathy of prematurity), that was rampant among premature infants. When she examined Beth, she confirmed that the child neither fixated nor followed objects. She examined Beth's retina with an ophthalmoscope and found a partial detachment of the retina in both eyes. Since no therapy was available then, all the pediatrician could do was advise the parents that the extent of Beth's loss of vision world become more apparent as she grew.

As was to be expected, Beth continued to develop slowly. She had floppy muscle tone and did not sit until 12 months of age. Her speech was also delayed, although her understanding of language was appropriate for her age.

By 2 years of age, Beth's behavior became a definite problem. She was very reluctant to try new things, and when frustrated, she would often hold her breath or scream. She also rocked and banged her head.

At this time, Beth's parents knew she had some perception of light and dark. She did move toward a bright light and would reach in the general direction of the light. But they also recognized that she could not reach toward a large object placed as close as 1 foot away from her.

Until this time, Beth's parents had been guilt-ridden and depressed over their child's affliction and had catered to her every whim. Beth, at 3 years of age, was a tyrant. Feeling that something had to be done, her parents consulted their pediatrician. She convinced them that their guilt feelings were felt by all parents of children with handicaps and were a normal reaction. At the same time, she encouraged them to be strict and consistent with Beth and not to give in to her demands. She also advised them to enroll Beth in a preschool program.

This was a turning point in Beth's life. Her parents' responses to her changed. When she screamed, they carried her to her room where they left her for a few minutes until she composed herself. When she started rocking and banging her head, her parents would ignore her or would involve her in other tasks. Soon this behavior stopped. She entered a small nursery school program with sighted children. Gradually, she adapted and became more independent. Her parents also attended classes designed to help them train Beth at home.

Things went smoothly until Beth was 8 years old. After a fall, her retinas completely detached. Her world became completely dark. Without light perception, Beth had to make new adaptations. For some time, she was terribly depressed. She tried using a seeing eye dog, but eventually gave him up because she felt this labeled her as being abnormal. Instead, she chose to use a cane and memorized the location of objects and steps in her home and her school.

In high school, Beth did very well. By this time, she had learned braille and also used talking books and tutors. Although she had to spend 4 to 5 hours a night doing homework, she graduated with honors.

SUMMARY

Our eyes help us perceive and understand our world. Indirectly, they also affect the development of muscle tone, language, and other developmental skills. The causes of blindness are many, ranging from cataracts to retinopathy of prematurity, and from infections to tumors. When the visual acuity is less than 20/200 with correction, the person is considered to be legally blind. A person with 20/200 vision can read large-type books, while a totally blind person must rely on braille or other aids. As an isolated disability, blindness is compatible with an independent and successful life-style. However, when combined with other developmental disabilities, the outcome is generally not good. To a great extent, the prognosis for a blind child depends on the child's and the parents' intelligence, courage, and the skill of his or her teachers.

REFERENCES

Ackroyd, R.S. (1984). Cortical blindness following bacterial meningitis: A case report with reassessment of prognosis and aetiology. *Developmental Medicine and Child Neurology, 26,* 227–230.

Alberman, E., Benson, J., & Evans, S. (1982). Visual defects in children of low birthweight. *Archives of Disease in Childhood, 57,* 818–822.

Ashton, N., Ward, B., & Serpell, G. (1953). Role of oxygen in the genesis of retrolental fibroplasia: A preliminary report. *British Journal of Ophthalmology, 37,* 513–520.

Atkinson, J., & Braddick, O. (1983). Assessment of visual acuity in infancy and early childhood. *Acta Ophthalmologica (Supplement), 157,* 18–26.

Belcher, T.L., Conetta, C., Cole, C., et al. (1982). Eliminating a severely retarded blind adolescent's tantrums using mild behavioral interruption: A case study. *Journal of Behavioral Therapy and Experimental Psychiatry, 13,* 257–260.

Beller, R., Hoyt, C.S., Marg, E., et al. (1981). Good visual function after neonatal surgery for congenital monocular cataracts. *American Journal of Ophthalmology, 91,* 559–565.

Beukelman, D.R., Traynor, C., Poblete, M., et al. (1984). Microcomputer-based communication augmentation system for two nonspeaking, physically handicapped persons with severe visual impairment. *Archives of Physical Medicine and Rehabilitation, 65,* 89–91.

Bloome, M.A., & Garcia, C.A. (1981). *Manual of retinal and choroidal dystrophies.* New York: Appleton-Century-Crofts.

Calhoun, J.H. (1983). Cataracts in children. *Pediatric Clinics of North America, 30,* 1061–1069.

Chew, E., & Morin, J.D. (1983). Glaucoma in children. *Pediatric Clinics of North America, 30,* 1043–1060.

Cooper, F.S., Gaitenby, J.H., & Nye, P.W. (1984). Evolution of reading machines for the blind: Haskins Laboratories research as a case history. *Journal of Rehabilitation Research & Development, 21,* 51–87.

Curtis, W.S., & Donlon, E.T. (1984). A ten-year follow-up study of deaf-blind children. *Exceptional Child, 50,* 449–455.

Daugherty, K.M., & Moran, M.F. (1982). Neuropsychological learning and developmental characteristics of the low vision child. *Journal of Visual Impairment & Blindness, 76,* 398–406.

Dobson, V., & Teller, D.Y. (1978). Visual acuity in human infants: A review and comparison of behavioral and electrophysiological studies. *Vision Research, 18,* 1469–1483.

Eichel, V.L. (1978). Mannerisms of the blind: A review of the literature. *Journal of Visual Impairment & Blindness, 72,* 125–130.

Eller, A.W., & Brown, G.C. (1983). Retinal disorders of childhood. *Pediatric Clinics of North America, 30,* 1087–1101.

Fox, R., Aslin, R.N., Shea, S.L., et al. (1980). Stereopsis in human infants. *Science, 207,* 323–324.

Fraiberg, S. (1971). Intervention in infancy: A program for blind infants. *Journal of the American Academy of Child Psychiatry, 10,* 381–405.

Fraiberg, S. (1977). *Insights from the blind.* New York: Basic Books.

Fraser, G.R., & Friedmann, A.I. (1967). *The causes of blindness in childhood: A study of 776 children with severe visual handicaps.* Baltimore: Johns Hopkins University Press.

Freiberger, H. (1974). Mobility and reading aids for the blind: Recent developments in rehabilitation devices. *Bulletin of the New York Academy of Medicine, 50,* 667–671.

Fulton, A.B., Hansen, R.M., & Manning, K.A. (1981). Measuring visual acuity in infants. *Survey of Ophthalmology, 25,* 325–332.

Goble, J.L. (1984). *Visual disorders in the handicapped child.* New York: M. Dekker.

Greenwald, M.J. (1983). Visual development in infancy and childhood. *Pediatric Clinics of North America, 30,* 977–993.

Hall, S.M., Pugh, A.G., & Hall, D.M. (1983). Vision screening in the under 5s. *British Medical Journal, 285,* 1096–1098.

Harcout, B. (1976). Squint. *British Medical Journal, 1,* 703–705.

Harley, R.D. (Ed.). (1983). *Pediatric ophthalmology* (2nd ed.). Philadelphia: W.B. Saunders Co.

Held, R., Birch, E., & Gwiazda, J. (1980). Stereoacuity of human infants. *Proceedings of the National Academy of Sciences USA, 77,* 5572–5574.

Helveston, E.M., & Ellis, F.D. (1984). *Pediatric ophthalmology practice* (2nd ed.). St. Louis: C.V. Mosby Co.

Hoyt, C.S. (1984). The clinical usefulness of the visual evoked response. *Journal of Pediatric Ophthalmology and Strabismus, 21,* 231–234.

Hubel, D.H. (1982). Exploration of the primary visual cortex, 1955–1978. *Nature, 299,* 515–524.

Hubel, D.H., & Wiesel, T.N. (1979). Brain mechanisms of vision. *Scientific American, 241,* 150–162.

Ing, M.R. (1981). Early surgical alignment for congenital esotropia. *Transactions of the American Ophthalmological Society, 79,* 625–627.

Jampolsky, A., Parks, M.M., & Robb, R.M. (1977). When should one operate for congenital strabismus? In R.J. Brockhurst, S.A. Boruchoff, B.T. Hutchinson, et al. (Eds.), *Controversy in ophthalmology.* Philadelphia: W.B. Saunders Co.

Jan, J.E., Freeman, R.D., & Scott, E.P. (Ed.). (1977). *Visual impairment in children and adolescents.* New York: Grune & Stratton.

Kanski, J.J. (1984). *Clinical ophthalmology.* St. Louis: C.V. Mosby Co.

Karavatos, A., Kaprinis, G., & Tzavaras, A. (1984). Hemispheric specialization for language in the congenitally blind: The influence of the Braille system. *Neuropsychologia, 22,* 521–525.

Kastein, S., Spaulding, I., & Scharf, B. (1980). *Raising the young blind child: A guide for parents and educators.* New York: Human Sciences Press.

Kelly, G.W., & Smith, J.L. (1984). A microprocessor-based large print reading/writing system for the visually impaired person. *Biomedical Scientific Instruments, 20,* 121–122.

Kraft, S.P., & Scott, W.E. (1984). Surgery for congenital esotropia—an age comparison study. *Journal of Pediatric Ophthalmology and Strabismus, 21,* 57–68.

Langman, J., & Sadler, T.W. (1985). *Langman's medical embryology* (5th ed.). Baltimore: Williams & Wilkins Co.

Lennerstrand, G., Andersson, G., & Axelsson, A. (1983). Clinical assessment of visual function in infants and young children. *Acta Ophthalmologica, 157,* 63–67.

Lennerstrand, G., Axelsson, A., & Andersson, G. (1983). Visual assessment with preferential looking techniques in mentally retarded children. *Acta Ophthalmologica, 61,* 183–185.

London, R. (1982). Optokinetic nystagmus: A review of pathways, techniques, and selected diagnostic applications. *Journal of the American Optometric Association, 53,* 791–798.

Maino, J.H. (1985). Computer low vision aids. *Journal of the American Optometric Association, 56,* 49–53.

Merin, S., & Crawford, J.S. (1972). Etiology of congenital cataracts. *Ophthalmology Digest, 34,* 16–23.

Miranda, S.B., Hack, M., Fantz, R.L., et al. (1977). Neonatal pattern vision: A predictor of future mental performance? *Journal of Pediatrics, 91,* 642–647.

Mohindra, I., Jacobson, S.G., Zwaan, J., et al. (1983). Psychophysical assessment of visual acuity in infants with visual disorders. *Behavioural Brain Research, 10,* 51–58.

National Society for the Prevention of Blindness. (1966). *Estimated statistics on blindness and vision problems.* New York: National Society for the Prevention of Blindness.

Nelson, L.B. (1984). *Pediatric ophthalmology.* Philadelphia: W.B. Saunders Co.

Newell, F.W. (1978). *Ophthalmology: Principles and concepts* (4th ed.). St. Louis: C.V. Mosby Co.

Olson, M.R. (1983). A study of the exploratory behavior of legally blind and sighted preschoolers. *Exceptional Children, 50,* 130–138.

Paakkala, A.M. (1982). Surgical treatment of strabismus. A retrospective investigation of results of surgical treatment of horizontal strabismus. *Acta Ophthalmologica, 156,* 1–107.

Pagon, R.A., Graham, J.M. Jr., Zonana, J., et al. (1981). Coloboma, congenital heart disease, and choanal atresia with multiple anomalies: CHARGE association. *Journal of Pediatrics, 99,* 223–227.

Parmelee, A.H., & Liverman, L. (1977). The blind infant and child. In M. Green & R.J. Hagerty (Eds.), *Ambulatory pediatrics II: Personal health care of children in the office* (2nd ed.). Philadelphia: W.B. Saunders Co.

Phelps, D.L. (1981). Retinopathy of prematurity: An estimate of vision loss in the United States—1979. *Pediatrics, 67,* 924–925.

Pirie, A. (1983). Vitamin A deficiency and child blindness in the developing world. *Proceedings of the Nutrition Society, 42,* 53–64.

Pring, L. (1984). A comparison of the word recognition processes of blind and sighted children. *Child Development, 55,* 1865–1877.

Robb, R.M. (1981). *Ophthalmology for the pediatric practitioner.* Boston: Little, Brown & Co.

Ronen, S., Nawratzki, I., & Yanko, L. (1983). Cortical blindness in infancy: A follow-up study. *Ophthalmologica, 187,* 217–221.

Scheiman, M.M. (1984). Optometric findings in children with cerebral palsy. *American Journal of Optometry and Physiological Optics, 61,* 321–323.

Schnittjer, C.J., & Hirshoren, A. (1981). Factors of problem behavior in visually impaired children. *Journal of Abnormal Child Psychology, 9,* 517–522.

Scott, E.P., Jan, J.E., & Freeman, R.D. (1977). *Can't your child see?* Baltimore: University Park Press.

Shields, J.A., & Augsburger, J.J. (1981). Current approaches to the diagnosis and management of retinoblastoma. *Surveys of Ophthalmology, 25,* 347–372.

Silverman, W.A. (1980). *Retrolental fibroplasia: A modern parable.* New York: Grune & Stratton.

Smith, V., & Keen, J. (1979). Visual handicaps in children. *Clinical Developmental Medicine, 73,* 44–55.

Sonksen, P.M., Levitt, S., & Kitsinger, M. (1984). Identification of constraints acting on motor development in young visually disabled children and principles of remediation. *Child: Care, Health and Development, 10,* 273–286.

Tasman, W. (1984). The natural history of active retinopathy of prematurity. *Ophthalmology, 91,* 1499–1503.

Teplin, S.W. (1983). Development of blind infants and children with retrolental fibroplasia: Implications for physicians. *Pediatrics, 71,* 6–12.

Tyler, C.W. (1982). Assessment of visual function in infants by evoked potentials. *Developmental Medicine and Child Neurology, 24,* 853–856.

Vander Kolk, C.J. (1981). *Assessment and planning with the visually impaired.* Baltimore: University Park Press.

Von Barsewisch, B. (1979). *Perinatal retinal haemorrhages: Morphology, aetiology, and significance.* Berlin: Springer-Verlag.

von Noorden, G.K. (1983). Practical management of amblyopia. *International Ophthalmology, 6,* 7–12.

Warburg, M. (1983). Why are the blind and severely visually impaired children with mental retardation much more retarded than the sighted children? *Acta Ophthalmologica (Supplement), 157,* 72–81.

Warburg, M., Frederiksen, P., & Rattleff, J. (1979). Blindness among 7700 mentally retarded children in Denmark. *Clinical Developmental Medicine, 73,* 56–67.

Wild, J.M., & Wolffe, M. (1985). The employment and education of the partially sighted in the period immediately after leaving special school. *Ophthalmic and Physiological Optics, 5,* 73–80.

Wood, T.A. (1981). Patterns of listening and reading skills in visually handicapped students. *Journal of Visual Impairment & Blindness, 75,* 215–218.

Zuckerman, D. (1984). Use of personal computing technology by deaf-blind individuals. *Journal of Medical Systems, 8,* 431–436.

Chapter 16

Hearing

Upon completion of this chapter, the reader will:
—be able to describe the anatomy of the ear
—know the different types of hearing losses and their causes
—be aware of the different hearing tests and their uses
—understand the ways to treat a child with hearing loss
—be able to discuss the prognoses for the different hearing impairments

---

Even when alone in the woods, a person is surrounded by meaningful sounds. The gurgling brook says that water is near. The chirping birds announce daybreak. The rustling leaves indicate the presence of wind or the approach of an animal or another person. Through hearing, we perceive and understand our surroundings. In this chapter, hearing problems, their treatment, and their effect on our ability to communicate are discussed.

DEFINING SOUND

When we hear a sound, we are actually interpreting a pattern of vibrations that originates somewhere in our surroundings. Similar to what happens when a stone is thrown into a pond, sound waves start at one point and spread out in circles of waves. The waves have both a *pitch,* or frequency, and an *intensity,* or loudness (Figure 16.1).

The closer the waves are to each other, the higher the frequency of the sound. To measure the frequency of a sound, the number of cycles per second is counted. One cycle is the distance from the top of one wave to the top of the next wave. Humans can hear frequencies ranging from 20 to 20,000 cycles per second, whereas dogs can hear frequencies above 40,000 cycles per second. The unit of measurement of frequency is called a hertz (Hz) and is equal to one cycle per second. Low-pitched sounds have a frequency less than 500 Hz and have a bass quality. High-pitched sounds, on the other hand, have a frequency above 2,000 Hz and a tenor quality. Middle C equals 256 Hz. Each octave above middle C doubles this frequency, and each octave below halves it (Jerger, 1984).

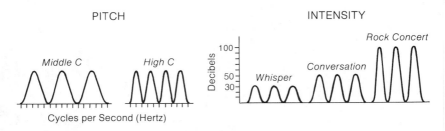

Figure 16.1. Pitch and intensity of sound waves. The pitch of a sound, its frequency, is expressed as cycles per second, or hertz (Hz). Middle C is 256 Hz; one octave above is 512 Hz. Intensity of sound is expressed in decibels (dB) and varies from a whisper at 30 dB to loud music at 100 dB or more.

While the frequency of the wave determines its pitch, intensity is defined by the height of the wave. The intensity produced by a sound is measured in decibels (dB). The softest sound a normal hearing person can perceive is defined as 0 dB hearing level (HL). The sound of a person whispering a few feet away would register 30 dB HL. The normal level of conversation measures 45–50 dB HL, and a rock concert would measure 100 dB HL or more. Sound at the latter level can cause temporary hearing loss (Northern & Downs, 1984).

ANATOMY OF THE EAR

Our mechanism for hearing, the ear, is a beautifully designed instrument. The external ear, also called the *auricle,* sticks out from the side of the head and stereophonically catches sound waves. After entering the external ear, the sound waves pass through the ear canal to the *tympanic membrane,* or eardrum (Figure 16.2).

The eardrum converts the sound waves to mechanical vibrations. Initially, the sound waves hit the eardrum and make it vibrate. The vibrations then pass along to a series of three small bones, or **ossicles**. The first of these bones is the *malleus,* or hammer. Then comes the *incus,* or anvil, followed by the *stapes,* or stirrup. The stapes lies next to the *oval window,* a membrane that is the gateway to the inner ear.

In the inner ear, sound is once again transformed, this time from mechanical to electrical energy. To understand how this happens, one must appreciate the complexity of the *labyrinth* in the inner ear. It contains two major structures, the **vestibular apparatus** and the **cochlea**. The vestibular apparatus helps maintain balance. The cochlea makes hearing possible; it is a membranous, snail-shaped structure that has three chambers. The outer and inner chambers are connecting canals that contain a fluid called *perilymph* (Figure 16.3). The middle chamber houses the **organ of Corti** and is bathed in a different fluid called *endolymph*. The organ of Corti consists of delicate hair cells that link up with the auditory or eighth cranial nerve, the nerve that carries sound to the brain. The hair cells near the oval window respond to high-frequency sounds, while those furthest away react to low-frequency sounds.

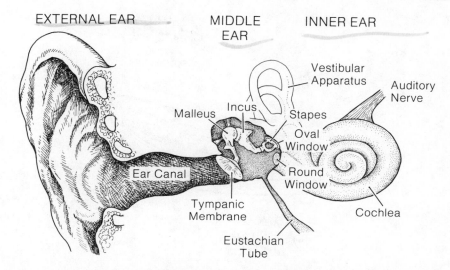

Figure 16.2. Structure of the ear. The middle ear is composed of the tympanic membrane, or eardrum, and the three ear bones, the malleus, the incus, and the stapes. The stapes lies next to the oval window, the gateway to the inner ear. The inner ear contains the cochlea and the vestibular apparatus, collectively called the labyrinth.

When the vibrations from the stapes in the middle ear hit the oval window, the window bulges slightly. This creates a change in pressure and sets off a wave in the perilymph that is transmitted to the endolymph. This, in turn, causes a slight movement of some of the hair cells; the extent of movement depends on the frequency and intensity of the stimulus. The mechanical energy generated by this movement is converted to electrical energy, and a nerve impulse is produced and carried to the temporal lobe of the brain. What then happens in the brain is discussed in Chapter 17.

HEARING LOSS

When some part of the hearing apparatus malfunctions, hearing loss results. Not only does this affect hearing, it may also hinder a person's ability to speak.

Types of Hearing Loss

Three types of hearing loss exist: *conductive, sensorineural,* and *mixed* (Ballantyne, 1977). Damage to either the external or the middle ear causes a conductive hearing loss, while a malfunctioning of the cochlea or auditory nerve results in a sensorineural loss. The mixed type occurs when the hearing loss has both a conductive and a sensorineural component.

Besides being defined according to the location of the damage, hearing loss is also categorized by its severity (Northern & Downs, 1984). A person who hears normally can distinguish sound intensities of 15 dB or less. A child with a *mild hearing impairment* can only hear sounds that are at least 15–45 dB. Speech is normal

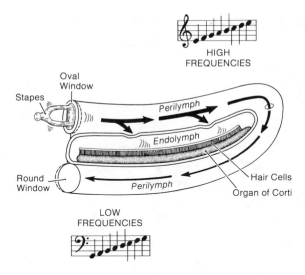

Figure 16.3. The cochlea. The cochlea has been "unfolded" for simplicity. Sound vibrations from the stapes are transmitted as waves in the perilymph. This leads to the displacement of hair cells in the organ of Corti. These hair cells lie above and attach to the auditory nerve, and the impulses generated are fed to the brain. Low-frequency sounds stimulate hair cells close to the oval window, while high-frequency sounds stimulate the end of the organ. The sound wave in the perilymph is rapidly dissipated through the round window, and the cochlea is ready to accept a new set of vibrations.

and conversation is easy, but the child will have difficulty hearing distant sounds. Early speech and language development may be somewhat delayed. An individual with a *moderate hearing loss* must have sounds register at least 45–70 dB to be audible. This amount of loss significantly affects the ability to hear normal conversation; articulation (the correct formation of speech) is also impaired. A child with a *severe* hearing loss requires sound to register at least 70–90 dB to be heard. With this degree of loss, the child cannot participate in conversations, although he or she may catch an occasional word. Hearing aids are most helpful for these individuals. A *profound* hearing impairment involves a loss greater than 90 dB. Although a child with this loss may react to very loud sounds, this hearing ability does not help in communication. A hearing aid may help, but he or she is usually unable to articulate normally.

Another way to describe hearing loss is to note whether one or both ears are affected. A *unilateral* loss involves one ear, whereas a *bilateral* hearing loss is present in both ears. A unilateral hearing loss, as would be expected, is less incapacitating than a bilateral one. Less than 20% of children with hearing impairment have unilateral losses (Ballantyne, 1977; Bess & Tharpe, 1984).

Causes of Hearing Loss

In approximately half of all children with a hearing loss, the cause is unknown. For the other half, a number of causes are identified (Bess, 1977). These include middle

ear infections, cleft palate, Down syndrome and other genetic causes, noise pollution, and infections.

Middle Ear Infections (Otitis Media) The most common type of hearing
impairment is a mild-to-moderate conductive hearing loss that results from chronic
middle ear infections. Middle ear infection, or otitis media, is most common in very
young children; 76%–95% of all children have at least one infection during their first
2 years of life (Northern & Downs, 1984). In most cases, fever or irritability is the
first sign of the illness. Frequently, the child will pull at his or her ears. On physical
examination, the eardrum looks red and opaque rather than white and translucent.
Fluid is usually present behind the eardrum. Ordinarily, treatment consists of an
antibiotic and a decongestant. However, controversy exists about the effectivenss of
these medicines. Most ear infections are viral in origin, and, therefore, they do not
respond to antibiotics (Paradise, 1980). Yet, because there is no easy way to
distinguish a viral from a bacterial infection, antibiotics are frequently given. A
decongestant is used to open up the **eustachian tube** and to equalize the pressure
between the middle ear and the throat, allowing the fluid to drain from the middle ear.
There is some question, however, as to whether this actually happens. Some
experimental studies suggest that decongestants make little difference in the duration
or outcome of a middle ear infection (Bluestone, 1982; Olson, Klein, Charney,
et al., 1978).

If hearing is tested during one of these infections, a conductive hearing loss is
frequently found. This usually clears up within a week. However, if the fluid buildup
persists or recurs, it may cause a persistent moderate hearing loss. This can affect
speech and language development (Downs & Blager, 1982; Friel-Patti, Finitzo-
Hieber, Conti, et al., 1982). Recurrent infections are often treated prophylactically
with antibiotics (frequently Bactrim) for a month. If this is not effective, an ENT (ear,
nose, and throat) surgeon may need to perform a **myringotomy**, an outpatient
surgical procedure in which the eardrum is cut. A small tube, called a PE tube, is then
inserted through the eardrum (Gebhart, 1981). This tube equalizes the pressure
between the middle ear and the ear canal and enables the fluid to drain. Over a period
of months, the tube gradually works its way into the ear canal and drops out or is
removed. The eardrum then closes over the incision. The use of these tubes has
significantly reduced the incidence of conductive hearing loss in children with
chronic otitis media (Fior & Veljak, 1984).

Cleft Palate Another condition associated with a conductive hearing loss is
cleft palate (Gopalakrishna, Goleria, & Raje, 1984). Children with this abnormality
are susceptible to severe and persistent middle ear infections (Hubbard, Paradise,
McWilliams, et al., 1985). The same malformation that affects the closure of the
palate also hinders middle ear drainage through the eustachian tubes. Without proper
drainage, infection is more likely. More than 30% of children with cleft palate
develop a conductive hearing loss because of repeated middle ear infections, and an
additional 25% have sensorineural or mixed-type hearing losses (Northern & Downs,
1984). To prevent hearing impairment in these children, myringotomies and PE tube
insertions are frequently performed.

Children with other cranial-facial abnormalities, for example, **Treacher-Collins syndrome**, have similar problems. Children with this syndrome have an unusual facial appearance, malformed ears, and abnormal ossicles and ear canals. As a result, these children have a conductive hearing loss. Plastic surgery often improves their physical appearance as well as the hearing loss (Northern & Downs, 1984).

Down Syndrome Children with Down syndrome have narrow ear canals and a strong tendency for middle ear infections. A majority of these children (78%) have some form of hearing loss; the most common is a conductive loss (Northern & Downs, 1984).

Noise Pollution Mild to moderate sensorineural hearing losses may result from "noise pollution," the most common source of which is heavy industry. Noise intensity levels greater than 120 dB have been recorded. Riveters, airplane maintenance personnel, and presspersons are particularly at risk for hearing loss and wear ear protectors to alleviate this hazard.

Another form of noise pollution may affect premature infants placed in incubators. The ambient noise level can range from 60–80 dB (Bess, Peek, & Chapman, 1979). It is still unclear whether this noise affects these infants' hearing and to what extent.

Genetic Causes Of the more severe sensorineural hearing losses, about half are caused by genetically inherited conditions. Often a child's sibling or parent is also affected. Over 70 types of hereditary deafness have been identified (Konigsmark & Gorlin, 1976). The vast majority of these are inherited as autosomal recessive disorders (see Chapter 2). Overall, the incidence of genetically inherited deafness is approximately 1 in 2,000 to 1 in 6,000 births (Konigsmark & Gorlin, 1976; Steele, 1981).

Infections Some severe sensorineural or mixed-type hearing losses are acquired rather than genetic in origin. Intrauterine infection is one cause. For example, a mother who contracts rubella during the first trimester of her pregnancy is very likely to have a malformed infant who has a severe, high-frequency sensorineural hearing loss (Gumpel, Hayes, & Dudgeon, 1971). Other viruses during pregnancy, including toxoplasmosis, herpesvirus, and cytomegalovirus (CMV), may cause similar hearing losses. The most prevalent of these is CMV, which may not result in malformations but may be responsible for a serious hearing impairment (Northern & Downs, 1984).

During infancy, certain bacterial infections can also lead to a hearing loss (Echeverria, Fina, Norton, et al., 1978). Meningitis, for instance, carries a 20% risk of hearing loss from damage to the auditory nerve (Eavey, Gao, Schuknecht, et al., 1985; MacDonald & Feinstein, 1984). In addition, the antibiotics given to treat an infection may be toxic to the auditory nerve (Assael, Parini, & Rusconi, 1982). Fortunately, physicians can now measure antibiotic blood levels during treatment to avoid the development of this toxic effect.

Perinatal Period During delivery or in the newborn period, a number of problems may bring about a hearing loss (Thiringer, Kankkunen, Liden, et al., 1984). Asphyxia may cause damage to the cochlea, resulting in hearing loss. Also, in the newborn period, kernicterus, an outcome of severe jaundice, is often associated with a high-frequency sensorineural loss (Ackerman, Dyer, & Leydorf, 1970). Premature infants are especially susceptible to both these problems (Bergman, Hirsch, Fria, et al., 1985).

Incidence of Hearing Loss

Hearing loss occurs in approximately 1% of all children. Among all individuals who have hearing problems, 40% have a mild loss, 20% a moderate loss, 20% a severe loss, and 20% a profound loss (Glorig & Roberts, 1977). Thus, a profound loss or deafness affects approximately 2 in 1,000 children; 65% of these children are born deaf. An additional 12% develop deafness during the first 3 years of life, and the rest become deaf later in life. Overall, more than 44,000 children in the United States receive their education in special programs for students with hearing impairments (Leske, 1981).

IDENTIFYING THE CHILD WITH HEARING IMPAIRMENT

The age at which children are identified as having a hearing problem varies. Most children with a profound hearing loss are recognized by 9–12 months of age when they stop babbling and do not follow spoken commands (Rutter & Martin, 1972). Deaf children coo and babble at about the same age as children who can hear. However, in normal children, the babbling becomes more specific and acquires meaning by 9 months of age. Progressing to this stage requires the ability to imitate, repeat, and associate sounds with meaning. Since the deaf child cannot hear the sounds and then copy them, he or she can go no further and stops babbling.

A similar situation exists for following verbal commands. From 6 to 9 months of age, most infants receive verbal instructions accompanied by gestures. The deaf child at this age can figure out the command by watching mouth movements and following the gestures. However, by 12 months, the child is expected to respond to words alone. The deaf child cannot.

In some children, deafness is discovered earlier than 9 months. Usually, such a child is identified because he or she was premature, jaundiced, or septic and so was at an increased risk for a hearing loss. These children are often watched more closely by their parents and their pediatricians. For instance, the parents may notice that the baby is not awakened by loud noises or seems uninterested in music. These early clues may lead to a hearing evaluation.

On the other hand, about 20% of children with hearing impairment are not identified until after 18 months of age (Gerber & Mencher, 1978). These children may have a moderate-severe hearing loss. The less severe the loss, the later it is usually discovered. Many children with mild to moderate hearing losses are first detected in a school hearing screening at 6 years of age. However, many children who fail this screening test do not have a persistent hearing impairment. Perhaps, these children were tested during or right after a middle ear infection when they had a short-term hearing loss. Actually, for every 10 children who fail a school hearing test, only one will turn out to have a permanent hearing loss (Fitzzaland & Zink, 1984).

HEARING TESTS

The usual way of identifying a child with a hearing loss is through the use of some kind of hearing test. The type of test used is determined by the age of the child (Fitzzaland & Zink, 1984).

For newborns, the effectiveness of screening for hearing loss is questionable. To get a rough idea of an infant's hearing ability, one may observe the baby's behavioral responses to different sounds. For instance, a bell or buzzer can be rung near the baby, and the observer can look for crying or arm and leg movements. However, even a strong response does not rule out a mild to moderate hearing loss because the sound of the bell is about 80 dB. At the same time, the absence of response to the sounds does not necessarily mean the child has a hearing loss. Infants rapidly adjust to the loud noises in a nursery. They may simply not respond to the bell because they associate these noises with the usual nursery sounds (Hodgson & Skinner, 1981). Thus, screening tests such as the Crib-o-Gram, in which a sound is automatically presented and subsequent body movement recorded, are often inaccurate (American Academy of Pediatrics, 1982).

In high risk infants, one can use a **brain stem auditory evoked response (BAER)** (described later in this chapter) to determine a hearing loss (Finitzo-Hieber, 1982; Jacobson, Morehouse, & Johnson, 1982; Stein, Ozdamar, Kraus, et al., 1983). However, this test is also often inaccurate. In one study, 18 of the 19 infants who failed this hearing test in the newborn period had normal hearing when tested again at 18 months of age (Shannon, Felix, Krumholz, et al., 1984).

After 6 months of age, a child can be tested using behavioral **audiometry** (Wong & Shah, 1979). One approach is the following: A Donald Duck mask is placed to the right of the child and a Mickey Mouse mask to the left. In the nose of each mask is a red light bulb. The child wears earphones, and the audiologist pairs a sound in the left ear with a lighting up of Mickey's nose and a sound in the right ear with Donald's nose. After a few trials, the child will consistently turn toward Mickey every time a sound is emitted through the left earphone. Then comes the trick. The audiologist turns on a sound in the left ear but does not light up Mickey's nose. If the child turns toward Mickey, the nose lights up, rewarding the child for turning toward the sound. If the child turns toward Donald or looks straight ahead, nothing happens. Using this technique, successively softer sounds of different frequencies are presented to each ear until the child stops turning in the correct direction. A fairly good measure of the child's hearing ability is determined with this technique.

A similar test without the behavioral component can be used for older children. Sounds ranging in intensity from 0 to 110 dB and in frequency from 125 to 8,000 Hz are presented (Figure 16.4). The right and left ears are tested separately to determine whether the hearing loss is unilateral or bilateral. The sounds are first presented through the earphones and then through a vibrator attached to the **mastoid** bone behind the ear. Administering the test both ways helps the audiologist distinguish between a conductive and sensorineural hearing loss. Children with a sensorineural loss will hear equally poorly in both tests; those with a conductive loss will show a

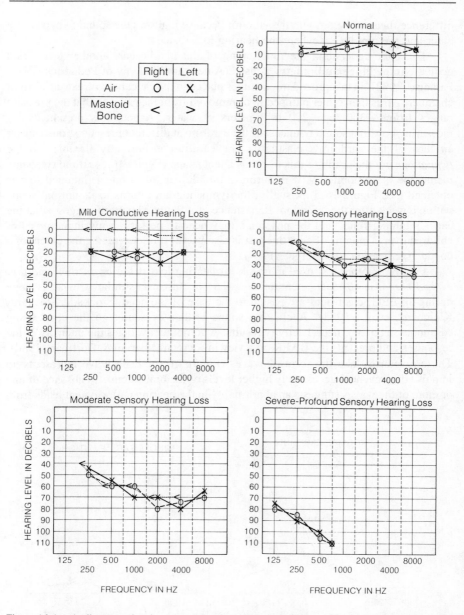

Figure 16.4. Audiograms showing normal hearing and various degrees of a loss. Note that, in most cases, both ears are equally affected. In a conductive hearing loss, bone conduction is found to be better than air conduction because it bypasses the outer and the middle ear where the damage lies. In sensorineural hearing loss, bone and air conduction produce similar results because the problem lies in the inner ear. The range of hearing loss is as follows: mild: 15–45 dB; moderate: 45–70 dB; severe: 70–90 dB; profound: greater than 90 dB. (Audiograms courtesy of Brad Friedrich, Ph.D., Hearing and Speech Department, Kennedy Institute for Handicapped Children, Baltimore.)

difference, hearing better with the vibrator because it allows the sound to bypass the outer and the middle ear where the hearing loss resides.

To better understand the functioning of the middle ear, another test called **acoustic impedance audiometry** is used (American Academy of Pediatrics, 1978; Paradise, 1982). In this procedure, a plug is placed in the ear canal to create an airtight chamber. Air is then either pumped in or removed from the canal so that the pressure ranges from −300 to +200 millimeters of water. A sound is presented. By measuring how that sound bounces off the eardrum at different pressures, one can get an idea of the eardrum's elasticity. The eardrum is normally flexible, so the *tympanogram,* the graph of this test, has a tent shape (Figure 16.5). If the tympanic membrane is immobile, as it is during a middle ear infection, a flattened line is obtained (see Figure 16.5). Usually, the tympanogram returns to its normal shape within a week after the infection. Persistence of a flattened pattern suggests that the ear is retaining fluid, and the physician may need to perform a myringotomy. For children over 7 months of age, this test is also useful for determining the extent of a conductive hearing loss (Jerger, 1984).

Finally, another test used to check for hearing loss is the *brain stem auditory evoked response (BAER),* mentioned earlier. In this test, similar to what is done during an EEG, electrodes are pasted to the base of the head (Stockard, Stockard, Kleinberg, et al., 1983). A clicking sound is then presented to the child using earphones; a burst of neural activity results. A computer averages the intensity of the responses and presents the BAER on a viewing screen (Mizrahi & Dorfman, 1980). These responses take the form of waves (Figure 16.6). Each wave represents an impulse that reaches successively higher levels of the brain stem. An absence of one or more of the waves suggests an abnormality in the hearing pathway that leads from

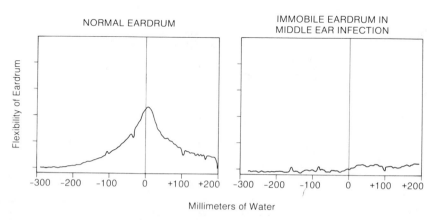

Figure 16.5.   Tympanogram. During otitis media (middle ear infection), the eardrum loses its elasticity and a flat-line tympanogram is recorded. Once the infection clears, a normal, tent-shaped tympanogram should be obtained. If it is not, a myringotomy and placement of PE tubes may be necessary to correct the impairment. (Courtesy of Brad Friedrich, Ph.D., Hearing and Speech Department, Kennedy Institute for Handicapped Children, Baltimore.)

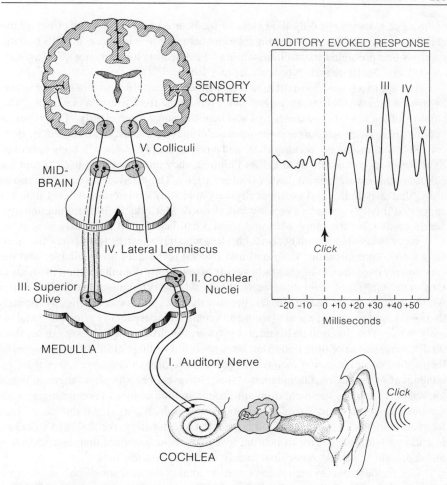

Figure 16.6. Brain stem auditory evoked response. The auditory nerve carries sounds to the medullary portion of the brain stem. Here most impulses cross over and ascend to the opposite sensory cortex, where the sound is perceived. The functioning of the brain stem can be measured by an auditory evoked response. Each wave corresponds to a different level of the brain stem (denoted by Roman numerals). The auditory evoked response has been used to test hearing in an infant or a child with severe handicaps.

the inner ear to the brain stem. In addition, the length of time between the click and the beginning of the wave indicates the rapidity of the conduction of the nerve impulse. A slow rate of conduction has been noted in disorders as diverse as attention deficit disorder and **multiple sclerosis**.

TREATMENT

Treatment for hearing loss primarily consists of aids for hearing and aids for speech (Mencher & Gerber, 1980). To decide on the proper form of treatment, the speech pathologist assesses not only the extent of the hearing loss but also its effect on the child's receptive and expressive language and behavior. For instance, a 10 dB hearing loss may be a problem for one child, while a 25 dB hearing loss may not affect another child (Lass, McReynolds, Northern, et al., 1982).

The approach used most often to help a child with a mild to severe hearing loss is to provide him with a hearing aid and place him in the front row of a classroom. The child can then read the teacher's lips and hear the voice more clearly. Two types of hearing aids exist: *body aids* and *ear-level aids* (Seewald, Ross, & Spiro, 1985). Both consist of a microphone, an amplifier, and a power supply. Although body aids used to be the most commonly used aid for children, they are now rarely used except for children with severe hearing losses (Rubin, 1976). The disadvantage of this type of aid is that it is bulky and cosmetically less appealing. Bilateral ear-level aids are suggested if both ears have a hearing loss (Bess & McConnell, 1981). Functionally, hearing aids raise the range of sound a child can hear by 10 to 80 dB.

Besides assistance with hearing, children who have hearing losses may also need help with communication. Both oral and manual techniques are available, and the controversy over the use of oral-only versus manual-only communication methods is long-standing. There is no disagreement over which technique to use with children who have mild-severe hearing losses, because they can still speak intelligibly. Speech therapy is used to improve articulation and syntax and is especially effective if started early in life. The situation is different, however, for children with losses greater than 90 dB; they may have little understandable speech. For these children, proponents of the manual communication method suggest the use of sign language rather than the attainment of verbal communication skills. However, because sign language is not known by everyone, these children are limited in their ability to communicate with the outside world. Proponents of the auditory approach play down the use of sign language and work toward developing speech. Unfortunately, the ability to articulate in children with this degree of hearing loss may be so abnormal that their speech is unintelligible to people other than family members and teachers.

Out of these two extremes has come a "total communication" philosophy that individualizes communication for each child (Thompson & Swisher, 1985). With this approach, a child's language program may consist of a combination of a hearing aid, natural gestures, pantomime, sign language, finger-spelling, lipreading, and body language with or without oral speech. In other words, the child learns to use whatever tools provide him or her with the best possible means of communication. The majority of speech pathologists use total communication techniques (Boothroyd, 1982; Rutter & Martin, 1972).

THE STORY OF AMY

At birth, Amy was an extremely pretty child with wide blue eyes, a rush of blonde hair, and dainty features. She had no difficulties during her newborn period, and she went home with her parents on the third day of her life. She fed well and looked around with interest. She also slept well no matter how much noise surrounded her.

She rarely awakened to her mother's voice but woke quickly if touched or picked up. She seemed to look at faces and to follow expressions closely. She smiled at 2 months and cooed at 3 months. Although her parents were concerned about her lack of response to noise, they felt relieved when Amy started to babble. Developmentally, she did fine. She sat at 6 months and crawled at 8 months; she also fed herself a cookie at 8 months. Yet, by 9 months, the babbling decreased. Her parents banged pans behind her, and she did not respond.

When her parents took Amy to the pediatrician, he, too, was concerned because she did not turn toward a loud bell noise. Otherwise, Amy's physical examination was normal. The pediatrician referred her to an audiologist. Testing revealed that Amy had a hearing loss of 90 dB across all frequencies in both ears. Her parents were distraught, but they were determined to help her. They were referred to a speech pathologist, who began a total communication approach with Amy.

By 2 years of age, Amy was able to communicate using many signs and gestures. At 5 years of age, she was in a special class for children with hearing impairment. Psychological testing showed an IQ of 120. She learned mathematics quickly and drew beautifully. Reading was much more difficult. Although she had a rich language of gestures and signs, her speech remained unintelligible. As she grew up, Amy became quite proficient in the use of her own communication methods.

PROGNOSIS

How successfully children like Amy will function is determined both by the severity of their hearing loss and by the presence of other disabilities (Mencher & Gerber, 1983). Most cases of hearing loss are unassociated with mental retardation or other developmental disabilities. For these children, the extent of their hearing problem and when it occurred are critical. Normally, children with conductive hearing losses do well. These children often attend college and have professional careers. They are able to communicate verbally and to understand speech with the use of a hearing aid. This is also true of children who have moderate-to-severe sensorineural losses.

For children with profound sensorineural hearing losses, the prognosis is different. Rarely can these children speak clearly. The one exception to this is the child who loses hearing after 3 years of age when he or she has already learned to talk. However, even this child will lose some speech skills. For children who are deaf from birth, the problem involves difficulty both in communication and in reasoning. The thinking pattern of the deaf child appears different from that of children who can hear. Education for these children must take this into account. For example, although deaf children may do well in mathematics and science, reading will remain a difficult task. Even bright deaf children may not be able to read beyond a sixth-grade level by the time they graduate from high school (Ballantyne, 1977).

SUMMARY

Among the senses, hearing is equaled only by vision in its importance to our understanding of the world around us. A hearing deficit, therefore, is a major disability. Hearing losses may be conductive, involving the outer or middle ear, or sensorineural, affecting the cochlea or auditory nerve. A hearing loss can range from mild to profound and may be unilateral or bilateral. Such a loss may exist alone or be part of a multiply handicapping condition. Defining the type of loss is important for treatment.

If a hearing loss is an isolated disability, the affected child tends to do well. This is true even for the profoundly deaf child, provided he or she is identified early and develops alternative methods of communication.

REFERENCES

Abramovich, S.J., Gregory, S., Slemick, M., et al. (1979). Hearing loss in very low birthweight infants treated with neonatal intensive care. *Archives of Disease in Childhood, 54,* 421–426.

Ackerman, B.D., Dyer, G.Y., & Leydorf, M.M. (1970). Hyperbilirubinemia and kernicterus in small premature infants. *Pediatrics, 45,* 918–925.

American Academy of Pediatrics. (1978). Use of acoustic impedance measurement screening for middle ear disease in children. *Pediatrics, 62,* 570–573.

American Academy of Pediatrics. Joint Committee on Infant Hearing. (1982). Position statement 1982. *Pediatrics, 70,* 496–497.

Assael, B.M., Parini, R., & Rusconi, F. (1982). Ototoxicity of aminoglycoside antibiotics in infants and children. *Pediatric Infectious Disease, 1,* 357–365.

Ballantyne, J. (1977). *Deafness* (3rd ed.). London: Churchill-Livingstone, Inc., 1977.

Bergman, I., Hirsch, R.P., Fria, T.J., et al. (1985). Cause of hearing loss in the high-risk premature infant. *Journal of Pediatrics, 106,* 95–101.

Bess, F.H. (Ed.). (1977). *Childhood deafness: Causation, assessment and management.* New York: Grune & Stratton.

Bess, F.H. (1982). Children with unilateral hearing loss. *Journal of the Academy of Rehabilitative Audiology, 15,* 131–144.

Bess, F.H., & McConnell, F.E. (1981). *Audiology, education and the hearing impaired child.* St. Louis: C.V. Mosby Co.

Bess, F.H., Peek, B.F., & Chapman, J.J. (1979). Further observations on noise levels in infant incubators. *Pediatrics, 63,* 100–106.

Bess, F.H., & Tharpe, A.M. (1984). Unilateral hearing impairment in children. *Pediatrics, 74,* 206–216.

Bluestone, C.D. (1982). Otitis media: To treat or not to treat. *New England Journal of Medicine, 306,* 1399–1404.

Boothroyd, A.L. (1982). *Hearing impairments in young children.* Englewood Cliffs, N.J.: Prentice-Hall.

Downs, M., & Blager, F.B. (1982). The otitis prone child. *Journal of Developmental and Behavioral Pediatrics, 3,* 106–113.

Eavey, R.D., Gao, Y.-Z., Schuknecht, H.F., et al. (1985). Otologic features of bacterial meningitis of childhood. *Journal of Pediatrics, 106,* 402–407.

Echeverria, P., Fina, D., Norton, S., et al. (1978). Ototoxicity of gentamicin: Clinical experience in a children's hospital. *Chemotherapy, 24,* 267–271.

Finitzo-Hieber, T. (1982). Auditory brainstem response: Its place in infant audiological evaluations. *Seminars in Speech, Language and Hearing, 3,* 76–87.

Fior, R., & Veljak, C. (1984). Late results and complications of tympanostomy tube insertion for prophylaxis of recurrent purulent otitis media in pediatric age. *International Journal of Pediatric Otorhinolaryngology, 8,* 139–146.

Fitzzaland, R.E., & Zink, G.D. (1984). A comparative study of hearing screening procedures. *Ear and Hearing, 5,* 205–210.

Friel-Patti, S., Finitzo-Hieber, T., Conti, G., et al. (1982). Language delays in infants associated with middle ear disease and mild fluctuating hearing impairment. *Pediatric Infectious Disease, 1,* 104–109.

Gebhart, D.E. (1981). Tympanostomy tubes in the otitis media prone child. *Laryngoscope, 91,* 849–866.

Gerber, S.E., & Mencher, G.T. (Eds.). (1978). *Early diagnosis of hearing loss.* New York: Grune & Stratton.

Glorig, A., & Roberts, J. (1977). *Hearing levels of adults by age and sex*. Series 11, No. 11. U.S. Vital and Health Statistics. Bethesda, MD: National Center for Health Statistics.

Gopalakrishna, A., Goleria, K.S., & Raje, A. (1984). Middle ear function in cleft palate. *British Journal of Plastic Surgery, 37*, 558–565.

Gumpel, S.M., Hayes, K., & Dudgeon, J.A. (1971). Congenital perceptive deafness: Role of intrauterine rubella. *British Medical Journal, 2*, 300–304.

Hodgson, W.R., & Skinner, P.H. (1981). *Hearing aid assessment and use in audiological habituation* (2nd ed.). Baltimore: Williams & Wilkins Co.

Hubbard, T.W., Paradise, J.L., McWilliams, B.J., et al. (1985). Consequences of non-remitting middle-ear disease in early life: Otologic, audiologic, and developmental findings in children with cleft palate. *New England Journal of Medicine, 312*, 1529–1534.

Jacobson, J.T., Morehouse, C.R., & Johnson, M.J. (1982). Strategies for infant auditory brain stem response assessment. *Ear and Hearing, 3*, 263–270.

Jerger, J. (Ed.). (1984). *Pediatric audiology*. San Diego: College-Hill Press.

Klein, J.O. (1984). Otitis media and the development of speech and language. *Pediatric Infectious Disease, 3*, 389–391.

Konigsmark, B.W., & Gorlin, R.J. (1976). *Genetic and metabolic deafness*. Philadelphia: W.B. Saunders Co.

Lass, N.J., McReynolds, L.V., Northern, J.L., et al. (1982). *Speech, language, and hearing*. Philadelphia: W.B. Saunders Co.

Leske, M.C. (1981). Prevalence estimates of communicative disorders in the U.S. Language, hearing, and vestibular disorders. *ASHA, 23*, 229–237.

MacDonald, J.T., & Feinstein, S. (1984). Hearing loss following hemophilus influenzae meningitis in infancy. Diagnosis by evoked response audiometry. *Archives of Neurology, 41*, 1058–1059.

Mencher, G., & Gerber, S. (1980). *Early management of hearing loss*. New York: Grune & Stratton.

Mencher, G.T., & Gerber, S.E. (Ed.). (1983). *The multiply handicapped hearing impaired child*. New York: Grune & Stratton.

Mizrahi, E.M., & Dorfman, L.J. (1980). Sensory evoked potentials: Clinical application in pediatrics. *Journal of Pediatrics, 97*, 1–10.

Northern, J.L., & Downs, M.P. (1984). *Hearing in children* (3rd ed.). Baltimore: Williams & Wilkins Co.

Olson, A.L., Klein, S.W., Charney, E., et al. (1978). Prevention and therapy of serous otitis media by oral decongestant: A double-blind study in pediatric practice. *Pediatrics, 61*, 679–684.

Palfry, J.S., Hanson, M.A., Pleszczynska, C., et al. (1980). Selective hearing screening for young children. *Clinical Pediatrics, 19*, 473–477.

Paradise, J.L. (1980). Otitis media in infants and children. *Pediatrics, 65*, 917–943.

Paradise, J.L. (1982). Tympanometry. *New England Journal of Medicine, 307*, 1074–1076.

Roeser, R.J., & Downs, M.P. (1981). *Auditory disorders in school children*. New York: Thieme-Stratton.

Rubin, M. (Ed.). (1976). *Hearing aids: Current developments and concepts*. Baltimore: University Park Press.

Rutter, M., & Martin, J.A.M. (1972). *The child with delayed speech*. Philadelphia: J.B. Lippincott Co.

Seewald, R.C., Ross, M., & Spiro, M.K. (1985). Selecting amplification characteristics for young hearing-impaired children. *Ear and Hearing, 6*, 48–53.

Shannon, D.A., Felix, J.K., Krumholz, A., et al. (1984). Hearing screening of high-risk newborns with brainstem auditory evoked potentials: A follow-up study. *Pediatrics, 73*, 22–26.

Stein, L., Ozdamar, O., Kraus, N., et al. (1983). Follow-up of infants screened by auditory brainstem response in the neonatal intensive care unit. *Journal of Pediatrics, 103*, 447–453.

Steele, M.W. (1981). Genetics of congenital deafness. *Pediatric Clinics of North America, 28*, 973–980.

Stockard, J.E., Stockard, J.J., Kleinberg, F., et al. (1983). Prognostic value of brainstem auditory evoked potentials in neonates. *Archives of Neurology, 40*, 360–365.

Thiringer, K., Kankkunen, A., Liden, G., et al. (1984). Perinatal risk factors in the aetiology of hearing loss in preschool children. *Developmental Medicine and Child Neurology, 26*, 799–807.

Thompson, M.D., & Swisher, M.V. (1985). Acquiring language through total communication. *Ear and Hearing, 6*, 29–32.

Wong, D., & Shah, C.P. (1979). Identification of impaired hearing in early childhood. *Canadian Medical Association Journal, 121*, 529–532.

Chapter 17

Speech and Language
Development and Disorders

with Sarah W. Blackstone

Upon completion of this chapter, the reader will:
—be able to define language and its different elements
—be aware of the normal development of speech and language in childhood
—understand the pathways of language in the brain
—know the main types of speech and language disorders
—recognize treatment approaches to speech and language disorders

---

Language is a code, a means of representing ideas using symbols. It is the major way we communicate with each other and is the primary skill that distinguishes human beings from lower animals. In young children, language is the best predictor of future intellectual functioning. A delay in the normal development of language may be a symptom of many disorders including mental retardation, cerebral palsy, language disorders, hearing impairment, and autism (Waterhouse & Fein, 1982). Such a delay should lead to early consultation between the child's pediatrician and a speech-language pathologist and audiologist. In this chapter, language development and the diagnosis and treatment of language and speech disorders are discussed.

THE DEVELOPMENT OF LANGUAGE

Through communication, we relate our needs and desires to those around us. While speech is our primary means of expression, gestures, facial expressions, and body language are all forms of communication. Before language develops, children

Sarah W. Blackstone, Ph.D., is Chief of Speech-Language Pathology at The Kennedy Institute for Handicapped Children in Baltimore and is an instructor in rehabilitation medicine at The Johns Hopkins University School of Medicine.

communicate using a variety of behaviors including crying, vocalizing, pointing, looking, and moving (De Villiers & De Villiers, 1978). In early infancy, a child grunts and cries. Parents interpret these vocalizations as expressions of discomfort, contentment, pain, or hunger. By 3 months, the infant is cooing and seems to be experimenting with the range of sounds that can be made. Oral motor skills continue to develop, and by 6 months of age, the child can better control jaw, tongue, and lip movements; this enables him or her to expand the repertoire of sounds. The child now makes consonant sounds and a variety of vowel sounds; he or she babbles.

Along with the expanding means to produce sounds is an ability to interpret patterns of sounds (Lass, McReynolds, Northern, et al., 1982). As a result, methods of communication gradually become more sophisticated and specific. A 1-month-old infant starts to differentiate speechlike sounds from other environmental noises (Bloom & Lahey, 1978). By 9 to 12 months, he or she will anticipate having a bath after hearing the water running. The child may even associate the word "bath" with that event. He or she is becoming a communicator as well as a listener (Stark, Tallal, Kallman, et al., 1983).

Expressive language evolves simultaneously with the understanding of language, called *receptive language*. By 11 months of age, the child understands a few familiar words. At 15 months, he or she responds to simple spoken commands. Sounds are combined to describe or request an object, to get attention, or to refuse to participate; the vocabulary expands. From this point, language progresses rapidly so that by 2 years of age, a child normally has learned how to communicate using a linguistic system (Bloom & Lahey, 1978).

PRINCIPLES OF LANGUAGE

Language has three components: *form, content,* and *use* (Bloom & Lahey, 1978). The form of language is its structure. In school, we learn about the form of language when we study grammar and **phonics**. Form is further broken down into **phonemes**, **morphemes**, and **syntax**. The phoneme is the smallest unit of sound that distinguishes one utterance from another. The vowel and consonant sounds are phonemes. The morpheme is the smallest unit of meaning, for instance, the -s at the end of the word that makes it plural or the -ed that denotes past tense. Syntax refers to the order in which words are put together to make phrases and sentences—for example, "We studied this problem" versus "This problem was studied by us."

Clearly, these elements relate closely to the meaning of language, the study of which is called *semantics*. It is our knowledge of the meaning of words that allows us to communicate effectively. A conversation that is completely accurate in syntax but devoid of meaning has little, if any, communicative value. An example of language that has form but no content is *echolalia,* where a person repeats automatically what is said to him or her without attaching any meaning to it.

Finally, how one uses language in a social context is important. Questions and statements can be posed simply and directly, or they may be obscure and roundabout, never getting to the point. Different language is used in different settings. For instance, one talks with friends in one way and in another way in a job interview. Proper use of language is needed for communication to impart information precisely and appropriately.

AN ADULT NEUROPATHOLOGICAL MODEL OF LANGUAGE

The brain mechanisms involved in language remain somewhat of a mystery. Most of what is known about these mechanisms comes from the neuropathological studies of brains of adults who have suffered strokes. Strokes cause damage to specific areas of the cortex. By correlating the loss of certain brain tissue with various language impairments, a model of language has been developed. Whether this model is correct for adults remains uncertain (Brown, 1972). Furthermore, one cannot extrapolate from this model to describe the development of normal language in children. Within these constraints, the neuropathological model provides some understanding of how the brain may process language.

In the adult brain, different regions seem to be primarily involved in expressive and receptive language (Manter, Gatz, Gilman, et al., 1982). Expressive language is controlled in the left frontal lobe in Broca's area (Figure 17.1). Receptive language is centered in Wernicke's area, located in the left temporal lobe. Connecting these two regions is a nerve tract called the **arcuate fasciculus** (see Figure 17.1).

During a conversation, the brain may work something like this. When a phrase is heard, impulses are sent along the auditory pathway to Wernicke's area, where they are interpreted. If a response is needed, signals are passed through the arcuate fasciculus to Broca's area. Here the correct words and phrases are formed and sent on to the motor strip, which controls the muscles of speech.

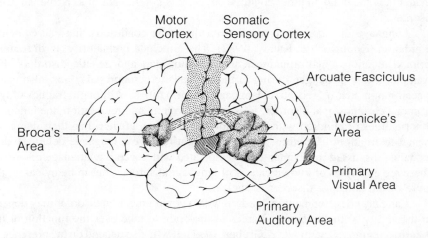

Figure 17.1.   An adult neuropathological model of language. Sounds are received in Wernicke's area and passed on to Broca's area via nerve fibers of the arcuate fasciculus. Expressive language is formed here, and the motor cortex is then stimulated to produce speech.

Damage to the language pathway may not only affect speech and understanding, it may also interfere with writing and reading. For writing, the stimulus is passed back to the visual area of the occipital lobe, where a visual pattern is formed. The visual image then goes to Broca's area, where the word is synthesized, and to the motor strip, where the word is spelled out. In reading, the reverse route is likely. The stimulus first comes to the occipital lobe and is passed on to the language areas of the temporal lobe. Thus, damage to the language pathway may affect all language-related activities, including speaking, understanding, writing, spelling, and reading.

In more than 90% of people, the control of language rests in the left hemisphere of the brain (Segalowitz & Gruber, 1977). This is why a stroke that affects the blood supply to the left cerebral hemisphere impairs language, while a stroke on the right side leaves language intact. Following a stroke, the deficit in language, called *aphasia,* is often permanent because of the loss of brain tissue. However, a person may gradually be better able to communicate over time as he or she recovers and learns how to compensate.

Although the cortex is where the spoken message originates, the actual control of speech resides in the brain stem. Here the mouth and tongue movements of articulation are directed. A message passes from the cortex to the motor neurons of the brain stem that activate the tongue and the mouth. An abnormality in the brain stem can lead to the various speech disorders that are discussed later in this chapter.

ETIOLOGY OF CHILDHOOD LANGUAGE PROBLEMS

Language problems can be divided into language delays and language disorders, which include communication and speech disorders. The most common cause of language delay is mental retardation (see Chapter 14). Unless the language delay is greater than the delay in other cognitive areas, it is not thought of as a true language disorder.

Language disorders may result from the same conditions that cause mental retardation (Knobeloch & Kanoy, 1982). These include prematurity, birth trauma, serious infections, malformations, and chromosomal and genetic disorders. For example, a loss of oxygen during birth that leads to cerebral palsy may also cause speech-motor and/or receptive language abnormalities. Although fragile-X syndrome, a chromosomal disorder, is associated with mental retardation, the language abnormalities of children with this syndrome are often greater than their degree of mental retardation. Therefore, they are thought to have a language delay. Hydrocephalus, discussed in Chapter 12, is associated with receptive language disorders. These are examples of known causes of language disorders, but in many cases, the cause of the language disorder is unclear.

Language development in children with a communication disorder may depend on the ability of the undamaged areas of the brain to take over the function of the abnormal regions (Segalowitz & Gruber, 1977). It will also depend on the presence or absence of other handicapping conditions as well as environmental and educational influences. The role of the speech and language pathologist is to identify the strengths and weaknesses of the child's communication skills and to plan appropriate therapy.

LANGUAGE DISORDERS IN CHILDHOOD

Language disorders include abnormalities in speech and in the expression and understanding of language (Ludlow, 1980). When both a child's expressive and receptive language are significantly delayed compared to other developmental milestones, he or she is said to have a *communication disorder*. This term is used to describe this disorder both in children with normal intelligence and in children with mental retardation (Kamhi & Johnston, 1982). Thus, a 4-year-old who has normal gross motor, visual-perceptual, and nonverbal cognitive skills, but whose language is at a 2-year-old level has a communication disorder. Likewise, an 8-year-old child with mental retardation whose reasoning abilities are at a 4-year-old level, but whose language ability is at a 2-year-old level, also has a language disorder.

Speech Disorders

Speech disorders can be isolated disabilities or part of a more complex developmental disorder such as cerebral palsy. Speech disorders are divided into problems of *articulation, rhythm,* and *resonance*. They may also include speech-motor problems.

Articulation problems are by far the most common speech disorder, occurring in 3% of all children (Fein, 1983; Mysak, 1976). Usual causes of articulation disorders include hearing loss and cleft palate. To articulate well, a child must progress through a series of milestones. For example, the "b" sound is spoken before the "t," and the "sh" and "th" sounds are some of the last sounds to be mastered. Normally, children are producing all of these sounds by 3 years of age (Van Dyke, Yeager, McInerney, et al., 1984). Most children who have articulation problems tend to improve without any treatment. However, the persistence of such problems indicates an articulation disorder (Sanders, 1972). Articulation disorders include the substitution of sounds ("wabbitt" for "rabbit"), the omission of sounds ("boo" for "book"), the addition of sounds ("ananamal" for "animal"), and the distortion of sounds.

Much less common, with an incidence of 0.7% of children, are defects in the rate and rhythm of speaking (Wilson, 1979). Stuttering is one example and is often seen in children with mental retardation or learning disabilities. However, it may also occur in an otherwise normal individual. In stuttering, the child's speech consistently has an abnormal rhythm, with hesitations, explosive words, and repetitions. The child's articulation, however, is normal. The stuttering becomes worse when the child is excited or anxious.

A defect in voice production is the least common speech disorder and affects only about 0.2% of children (Travis, 1971). The quality of speech is altered. Speech is either too low pitched, too high pitched, too loud, or too soft. A nodule on a vocal cord may affect voice resonance, making it low and raspy.

Finally, speech-motor disorders, classified both as speech and as expressive language disorders, include **dysarthria** and speech **dyspraxia**. In dysarthria, the child's articulation is impaired because of poor muscle control. Extrapyramidal cerebral palsy is often associated with dysarthria. In this form of cerebral palsy, areas of the brain that normally control speech-motor activity are damaged. On the other hand, in dyspraxia, there is no muscle damage or weakness. Yet, the child has trouble positioning the structures involved in speech—for instance, the tongue, lips, pharynx—and has difficulty producing phonemes (Aram & Horwitz, 1983).

For all types of speech disorders, speech therapy is invaluable. In some cases, such as cleft palate, surgery also may be necessary to improve speech. In most instances, speech defects affect development less than communication disorders do. However, a child whose speech dysfunction is so severe that it interferes with his or her ability to communicate will also experience developmental problems.

Communication Disorders

When an individual has difficulty expressing him- or herself despite having adequate speech abilities, that person has an *expressive language disorder* (Silva, 1980). If the processing of language is abnormal, he or she has a *receptive language disorder* (Flower, 1981). When the communication disorder is profound and is associated with mental retardation and bizarre behavior, the child has what is called *infantile autism*, discussed in Chapter 18.

Expressive Language Disorders The classic example of an expressive language disorder is the adult who becomes aphasic after a stroke. If the person is able to speak at all, the speech is slow and labored; articulation is primitive. Sentences are spoken in a telegraphic style—for example, "coffee—hot—burn." In addition, the person has difficulty finding words. For instance, he or she may be shown a key and asked, "What is this?" Rather than answering with the right word, the individual responds with a description, "Open door, metal, round." Yet, when given a choice of words, he or she will invariably choose "key" (Brown, 1972).

A child's expressive language problems are different from those of an adult, both in cause and characteristics. Such problems range from mild, in children with learning disabilities, to severe, as in developmental aphasia. A child with learning disabilities seems to acquire expressive language according to developmental norms. Yet, subtle deficits emerge. Such a child may talk in circles and be verbose; he or she may have difficulty using language properly and accurately. For example, instead of asking for a glass of water when thirsty, the child with learning disabilities might ask if there is water in the house. The listener then has to interpret what the child means. In other words, the child lacks a complete functional use of language (Bishop, 1979).

When a child has developmental aphasia, he or she has problems with syntax, semantics, and the flow of language. Often, articulation is normal, but the development of speech is significantly delayed (Bloom & Lahey, 1978). Children who have been in a coma after suffering severe head trauma, usually after a car accident, may exhibit a secondary form of aphasia. These children generally improve significantly, although many are left with mild expressive language problems for years after their accident (Johnston & Mellitis, 1980).

Receptive Language Disorders In this group of disorders, understanding of language is impaired. The classic example is the adult who has suffered damage in Wernicke's area and develops receptive aphasia. This person is unable to process the information he or she hears. Although this individual will speak with the correct rhythm, grammar, and articulation, he or she will not be able to carry on a conversation.

In children, receptive language disorders range from mild, in children with learning disabilities, to moderate, in children with hearing impairment and in those with hydrocephalus, to profound in deaf and autistic children. An isolated receptive language disorder is rare; it is usually accompanied by some expressive language problem (Lass, McReynolds, Northern, et al., 1982). For example, the expressive component of a language disorder in children with learning disabilities may be a delay in learning certain grammatical forms such as the verb "to be," while in a child with hydrocephalus, speech might consist of "cocktail party language" (Bloom & Lahey, 1978). In the latter case, the child's speech, although articulate, lacks meaning or, at best, is only slightly related to the subject. A deaf child, who cannot hear sounds and has a severe receptive language problem, will also have impaired expressive language.

DIAGNOSIS

Early identification of speech and language disorders is essential to avoid frustrating the child and to facilitate early treatment (Nation & Aram, 1984). When a child does not progress through the developmental milestones for language but develops normally in other areas, he or she may have a communication disorder. Such milestones include babbling at 6 months, producing single words by 12 months, having a 5-word vocabulary by 20 months of age, and being able to speak 2-word phrases after 24 months and sentences after 3 years. Also, inability to distinguish verb tenses or to tell one's experiences after 5 years of age indicates a noteworthy delay in language development.

As is true of mental retardation, a language disorder may be diagnosed early on in a severely affected child, while it may be missed for many years in a child with milder deficits. A thorough developmental history, with special attention paid to language milestones, is helpful in making the diagnosis (see Table 14.1 in Chapter 14). Mild articulation delays are only evident after the child is at least 4 years old.

To evaluate the form, use, and content of language, a number of tests are available. Communication is very complex, and no single test adequately evaluates all the components. Some commonly used tests are discussed next.

Among the language screening tests used by pediatricians is the Clinical Linguistic and Auditory Milestones Scale (CLAMS), which lists 1–3 tasks that should be accomplished at each month of development between 2 and 24 months of age (Capute & Accardo, 1978). Another screening scale for young children is the Receptive-Expressive Emergent Language (REEL) Scale, which evaluates the child's verbal abilities through a parent interview. For older children, it is advisable to use a battery of standardized tests to assess different areas of language abilities. These abilities include: 1) understanding and expressing single words; 2) comprehending and using grammar and syntax; 3) handling language as it increases in complexity and length, and 4) reading and writing.

To evaluate these items, certain tests are used (Wodrich, 1984). One of these is the Illinois Test of Psycholinguistic Abilities (ITPA). This includes a battery of tests that assesses a multitude of language abilities (see Chapter 20). Another test, the Wepman Auditory Discrimination Test, asks the child to discriminate between the sounds of two similar words. The Peabody Picture Vocabulary Test (PPVT) deals with single-word recognition. And, finally, the verbal subtests of the various IQ tests—for example, the Wechsler Preschool and Primary Scale of Intelligence (WPPSI) and the Stanford-Binet Intelligence Scale—measure some aspects of language comprehension and use. Using these tests combined with an interview and direct observation of a child's communication patterns, a speech-language pathologist can obtain a profile of a child's strengths and weaknesses.

SPEECH AND LANGUAGE THERAPY

Once identified, a child who has a speech and language disorder needs an individualized treatment program aimed at his or her developmental level. This program must be integrated with the other educational, physical, and occupational therapy needs of the child. For most children, treatment results in improved speech and language; rarely is a cure possible. Treatment approaches are varied and complex. The goals of therapy are to teach the child to use existing language more effectively and to provide other techniques to compensate for any remaining deficits.

Some of the approaches used to treat speech disorders include articulation therapy, the neurodevelopmental approach, the motor-kinesthetic approach, and biofeedback techniques. In articulation therapy, the child is trained to produce phonemes, words, phrases, and sentences. The child practices by repeating sounds; learning theory is used in this form of treatment. For children with an isolated articulation disorder, this approach works well. It is less effective, however, in children with multiple handicaps—for example, those with cerebral palsy, a severe hearing loss, or mental retardation (Blackstone & Painter, 1985).

For children with cerebral palsy, the neurodevelopmental approach developed by Bobath and Bobath (1972) is more effective. The purpose here is to inhibit the persistent primitive reflexes (see Chapter 21) and to facilitate normal movement. Improvement in muscle tone and in neuromuscular control benefits speech as well as gross motor activity. A motor-kinesthetic approach aims to enhance oral and speech-motor movements (Mysak, 1980) so that accuracy and speed are improved.

Biofeedback techniques are used to give immediate feedback on errors or successes when a child is learning speech sounds. These are combined with other teaching techniques to reinforce the correct formation of these sounds.

For the treatment of expressive and receptive language disorders, some combination of language facilitation and direct teaching of vocabulary, grammar, and language usage seems to work best (Conant, Budoff, & Hecht, 1983; Conant, Budoff, Hecht, et al., 1984; Lombardino & Mangan, 1983; Ochs & Schieffelin, 1979).

Children with severe communication impairments may require alternative means of communication, such as manual signing, communication boards, or computer synthesized speech (Ferry & Cooper, 1978). These additional tools are also helpful for children with severe retardation who may be frustrated by their lack of speech. A few functional signs can enable these children to communicate daily needs, such as hunger, a wish to go outside, and so forth. Communication boards (Figure 17.2) and computers have been particularly helpful for the neurologically impaired person. These aids help the child to interact more effectively with those around him or her and may provide significant educational and vocational benefits.

SUMMARY

The spectrum of language disorders ranges from mild speech defects to severe communication disorders that affect both expressive and receptive language. Children with other developmental disabilities such as cerebral palsy, hydrocephalus, and learning disabilities also tend to have speech and language problems. Early identification is important to facilitate the beginning of effective treatment and to allow the child to develop fully.

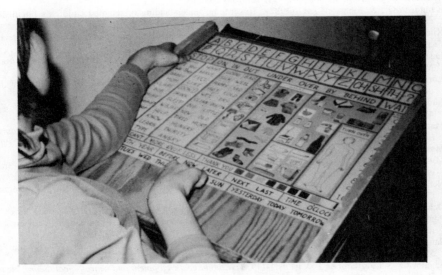

Figure 17.2.   A communication board is being used by a child with cerebral palsy. A combination of pictures, letters, and words is used to allow the child to communicate with others.

REFERENCES

Aram, D.M., & Horwitz, S.J. (1983). Sequential and non-speech praxic abilities in developmental verbal apraxia. *Developmental Medicine and Child Neurology, 25,* 197–206.

Bishop, D.V.M. (1979). Comprehension in developmental language disorders. *Developmental Medicine and Child Neurology, 21,* 225–238.

Blackstone, S.W., & Painter, M.J. (1985). Speech problems in multihandicapped children. In J.K. Darby (Ed.), *Speech and language evaluation in neurology: Childhood disorders.* New York: Grune & Stratton.

Bloom, L., & Lahey, M. (1978). *Language development and language disorders.* New York: John Wiley & Sons.

Bobath, K., & Bobath, B. (1972). The neurodevelopmental approach to treatment. In P.H. Pearson & C.E. Williams (Eds.), *Physical therapy services in the developmental disabilities.* Springfield, IL: Charles C Thomas.

Brown, J.W. (1972). *Aphasia, apraxia, and agnosia: Clinical and theoretical aspects.* Springfield, IL: Charles C Thomas.

Capute, A.J., & Accardo, P.J. (1978). Linguistic and auditory milestones during the first 2 years of life. A language inventory for the practitioner. *Clinical Pediatrics, 17,* 847–853.

Conant, S., Budoff, M., & Hecht, B. (1983). *Teaching language-disabled children. A communication games intervention.* Brookline, MA: Brookline Press/Books.

Conant, S., Budoff, M., Hecht, B., et al. (1984). Language intervention: A pragmatic approach. *Journal of Autism and Developmental Disorders, 14,* 301–317.

De Villiers, J.G., & De Villiers, P.A. (1978). *Language acquisition.* Cambridge, MA: Harvard University Press.

Fein, D.J. (1983). The prevalence of speech and language impairments. *ASHA, 25,* 37.

Ferry, P.C., & Cooper, J.A. (1978). Sign language in communication disorders of childhood. *Journal of Pediatrics, 93,* 547–552.

Flower, R.M. (1981). Neurodevelopmental disorders in childhood. In J.K. Darby (Ed.), *Speech evaluation in medicine.* New York: Grune & Stratton.

Johnston, R.B., & Mellitis, E.D. (1980). Pediatric coma: Prognosis and outcome. *Developmental Medicine and Child Neurology, 22,* 3–12.

Johnston, R.B., Stark, R.E., Mellitis, E.D., et al. (1981). Neurological status of language-impaired and normal children. *Annals of Neurology, 10,* 159–163.

Kamhi, A.G., & Johnston, J.R. (1982). Towards an understanding of retarded children's linguistic deficiencies. *Journal of Speech and Hearing Research, 25,* 435–445.

Knobeloch, C., & Kanoy, R.C. (1982). Hearing and language development in high risk and normal infants. *Applied Research in Mental Retardation, 3,* 293–301.

Lass, N.J., McReynolds, L.V., Northern, J.K., et al. (Eds.). (1982). *Speech, language, and hearing: Normal processes and clinical disorders.* Philadelphia: W.B. Saunders Co.

Lombardino, L., & Mangan, N. (1983). Parents as language trainers: Language programming with developmentally delayed children. *Exceptional Children, 49,* 358–361.

Ludlow, C.L. (1980). Children's language disorders: Recent research advances. *Annals of Neurology, 7,* 497–507.

Manter, J.T., Gatz, A.J., Gilman, S., et al. (1982). *Manter and Gatz's essentials of clinical neuroanatomy and neurophysiology* (6th ed.). Philadelphia: F.A. Davis Co.

Mysak, E.D. (1976). *Pathologies of speech systems.* Baltimore: Williams & Wilkins Co.

Mysak, E.D. (1980). *Neurospeech therapy for the cerebral palsied: A neuroevolutional approach.* (3rd ed.). New York: Teachers College Press, Columbia University.

Nation, J.E., & Aram, D.M. (1984). *Diagnosis of speech and language disorders* (2nd ed.). San Diego: College-Hill Press.

Ochs, E., & Schieffelin, B. (Eds.). (1979). *Developmental pragmatics.* New York: Academic Press.

Poulton, K.T., & Algozzine, B. (1980). Manual communication and mental retardation: A review of research and implications. *American Journal of Mental Deficiency, 85,* 145–152.

Sanders, E.K. (1972). When are speech sounds learned? *Journal of Speech and Hearing Disorders, 37,* 55–63.

Segalowitz, S.J., & Gruber, F.A. (Eds.). (1977). *Language development and neurological theory.* New York: Academic Press.

Silva, P.A. (1980). The prevalence, stability, and significance of developmental language delay in preschool children. *Developmental Medicine and Child Neurology, 22,* 768–777.

Stark, R.E., Tallal, P., Kallman, C., et al. (1983). Cognitive abilities of language-delayed children. *Journal of Psychology, 114,* 9–19.

Travis, L.E. (Ed.). (1971). *Handbook of speech pathology and audiology.* Englewood Cliffs, NJ: Prentice-Hall.

Van Dyke, D.C., Yeager, D.J., McInerney, J.F., et al. (1984). Speech and language disorders in children. *American Family Physician, 29,* 257–268.

Waterhouse, L., & Fein, D. (1982). Language skills in developmentally disabled children. *Brain and Language, 15,* 307–333.

Wilson, D.K. (1979). *Voice problems of children* (2nd ed.). Baltimore: Williams & Wilkins Co.

Wodrich, D.L. (1984). *Children's psychological testing: A guide for nonpsychologists.* Baltimore: Paul H. Brookes Publishing Co.

Chapter 18

Autism

Upon completion of this chapter, the reader will:
—be able to define autism
—understand the characteristics of this disorder
—know how to distinguish autism from other developmental disabilities
—be acquainted with the various treatment approaches to this disorder

Autism, a rare disorder that occurs in about 4 in 10,000 children, has been the focus of considerable study (American Psychiatric Association, 1980; Lotter, 1966). Perhaps this attention has been prompted by the bizarre behavior of autistic children, or possibly it is attributable to the frequent confusion of autism with the more common forms of mental retardation that have autistic characteristics (Capute, Derivan, Chauvel, et al., 1975). Many have questioned whether autism is a distinct entity. This chapter reviews the characteristics of autism and the attempts at treatment.

For a child to be diagnosed as having "infantile autism," the onset of the disorder must occur before he or she is 30 months of age (American Psychiatric Association, 1980). In a child with autism, thinking, language, and behavior are all disturbed (DeMyer, 1982). The disorder is about two to four times more common in males than females (Schwartz & Johnson, 1981), and there is also a genetic influence. A 2% risk of having autism exists in the siblings of an autistic child (Folstein & Rutter, 1977).

IDENTIFICATION OF AUTISM

Dr. Leo Kanner at The Johns Hopkins Hospital first described infantile autism in 1943. He identified a group of children who exhibited symptoms that isolated them from their environment, and who either had abnormal language or did not speak at all. He noted that these children did not bond to their mothers and treated people as objects, rarely making eye contact. In addition, they required such a sameness in their environment that even a minor change—for example, the repositioning of a chair—threw them into a rage. Self-stimulatory and self-injurious behaviors, such as spinning, rocking, and head banging, were common. At times, the children appeared to be deaf, not responding to commands or loud noises. Their play was repetitive and stereotyped, with little genuine use of toys and other objects (Kanner, 1943). Dr. Kanner decided to call this collective group of symptoms *infantile autism*.

Since the identification of this syndrome, there has been an evolution in the way it is perceived. In the 1950s, the psychosocial aspect of these children's lives was emphasized. Parental problems received a great deal of attention, and parents were often told they were responsible for the child's problems. Now, autism tends to be viewed mainly as a severe language disorder associated with brain damage.

CHARACTERISTICS OF AUTISM

In general, autistic children have a language disorder, display abnormal intellectual and neurological functioning, exhibit bizarre behaviors, and have impaired social interactions.

Language Disorder

In autistic children, language is both delayed and deviant, and both expressive and receptive communication are affected (Ferrari, 1982). About half of these children remain mute throughout their lives and may even be unable to use gestures or signs to communicate (Schwartz & Johnson, 1981). Those who do develop language do not use it effectively. Their voices are often high pitched and strange sounding. They tend to use language in a very stereotyped, rote fashion, exhibiting excellent memorization skills but actually communicating very little, if any, meaning. They tend to repeat phrases (echolalia) and long commercial jingles. It may seem that they are understanding what they are saying, but they are usually simply parroting what they have heard. Rarely is an autistic child able to compose a spontaneous sentence that has meaning to him or her or to others. Despite good articulation and an adequate vocabulary, these children have a more severe expressive language disorder than the children discussed in Chapter 17. Receptive language is also affected. Autistic children may respond to brief, memorized phrases, but they find it very difficult to understand more complex commands. They learn better with visual rather than auditory cues. Thus, these children appear to have a form of global aphasia that affects all aspects of their language and communication (Bettelheim, 1967).

Intellectual and Neurological Functioning

Most autistic children have mental retardation, although the extent of retardation varies. About 40% of these children have IQs below 50 (American Psychiatric Association, 1980; Rutter, 1983; Schwartz & Johnson, 1981). Less than 10% score in the normal range on nonverbal intelligence tests (Baker, 1983). Some studies have shown a low level of abstract or symbolic reasoning ability, while rote memory skills are good. To add to the puzzle, some of the children have amazing isolated skills. For example, they may be able to assemble complex puzzles, multiply as quickly as pocket calculators, and read the *New York Times* with expression but no understanding.

In addition to intellectual impairment, neurological abnormalities often exist. The electroencephalogram is unusual in half of these children, and 20% have seizures (Rutter & Schopler, 1978). Computerized brain scans (CT scans) often show evidence of atrophy or shrinkage, primarily in the language regions of the brain (Campbell, Rosenbloom, Perry, et al., 1982; Damasio, Maurer, Damasio, et al., 1980). Gross motor skills are usually intact.

Bizarre Behaviors

The autistic child often exhibits behavior that is uncommon or nonexistent in normal children or in children with other developmental disabilities (Freeman, Ritvo, Tonick, et al., 1981). For example, as already mentioned, the child often has a tantrum when any change is made in the environment, however small. In addition, the child with autism is often very attached to some specific, inanimate object. For instance, he or she might insist on carrying around a string, blanket, or rubber band at all times (American Psychiatric Association, 1980). Often, these children exhibit ritualistic hand movements or other rhythmic movements such as rocking. They may suddenly cry or laugh with no apparent cause. Sometimes they also display self-injurious behavior such as head-banging or eye-gouging. Finally, they frequently have eating problems and refuse food or eat only one or a few kinds of food.

Social Interactions

One of the most outstanding characteristics of autistic children is their social isolation (Cantwell, Baker, & Rutter, 1979). As infants, autistic children do not seem to enjoy being held or cuddled. They neither respond to nor appreciate the feelings and needs of others (Rutter & Schopler, 1978; Schwartz & Johnson, 1981). The autistic child actively avoids contact with strangers and family members alike. Socially, therefore, the autistic child is very awkward and ill at ease.

CAUSES OF AUTISM

Theories have abounded as to the causes of infantile autism. They have ranged from inherited metabolic defects to maternal neglect. Most of these theories remain unsupported. For example, studies of twins suggest that heredity plays some role in this disorder, while studies that initially showed all parents of autistic children to be cold and unemotional have proved to be incorrect (Knobloch & Pasamanick, 1975). What does seem likely is that these children are brain damaged. The incidence of prematurity, birth trauma, and central nervous system infections is very high in autistic children. Also, some patients with untreated PKU (phenylketonuria) and fragile-X syndrome (Blomquist, Bohman, Edvinsson, et al., 1985) have been diagnosed as autistic. This suggests a possible link between metabolic and chromosomal disorders and autism. Thus, the same problems that lead to mental retardation and cerebral palsy may also produce autism (Lobascher, Kingerlee, & Gubbay, 1970) by damaging certain areas of the brain.

DISTINGUISHING AUTISM FROM OTHER DEVELOPMENTAL DISABILITIES

Since treatment and prognosis vary according to the diagnosis, it is important to distinguish autism from other developmental disabilities. The most common disorders that are mistaken for autism are mental retardation, childhood psychiatric disorders, sensory impairments, and degenerative nervous system disorders.

Considering the generally low IQ scores of these children, one could legitimately ask whether autism is not simply another form of mental retardation. Yet, the combination of social isolation, bizarre behavior, and language disorder makes it distinguishable from mental retardation. The autistic child remains narcissistic, like a newborn infant. He or she does not maintain eye contact and treats everyone, even parents, as objects. On the other hand, the child with severe retardation, while often displaying self-stimulatory behaviors and other autistic features, shows affection and interest in others, especially parents.

A second distinguishing feature is language. Unlike the autistic child, a child with retardation usually has an equal delay in language and visual-perceptual skills. Yet, an autistic child may have wondrous memory skills and be very agile while remaining mute (American Psychiatric Association, 1980; O'Connor & Hermelin, 1967).

Comparing incidence, the child with severe retardation and autistic features outnumbers the child with infantile autism by more than 10 to 1 (Capute, Derivan, Chauvel, et al., 1975). Yet, many children with severe retardation, who have some autistic features, are misdiagnosed as being autistic. For example, when Capute, Derivan, Chauvel, and colleagues (1975) applied the Clancy Scale of Autistic Features (Clancy, Dugdale, & Rendle-Short, 1969) to a randomly selected group of 200 children with severe mental retardation, 48 of these children had enough autistic features to be designated autistic, but only one of them actually had infantile autism.

In addition to children with mental retardation having some autistic characteristics, children with psychiatric disorders such as pervasive developmental disorder and **schizophrenia** may also present similar symptoms (American Psychiatric Association, 1980; Creak, 1963). Pervasive developmental disorder involves the presence of sudden excessive anxiety, disturbances in affect, resistance to change, and self-injurious behavior. Although this disorder shares a number of the characteristics of autism, its onset is later, occurring between the ages of 30 months and 12 years of age. In comparing autism to schizophrenia, one finds noticeable differences. Whereas the autistic child shows a lack of imagination, the schizophrenic child may live in a fantasy world. Also, autistic children do not have the hallucinations and delusions found in children with schizophrenia (Rapoport & Ismond, 1984). In addition, schizophrenic children do not usually have mental retardation.

Children with sensory impairments may also show autistic features. Children who are blind and those who have hearing impairment often exhibit self-stimulatory behavior and poor interpersonal interactions. However, they lack the global language disorder that distinguishes autistic children, and their intelligence is usually normal. In these children, when their sensory function improves, the autistic features disappear. This makes it extremely important for the vision and hearing of children with autistic behaviors to be tested before their diagnosis is confirmed.

Finally, a group of degenerative nervous system diseases may initially be misdiagnosed as autism. These are extremely rare disorders with an incidence of about 1 in 30,000 (Menkes, 1985). Children with these disorders develop normally in infancy and then start to lose skills and fall behind. By 2 years of age, most have severe retardation. By 5, most have died. Tay-Sachs disease is one example of this group. Early in the course of Tay-Sachs disease, the child may have autistic features. The real diagnosis, however, becomes tragically apparent over a few months as the child continues to regress, losing both gross motor and language skills. By the time of death, the child is usually in a severely debilitated state, being deaf, blind, and unable to move.

TREATMENT OF AUTISM

Once a child is identified as having infantile autism, the next question is how to treat that child. The large number and variety of treatment approaches illustrate that no one approach has been found to be entirely satisfactory. Inadequate therapies have ranged from the administration of megavitamins to psychotherapy, with a whole range of treatments in between. At present, an interdisciplinary treatment program seems to be most helpful (Bachrach & Swindle, 1984; Rutter, 1985; Wing, 1985). This includes an appropriate educational placement, language therapy, behavioral modification, parental support, and possibly medication.

The educational program should be suited to the child's cognitive abilities (Everard, 1976; Koegel, Rincover, & Egel, 1982). Most autistic children do not do well as part of a regular class. Although specific schools and classes for autistic children exist, many of these children will learn effectively in a public school special education class with children who function at similar mental ages. The environment should be very structured, and instructions must be very simple.

A speech and language pathologist is most helpful for treating the language disorder in these children (Conant, Budoff, Hecht, et al., 1984). Stimulating the development of language is important, but the child may also need to learn alternative forms of communicating. Signing and communication boards may improve expression and behavior.

To help the child improve social skills and to decrease the incidence of self-injurious behaviors, behavior modification techniques are used. Behavioral techniques have included time-out and overcorrection procedures (see Chapter 14).

The value of medication is controversial. Often, antipsychotic drugs such as Mellaril or Haldol are given to decrease the child's bizarre behavior (Campbell, Anderson, Meier, et al., 1978). In one study of autistic children, Haldol resulted in a significant decrease in behavioral symptoms and improved retention of learned tasks (Anderson, Campbell, Grega, et al., 1984). Recently, the use of fenfluramine, a neurochemical that was initially developed to help people lose weight, has been suggested for the treatment of autism (August, Raz, & Baird, 1985; Ritvo, Freeman,

Yuwiler, et al., 1984). Fenfluramine works for weight control because it affects serotonin, a neurochemical that is involved with our feelings of hunger. Some autistic children have increased levels of serotonin in their blood. In a pilot study, Ritvo, Freeman, Yuwiler, et al. (1984) found that treatment with this drug decreased hyperactivity, increased social awareness, and improved communication in a group of 14 autistic children. Fenfluramine is currently considered an experimental drug for the treatment of autism.

Although psychotherapy for the autistic child is rarely possible because of his low intelligence and poor communication skills, counseling for other family members is important. This may help to decrease their anxiety and guilt feelings and assist them in coping more effectively (see Chapter 24).

KENNY, A CHILD WITH AUTISM

Kenny had problems from birth. He was premature and suffered hypoglycemia and respiratory distress syndrome during the first weeks of life. He was hospitalized for 2 months, and when he came home, he was neither alert nor active. His early development was delayed, and his parents were quite concerned that Kenny would have mental retardation. Soon, his motor development picked up. He sat up by 8 months and walked by 15 months. His parents became hopeful that he had suffered no brain damage. He also showed good visual-perceptual skills, being able to put together simple puzzles by 2 years of age and to build intricate block towers by 2½.

Yet, his parents remained concerned about his language, behavior, and relationships with other people. By 2 years of age, he neither spoke nor consistently followed one-step commands. He was a loner. He showed no interest in playing with other children and barely acknowledged his parents. He also would not allow anyone to hold him. Kenny exhibited no warmth and maintained no eye contact with others. He had many strange, ritualistic behaviors. He spun around, rocked, and constantly played with a string. He would fly into a rage when the furniture was moved or when he was placed in a new situation.

By 4 years of age, Kenny had developed some language, but it was very strange. He had an extraordinary memory for numbers and commercials. He would constantly carry a detergent bottle around the house singing its advertising jingle, and he would endlessly repeat strings of numbers. However, he still basically communicated with no one. He could not follow two-step commands and spoke in only one- or two-word phrases. More often than not, he pointed to what he wanted.

At this time, psychological testing was performed. Kenny's IQ was 37, indicating he functioned around the level of an 18-month-old. However, he could build block towers and solve puzzles at a 4-year-old level. Because of his strange behavior, withdrawal, and reactions of rage, he was referred to a child psychiatrist. These symptoms, combined with good gross motor and visual-perceptual skills and severe mental retardation, led to a diagnosis of infantile autism. His parents, in a sense, were relieved. At last they had a diagnosis, some place to start.

Even more important, Kenny was enrolled in a treatment program. He received the drug, Haldol, to decrease his anxiety. His reactions of rage decreased. He entered a special school program where language and other reasoning skills were taught at an 18-month-old level. Behavior modification techniques were used to help Kenny with new social situations and to reduce his self-stimulatory behavior. At the same time, Kenny's parents received counseling from a social worker, and they instituted a behavior modification program set up by a behavioral psychologist.

By 6 years of age, Kenny had improved substantially. He could now form three-word sentences, and the automatic repetition of words decreased. His behavior was better, and he could be brought into new situations without difficulty. Even with this progress, however, on repeated psychological tests, his IQ stayed about the same.

Kenny has been able to remain at home; he has made progress. Yet, it is unlikely he will ever be self-sufficient. He will continue to function as a child with severe mental retardation. In addition, his bizarre behavior will persist, making it more difficult for society to accept him.

PROGNOSIS

For some reason, parents seem to prefer the diagnosis of autism to that of mental retardation. Perhaps it carries less of a stigma and somehow suggests the hope of a cure. Unfortunately, this is not true. Usually, the autistic child has a worse prognosis than the child with mental retardation with the same IQ (Gillberg, 1984; Knobloch & Pasamanick, 1975; Rutter, Greenfeld, & Lockyer, 1967; Schopler & Mesibov, 1983).

In follow-up studies of autistic children, fewer than 5% were found to function effectively in society and to hold a paying job as an adult. Approximately half ended up institutionalized (Rutter, Greenfeld, & Lockyer, 1967). As adults, individuals with autism do lose some of their aberrant behavior patterns. Yet, vestiges of the autism remain. If speech has not developed by 6 years of age, it is unlikely to develop later.

SUMMARY

Autism appears to be a distinct syndrome. Its principal characteristics are a global language disorder, abnormal behavior patterns, social isolation, and, usually, mental retardation. The causes are many and unclear. Differentiation from other disabilities such as mental retardation, psychiatric illness, sensory impairments, and progressive neurological disorders is essential for proper therapy to be possible. Therapy consists of an interdisciplinary approach with psychiatry, pediatrics, speech pathology, behavioral psychology, and social work all playing a role. At this point, the value of medication is uncertain. Prognosis is generally poor. The children with the best hope for the future are those with the higher IQ scores. As adolescents and adults, the bizarre behavior becomes less apparent.

REFERENCES

American Psychiatric Association. (1980). *Diagnostic and statistical manual of mental disorders (DSM III)* (3rd ed.). Washington, DC: American Psychiatric Association.

Anderson, L.T., Campbell, M., Grega, D.M., et al. (1984). Haloperidol in the treatment of infantile autism: Effects on learning and behavioral symptoms. *American Journal of Psychiatry, 141,* 1195–1202.

August, G.J., Raz, N., & Baird, T.D. (1985). Brief report: Effects of fenfluramine on behavioral, cognitive and affective disturbances in autistic children. *Journal of Autism and Developmental Disorders, 15,* 97–107.

Bachrach, A.W., & Swindle, F.L. (1984). *Developmental therapy for young children with autistic characteristics.* Austin: PRO-ED.

Baird, T.D., & August, G.J. (1985). Familial heterogeneity in infantile autism. *Journal of Autism and Developmental Disorders, 15,* 315–321.

Baker, A.F. (1983). Psychological assessment of autistic children. *Clinical Psychology Review, 3,* 41–59.

Bettelheim, B. (1967). *The empty fortress: Infantile autism and the birth of the self.* New York: Free Press.

Blomquist, H.K., Bohman, M., Edvinsson, S.O., et al. (1985). Frequency of the fragile X syndrome in infantile autism. A Swedish multicenter study. *Clinical Genetics, 27,* 113–117.

Campbell, M., Anderson, L.T., Meier, M., et al. (1978). A comparison of haloperidol and behavior therapy and their interaction in autistic children. *Journal of American Academy of Child Psychiatry, 17,* 640–655.

Campbell, M., Rosenbloom, S., Perry, R., et al. (1982). Computerized axial tomography in young autistic children. *American Journal of Psychiatry, 139,* 510–512.

Cantwell, D.P., Baker, L., & Rutter, M. (1979). Families of autistic and dysphasic children. I. Family life and interaction patterns. *Archives of General Psychiatry, 36,* 682–687.

Capute, A.J., Derivan, A.T., Chauvel, P.J., et al. (1975). Infantile autism. I: A prospective study of the diagnosis. *Developmental Medicine and Child Neurology, 17,* 58–62.

Clancy, H., Dugdale, A., & Rendle-Short, J. (1969). The diagnosis of infantile autism. *Developmental Medicine and Child Neurology, 11,* 432–442.

Conant, S., Budoff, M., Hecht, B., et al. (1984). Language intervention: A pragmatic approach. *Journal of Autism and Developmental Disorders, 14,* 301–317.

Creak, E.M. (1963). Childhood psychosis: A review of 100 cases. *British Journal of Psychiatry, 109,* 84–89.

Damasio, H., Maurer, R.G., Damasio, A.R., et al. (1980). Computerized tomographic scan findings in patients with autistic behavior. *Archives of Neurology, 37,* 504–510.

DeMyer, M.K. (1979). *Parents and children in autism.* Washington, DC: V.H. Winston.

DeMyer, M.K. (1982). Infantile autism: Patients and their families. *Current Problems in Pediatrics, 12,* 1–52.

DeMyer, M.K., Hingtgen, J.N., & Jackson, R.K. (1981). Infantile autism reviewed: A decade of research. *Schizophrenia Bulletin, 7,* 388–451.

Everard, M.P. (Ed.). (1976). *An approach to teaching autistic children.* Oxford, NY: Pergamon Press.

Ferrari, M. (1982). Childhood autism: Deficits of communication and symbolic development. I. Distinctions from language disorders. *Journal of Communication Disorders, 15,* 191–208.

Folstein, S., & Rutter, M. (1977). Infantile autism: A genetic study of 21 twin pairs. *Journal of Child Psychology and Psychiatry, 18,* 297–321.

Freeman, B.J., Ritvo, E.R., Tonick, I., et al. (1981). Behavior observation system for autism: Analysis of behaviors among autistic, mentally retarded, and normal children. *Psychological Reports, 49,* 199–208.

Gillberg, C. (1984). Autistic children growing up: Problems during puberty and adolescence. *Developmental Medicine and Child Neurology, 26,* 125–129.

Gillberg, C., & Svendsen, P. (1983). Childhood psychosis and computed tomographic brain scan findings. *Journal of Autism and Developmental Disorders, 13,* 19–32.

Greenfeld, J. (1978). *A place for Noah.* New York: Holt, Rinehart & Winston.

Harris, S.L., Handleman, J.S., & Palmer, C. (1985). Parents and grandparents view the autistic child. *Journal of Autism and Developmental Disorders, 15,* 127–139.

Kanner, L. (1943). Autistic disturbances of affective contact. *Nervous Child, 2,* 217–250.

Kanner, L. (1971). Follow-up study of 11 autistic children originally reported in 1943. *Journal of Autism and Childhood Schizophrenia, 2,* 119–145.

Knobloch, H., & Pasamanick, B. (1975). Some etiologic and prognostic factors in early infantile autism and psychosis. *Pediatrics, 55,* 182–191.

Koegel, R.L., Rincover, A., & Egel, A.L. (1982). *Educating and understanding autistic children.* San Diego: College-Hill Press.

Lobascher, M.E., Kingerlee, P.E., & Gubbay, S.S. (1970). Childhood autism: An investigation of aetiological factors in 25 cases. *British Journal of Psychiatry, 117,* 525–529.

Lotter, V. (1966). Epidemiology of autistic conditions in young children. I. Prevalence. *Social Psychiatry, 1,* 124–137.

Menkes, J.H. (1985). *Textbook of child neurology* (3rd ed.). Philadelphia: Lea & Febiger.

O'Connor, N., & Hermelin, B. (1967). Auditory and visual memory in autistic and normal children. *Journal of Mental Deficiency Research, 11,* 126–131.

Paluszny, M.J. (1979). *Autism: A practical guide for parents and professionals.* Syracuse, NY: Syracuse University Press.

Rapoport, J.L., & Ismond, D.R. (1984). *DSM-III training guide for diagnosis of childhood disorders.* New York: Brunner/Mazel.

Ritvo, E.R., Freeman, B.J., Yuwiler, A., et al. (1984). Study of fenfluramine in outpatients with the syndrome of autism. *Journal of Pediatrics, 105,* 823–828.

Rutter, M. (1983). Cognitive deficits in the pathogenesis of autism. *Journal of Child Psychology and Psychiatry, 24,* 513–531.

Rutter, M. (1985). The treatment of autistic children. *Journal of Child Psychology and Psychiatry, 26,* 193–214.

Rutter, M., Greenfeld, D., & Lockyer, L. (1967). A five to fifteen year follow-up study of infantile psychosis. II. Social and behavioural outcome. *British Journal of Psychiatry, 113,* 1183–1199.

Rutter, M., & Schopler, E. (Eds.). (1978). *Autism: A reappraisal of concepts and treatment.* New York: Plenum Press.

Schopler, E., & Mesibov, G. (1983). *Autism in adolescents and adults.* New York: Plenum Publishing Corp.

Schwartz, S., & Johnson, J.H. (1981). *Psychopathology of childhood: A clinical-experimental approach.* New York: Pergamon Press.

Steffen, J.J., & Karoly, P. (Eds.). (1982). *Autism and severe psychopathology.* Lexington, MA: Lexington Books.

Webster, C.D., & Konstantareas, M. (Eds.). (1980). *Autism: New directions in research and education.* New York: Pergamon Press.

Wing, L. (1985). *Autistic children: A guide for parents and professionals* (2nd ed.). New York: Brunner/Mazel.

Chapter 19

Attention Deficit Disorder and Hyperactivity

Upon completion of this chapter, the reader will:
—be able to define attention deficit disorder
—recognize some of the problems associated with this syndrome
—understand what is known about the various causes of hyperactivity
—know the different approaches to treatment

When a child has a short attention span coupled with hyperactivity, it is exhausting for both the family and the child. These types of difficulties are symptoms rather than diseases and are common to many different disorders. A child may have attention deficit disorder with hyperactivity (ADD-H) or without (ADD) as a primary condition. Or these symptoms might occur because of brain damage, an emotional disturbance, a hearing deficit, or mental retardation. This chapter focuses mainly on children diagnosed as having ADD and ADD-H and discusses the treatment and prognosis for these children.

MATTHEW: A HYPERACTIVE CHILD

The story of Matthew provides a typical illustration of a child with attention deficit disorder with hyperactivity. Matthew was the third child in his family. Although the labor and delivery were uncomplicated, Matthew, as an infant, did not feed well. He would suck greedily at his mother's breast for a few minutes and then lose interest. He did not like being held or cuddled, and he slept fitfully. During the first 3 months of his life, Matthew had colic, crying as if in pain after each feeding. He was a cranky, unhappy infant.

Developmentally, Matthew reached the various milestones at normal times, although his development was somewhat slower than that of his two siblings. Both his sister and his brother had spoken in phrases by 2 years of age, but Matthew did not do this until several months later.

By the time he was 2 years old, Matthew's parents were quite concerned about his marked hyperactivity. He was not merely curious; he was a terror, running aimlessly from one room to the next. He would pull out all the pots and pans, tear the curtains, and write on the walls. Matthew would cover three or four rooms in a matter of minutes, wrecking each as he passed through. His parents, always worn out, nicknamed him "The Little Hurricane."

As he grew up, Matthew knew no fears. He could not be left alone, even for a few moments. He was just as likely to turn on the stove as he was to run outside and cross the street without looking. Matthew also hated sharing things. He showed little interest in playing cooperatively and was easily frustrated in his dealings with other children. He was soon recognized as a loner.

In first grade, Matthew failed academically. His handwriting was messy, and many letters were reversed. He did not know the alphabet. His memory for numbers was poor, and he frequently forgot lessons he had just been taught. Socially, he was ostracized by the other children, who called him "retarded." At home, he did no better. He was constantly punished for his uncontrollable behavior and poor school performance. Matthew was unhappy most of the time and had many mood swings.

Fortunately, at the end of the first grade, Matthew was evaluated for a special education placement. On the Wechsler Intelligence Scale for Children–Revised (WISC–R), Matthew scored a verbal IQ of 105 and a performance IQ of 85. A neurological examination showed clumsiness and other "soft neurological signs" (discussed later in this chapter). Special education testing found visual-perceptual problems and a scattering of scores ranging from a 4- to a 7-year-old level. Matthew was particularly poor at remembering numbers and instructions that were spoken to him. His ability to pay attention was markedly decreased. Also, it was clear Matthew had a poor self-image and expected to fail at anything he tried.

The sum of this information led to a diagnosis of attention deficit disorder with hyperactivity and the beginning of a coordinated effort to help Matthew. The treatment program involved: 1) enrollment in a small, self-contained learning disability class, 2) behavior modification therapy, and 3) stimulant medication. The results of this effort are reviewed later in this chapter.

WHAT IS ATTENTION DEFICIT DISORDER?

Matthew's problem has been called by many names: *minimal cerebral dysfunction, minimal brain damage, minimal cerebral palsy, hyperactive child syndrome,* and *attention deficit disorder with hyperactivity.* As is often the case, these large terms mask a scarcity of knowledge. ADD is a symptom complex rather than a disease. In other words, it represents a group of symptoms that receive a specific label when they occur together. The value of this label is its use in deciding on a treatment program.

As already noted, ADD can occur either with or without hyperactivity. The overall incidence of ADD is at least 8% and that of ADD-H about 3% (American Psychiatric Association, 1980). As a toddler, the child with ADD-H is in constant motion, getting into everything from dawn to dusk (Kohler, Kohler, & Regefalk,

1979). The child remains hyperactive as he or she grows older. In elementary school, the child fidgets so much in the chair that he or she often falls out of it. The child will walk around the classroom and disrupt the other students. This hyperactivity frequently decreases or disappears by adolescence.

In ADD and in ADD-H, the child also has a decreased attention span. Unlike the hyperactivity, this persists throughout life. The child moves from one project to another, rarely staying with one task any longer than 5–10 minutes. In school, he or she has trouble concentrating on work, is easily distracted, does not seem to listen, and often fails to finish tasks (Rapoport & Ismond, 1984). This short attention span makes it difficult for the child to follow more than one command at a time.

Associated with poor attention are perceptual problems that further hinder school performance (Figure 19.1). Generally, the child with ADD or ADD-H has widespread learning problems that are apparent in all subjects. He or she may reverse letters, have poor penmanship and spelling, and find it difficult to trace letters. The combination of hyperactivity, poor attention span, and auditory and visual-perceptual learning problems causes the child to fail in school.

These learning difficulties are compounded by the child's poor impulse control and low tolerance of frustration. Children with ADD or ADD-H are often impulsive in everything they do. They are quick to anger and get into frequent fights. Because of their impulsiveness, these children are prone to accidents and injuries. In learning situations, they are also reckless and will take a wild guess at a word after simply looking at the first letter. Gradually, as they continue to have difficulty learning, they cease trying.

To compound their sense of frustration, many of these children do poorly in physical activities because of their clumsiness. Upon physical examination, a physician finds so-called soft neurological signs (Rapoport & Ismond, 1984). For example, the child might not be able to stand on one foot without falling, or he or she may have a hard time distinguishing the right from the left hand or moving the fingers of one hand while keeping the fingers of the other hand still. Left-handedness is more

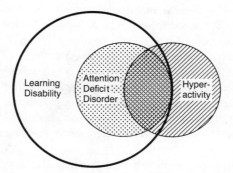

Figure 19.1.   Interrelationships between attention deficit disorder, learning disabilities, and hyperactivity. All children with ADD have learning disabilities; some are also hyperactive. However, not all children with hyperactivity or learning disabilities have ADD.

common in these children than in the general population. These difficulties indicate impaired coordination and make the child appear clumsy.

Thus, children with ADD or ADD-H are beset with many difficulties. They may think of themselves as being "retarded" because they have such difficulty in school. They also fail in social relationships and in physical activities such as sports. And they receive little encouragement at home because of their hyperactive and aggressive behavior. Eventually, these children develop a poor self-concept, expect to fail at anything they try, and stop trying (Weiss & Hechtman, 1979).

Yet, these children do have good potential. Although they may develop at a slightly slower pace than other children, their intelligence falls within the normal range or may even be superior. Often, however, this may not be apparent because of their wide variability of performance in different areas of intellectual functioning. This is in contrast to an average child's IQ test results, which are usually similar in each area that is tested. For example, ADD-H children often receive the lowest scores on the subtests that require close attention and concentration such as arithmetic coding, information, and digit span. Yet, they may do well on verbal tasks such as comprehension. On the WISC–R, therefore, such a child may have a 20-point or more discrepancy between the verbal and performance areas. Educational testing of these children helps to reveal their current level of academic achievement, areas of strengths and weaknesses, and how they respond to various teaching techniques. The results of these tests help special educators to develop a school program that can best meet the needs of the child.

CAUSES AND INCIDENCE OF ADD

Exactly what causes ADD is unknown. Sometimes, there is a genetic component (Safer, 1973). For example, the father of an ADD child may have done poorly in school and may have been hyperactive as a child. It is known that ADD occurs much more frequently in boys than in girls (American Psychiatric Association, 1980). Also, ADD is more of a problem in upper middle class families who have high academic expectations than it is in families who do not have such expectations (Johnson & Prinz, 1976; Lambert, Sandoval, & Sassone, 1978). This disorder is not seen in developing countries.

Although the term *minimal brain damage* has been used to describe this disorder, children with ADD do not usually have a history of birth trauma or brain damage. However, certain conditions may predispose a child to develop this disorder. Premature infants and those who are small for gestational age seem to be most likely to have ADD. Other risk factors include prenatal exposure to excessive alcohol (Abel, 1984), exposure to lead after birth (Bellinger & Needleman, 1983), and brain infections.

In addition to not knowing exactly what causes ADD, little is understood about the brain mechanisms that underlie this syndrome. The following is known. The area of the brain called the **reticular activating system/locus ceruleus** helps control attention (Kalat, 1976; Raskin, Shaywitz, Shaywitz, et al., 1984). It works by screening out distracting sounds and images so we can concentrate on a particular task. For example, a person in a theater is able to listen to his or her neighbor's conversation only when he or she blocks out the conversations of the other people. In a similar way, a child can learn effectively only if he or she pays attention to the teacher and is not distracted by every other image that comes into his or her line of vision. In effect, the reticular activating system puts "mental blinders" on a person, allowing him or her to pay attention. As is true of every other part of the brain, the stimulation of this system requires neurochemicals. Recent research suggests that children with ADD have neurochemical deficits (Shaywitz, Cohen, & Shaywitz, 1978). This underlies the rationale for using amphetamines to treat ADD, since these drugs may modify these abnormalities.

OTHER CAUSES OF HYPERACTIVITY

Before discussing the various treatment approaches for ADD, it is important to note that there are other disorders connected with hyperactivity besides ADD. For example, children who have mental retardation may also be hyperactive. In this instance, the combination of hyperactivity, short attention span, impulsive behavior, frustration intolerance, and poor school performance is associated with an IQ below 70. Generally, medications used to treat children with ADD are less effective in treating children with mental retardation who are also hyperactive.

Inattentiveness and hyperactivity may also be apparent in a child who has a seizure disorder. Here, the problem behavior occurs either when excessive seizure activity is going on or as a side effect of an anticonvulsant medication. A child who has poorly controlled seizures will be inattentive both during the seizure and for a while after it. Reactions to toxic levels of phenobarbital or to any other anticonvulsant may include behavior problems. Twenty percent of the children who take phenobarbital to control their seizures become hyperactive (Livingston, 1972).

Children with hearing impairment may also be hyperactive or have other behavior problems. These problems may be due to some form of brain damage or result from an inadequately corrected or undiagnosed hearing impairment.

Finally, children with psychiatric disorders are sometimes hyperactive. These children are the most difficult to differentiate from children with ADD, because their symptoms are extremely similar. However, in psychological testing, children with psychiatric problems do not have the variability of scores that children with ADD do, and no soft neurological signs are evident. Also, while children with ADD may have emotional problems related to their poor self-image and insecurity, the child with a psychiatric disorder usually has more severe symptoms that may include overwhelming anxiety, quick mood swings, and lack of responsiveness to others.

DIAGNOSIS OF ADD AND ADD-H

Unfortunately, no test exists that specifically diagnoses ADD or ADD-H. Brain wave tests, called electroencephalograms or EEGs, are mildly abnormal in about half of these children, but these alterations are also seen in about a quarter of normal children (Caresia, Pugnetti, Besana, et al., 1984). Computerized brain scans have failed to reveal any abnormalities (Shaywitz, Shaywitz, Byrne, et al., 1983). As mentioned earlier, soft neurological signs often exist, but their absence does not rule out the possibility of this disorder (Camp, Bialer, Sverd, et al., 1978; Gillberg, 1985). Finally, psychological testing may show a significant discrepancy between verbal and visual-perceptual performance; educational testing usually reveals evidence of attention problems and a learning disability. Ultimately, the diagnosis of ADD relies on the exclusion of the other diagnoses noted above and the presence of the clinical symptoms of attention deficit, impulsivity, and, often, hyperactivity. Proper diagnosis is important because the diagnosis dictates the type of therapy used.

TREATMENT OF ADD

Treating children with ADD normally demands a combination of approaches, including a special education program, behavior modification, medication, and counseling. These approaches are discussed separately below. Controversial approaches have included the use of a special diet and other drugs and vitamins; these are considered briefly.

Educational Approach

An appropriate school placement and program are extremely important in the treatment of a child with ADD. Children with ADD have learning disabilities that are accentuated by their hyperactivity, impulsiveness, and decreased attention span (Strauss & Lehtinen, 1955). There is no substitute for a well-trained and caring teacher who will provide special help to a child and a program suited to his or her needs. Assistance in the form of structured or self-contained special education classrooms and resource help may also be necessary.

Behavior Modification Techniques

One of the most effective approaches to treating ADD-H appears to be behavior modification. This method involves consistent management, a structured environment, and the reinforcement of appropriate behavior along with the discouragement of inappropriate behavior.

The basic premise in behavior modification is that behavior is controlled by its consequences. Thus, if a behavior results in a reward, it will occur with a greater frequency in the future. If the behavior is unrewarded, it is less likely to recur. This premise leads to three basic methods of controlling behavior: reinforcement, punishment, and extinction.

Reinforcement In reinforcement, one tries to increase the frequency of a desirable behavior. As is true in all behavior modification techniques, this is done by establishing the relationship between a certain behavior and the events that follow that behavior (Craighead, Kazdin, & Mahoney, 1981). Reinforcement may be either positive or negative.

The most effective approach with ADD-H children is positive reinforcement. The example in Figure 19.2A illustrates the way positive reinforcement works. To improve attention in a classroom, a teacher might tell a student to keep his or her eyes on her. If the student does this for a given period of time, he or she is reinforced in some way. The reinforcement might be social in the form of approval or a hug, or it might be material, such as candy or a happy face symbol. Also, an accumulative type of reinforcement may be used. The child may receive a token or a star each time he or she exhibits the desired behavior. Then, after a certain number of tokens are collected, the child can trade them in for a privilege or a gift.

Sometimes, an even more formal type of positive reinforcement, involving an oral or written contract, is used. The child may agree to do certain things—for example, remain in a seat, learn certain mathematical facts, or complete homework assignments. At the end of a week, he or she receives a special reward for adhering to the contract. The child's parents, for instance, might take him or her out to a restaurant or a movie or might buy the child a gift. Such a contract usually runs for a fairly short period of time so that the reinforcement is not too delayed. Because hyperactive children are so infrequently rewarded and so often punished, this approach is especially helpful. Not only does the behavior improve, but the child also learns to succeed.

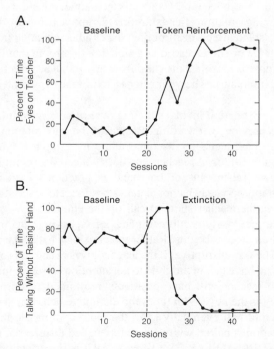

Figure 19.2.   Effects of two behavior modification techniques on changing the frequency of a behavior. A) Positive reinforcement results in an increase in the percentage of time a child keeps his or her eyes on the teacher. B) An extinction procedure results in a decrease in the percentage of time a child talks out of turn.

Contrary to positive reinforcement, negative reinforcement increases the frequency of a desirable behavior by removing an unpleasant consequence. The classic example is the man who forgets to put on an overcoat when he goes outside in 20° weather. When he walks out without a coat, he gets very cold. To avoid this, he puts on the coat. In the future, he is likely to put on his coat each time he goes out into such cold temperatures (Craighead, Kazdin, & Mahoney, 1981). An analogous situation is one in which a hyperactive child is constantly being yelled at by his or her parents and teachers for not sitting still. When the child does sit still for awhile, he or she notices that the screaming stops. Therefore, the youngster may increase the length of time spent sitting still to decrease the amount of yelling. However, this type of reinforcement is less effective than positive reinforcement because the reward is the removal of punishment rather than the gaining of a privilege.

Punishment Punishment differs from reinforcement in that the goal is to reduce the frequency of a behavior rather than increase it, either by the use of adverse consequences or by the withdrawal of positive reinforcement (Bellack & Hersen, 1977).

Punishment, ranging from scolding to spanking, generally does not work well with hyperactive children. It often results in an increase in aggressive behavior, or the child may attempt to physically escape the punishment. This technique is also open to potential abuse by the practitioner. A more effective form of punishment for these children is the time-out procedure. Using this technique, the child is removed from a positively reinforcing situation after exhibiting disruptive behavior. In a modification of the traditional "stand in a corner" routine, the child is separated from opportunities of reinforcement. He or she is placed in a situation or a room that lacks anything of interest. The purpose is to isolate the child from any social activity for a period of not more than 5 to 10 minutes. The youngster is soon ready to reenter the reinforcing social situation.

Extinction Extinction involves the removal of positive reinforcement from a situation that was previously rewarding. Basically, the prior relationship between the behavior and the consequence is disconnected. An example is ignoring disruptive behavior (see Figure 19.2B). A teacher who does not call on a child who consistently speaks out without raising his or her hand is practicing extinction. The child eventually learns appropriate behavior to gain attention. He or she stops speaking out, raises a hand, and the teacher starts to call on the child.

Usually, the previously reinforced behavior (speaking out) initially increases when the extinction process begins. Rather than raising a hand, the child may yell or scream more and be very disruptive. If the teacher gives in and calls on the child at this point, he or she will have taught the child to get attention by screaming and yelling. In other words, the teacher will have positively reinforced inappropriate behavior. Thus, consistency is the key. With time, the disruptive behavior should diminish or disappear. The child will eventually learn the more appropriate thing to do.

Often extinction is paired with a procedure called differential reinforcement of other behaviors (DRO) (O'Leary & O'Leary, 1976). In extinction with DRO, the elimination of the disruptive behavior (talking out of turn) is combined with the positive reinforcement of another and often incompatible behavior (raising the hand).

Because of the added reinforcement, the technique is stronger and more apt to succeed.

How to Implement Behavior Modification Knowing the theory behind behavior modification is simpler than putting it into practice. It is helpful to keep in mind some guidelines. First of all, one must obtain baseline data. The only way of knowing if a procedure works is to have data before the treatment procedure is begun. An initial period of nonintervention should be observed during which one keeps a record of the frequency of the inappropriate behavior (see Figure 19.2). Then, a treatment method is begun. If this method works, and the child's behavior improves, the procedure can then be used on a long-term basis. Another major point is that the technique must be administered consistently and immediately after the inappropriate behavior takes place. This is the only way to guarantee that the child makes the proper connection between the behavior and its consequence (Patterson, 1975).

Shaping and Generalization Often, good behavior does not occur spontaneously. Any child, and especially a hyperactive child, must learn a series of behaviors that make him or her more socially acceptable and better able to learn. These behaviors are acquired in much the same way that a new play in sports is learned. Step by step, a coach goes over the component parts of the play and rewards an athlete when each step is perfected. Eventually, the athlete masters all the steps and combines them into the complete play. This process of teaching behavior step by step is called *shaping*. Shaping can be equally effective with hyperactive children. One rewards the behavior that most closely approximates what is socially acceptable or what improves attention. As this behavior occurs more often, it can be shaped into even more appropriate responses.

Besides shaping, one needs to use techniques that help the child to generalize his or her learned behaviors, transferring them from the school situation to the home, playground, and other environments. By applying the techniques of behavior modification, the teacher and parents can teach the child to continue to be less hyperactive and impulsive and more attentive as he or she moves from one situation to another.

Medication

In the beginning of treatment, the combination of behavior modification and medication may work better than either approach alone. Later, the child may be able to stop taking the drug (Christensen, 1975). The main group of drugs used to treat children with ADD-H is amphetamines. Other less effective drugs include pemoline, antidepressants, and phenothiazines. These drugs are likely to decrease motor activity, impulsivity, and enhance attention, but they will not remedy the other problems associated with ADD—for example, learning disabilities and poor self-image.

Amphetamines It was by chance that amphetamines were first used to treat hyperactivity. In 1937, Dr. Charles Bradley used amphetamines to treat children with various behavior disorders and found that these drugs reduced hyperactivity and increased attention span. Over the next 30 years, the use of amphetamines proliferated. By the late 1960s, one study estimated that about 10% of children attending public schools were taking amphetamines (Krager & Safer, 1974). Not only were amphetamines being prescribed for hyperactivity, but they were also being used in the treatment of many other kinds of behavioral and psychiatric problems. In addition to treatment-related uses, amphetamines were being taken by college students to "pull all-nighters," by truckers to maintain vigilance while driving, and by dieters to curb their appetites. The high levels of misuse eventually led to the passage of federal legislation that classified these drugs as "controlled substances." This legislation also limited the use of amphetamines to the treatment of hyperactivity and narcolepsy, a rare neurological disorder with sudden, uncontrolled bouts of sleeping during the day. Now, fewer than 4% of school children receive amphetamines (Krager & Safer, 1974).

In both hyperactive and normal children, amphetamines reduce the extent of physical activity, decrease impulsivity, and improve the attention span. Although no drug exists that can alleviate all the problems associated with ADD-H, the effects of the amphetamines certainly can give these children some short-term help.

The two most commonly used amphetamines are methylphenidate (Ritalin) and dextroamphetamine (Dexedrine). The usual dosage for Ritalin ranges from 10 to 80 milligrams/day. This may be divided into two or three doses (Shaywitz, Hunt, Jatlow, et al., 1982; Sleator & Von Neumann, 1974; Swanson, Sandman, Deutsch, et al., 1983), or it can be given as a single, time-release tablet. For Dexedrine, the daily dosage is about half that amount and comes as a liquid, tablet, or sustained release tablet. Generally, these drugs begin working within 30 to 45 minutes. The effects of the regular tablets last about 4 hours, and the sustained release type works for 6–8 hours.

As with other drugs, there are side effects, but they are not dangerous. A child may lose his appetite within 30 minutes after taking the medication. (This explains why dieters have used these drugs.) Children may also experience some decrease in weight and height gain during treatment. However, this is followed by a rapid gain of weight and height when the medication is stopped (Kalachnik, Sprague, Sleator, et al., 1982). There is no evidence that amphetamines affect eventual growth outcome (Satterfield, Cantwell, Schell, et al., 1979). Besides the impact on appetite and growth pattern, these drugs may cause insomnia if they are taken within 3 hours of bedtime. In addition, about 10% to 20% of the children who take these drugs develop stomach cramps or irritability (Golinko, 1984).

While these are the known side effects, other potential disadvantages are more difficult to evaluate. One concern is that amphetamines may become "magic pills" for the child. The child may believe that the drug controls behavior and that, consequently, if he or she forgets to take a pill, any naughty behavior can be blamed on the absence of the medicine. It is very important for the child to learn that this is not so and that he or she, not the medication, is responsible for what happens.

Another concern is whether or not the use of amphetamines leads hyperactive children to future drug abuse. Amphetamines have street names such as "speed" and "uppers" and are commonly abused drugs. Most long-term follow-up studies have not supported this concern (Hechtman, Weiss, & Perlman, 1984a, 1984b; Weiss, Kruger, Danielson, et al., 1975). Although amphetamines cause a euphoric effect in normal individuals, they do not produce such a "high" in children with ADD-H. By adolescence, the hyperactivity has usually decreased enough so that this medication is no longer necessary.

Before starting the medication, the pediatrician may use a teacher/parent behavior report to document the problem behaviors. Changes in behavior can then be followed during treatment. To minimize the adverse effects, many physicians suggest that the child be given the medication only on weekdays during the school year. For most children, this works fine. However, for some, the hyperactivity is so severe that the parents cannot handle the child at home without the assistance of the medication (Gadow, 1983). No blanket rule can be written on who should receive these drugs and when. The decision must be made according to the needs of the individual child and the family. However, every year, the child should be given a drug "holiday" to determine if medication is still needed.

Evaluating the long-term benefits of amphetamine treatment is extremely difficult. For the most part, only short-term follow-up has been done. These studies have shown improvement in over 80% of the children treated with this type of medication (Abikoff & Gittelman, 1985). Teachers rated both the children's behavior and their attention span as improved. These children also performed better on visual-motor tasks, such as puzzles and penmanship. The few long-term studies suggest, however, that these benefits may be short-lived (Charles, Schain, & Guthrie, 1979; Milman, 1979; Weiss, Hechtman, Perlman, et al., 1979). In comparing one group of ADD-H children who were treated for 2 years or more with amphetamines with another group not treated with amphetamines, no difference in achievement between the two groups existed 10 years later (Hechtman, Weiss, & Perlman, 1984b; Weiss, Hechtman, Perlman, et al., 1979). However, the medication may have helped the children to be better accepted by their peers and, thus, improved their self-images and their feelings about others.

Trying to assess the merits of these kinds of studies raises numerous questions and problems. Since it is very difficult to match for variables such as severity of hyperactivity or the effect of behavior modification at home, a comparison of results across studies may not be valid. Nonetheless, a number of studies do point out that acute control of hyperactivity and attention does not necessarily ensure academic improvement. One study, in fact, suggests that high levels of stimulants may have an adverse effect on learning (Sprague & Sleator, 1977). In that experiment, investigators measured both the teacher's ratings of the hyperactive children's behavior and the children's actual performance on academic tasks at various doses of amphetamines. They found the higher the dosage of medication, the quieter the child became. Above a certain dosage, however, the child started to slide in academic performance even though he or she was better behaved (Figure 19.3). While a single dose of 0.3 milligrams/kilogram of Ritalin was effective both in improving learning and controlling behavior, a 1.0 milligram/kilogram dose was better for behavior and worse for academic performance. Therefore, the amount of medication must be carefully monitored, with the smallest effective dose possible being the one that is

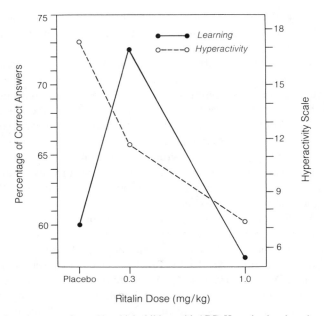

Figure 19.3.   A study was performed in which children with ADD-H received various doses of Ritalin and their degree of hyperactivity and academic performance were measured. At a dose of 0.3 milligrams/kilogram, there was improvement in both hyperactivity and learning compared with a placebo trial. A further increase to 1.0 milligrams/kilogram dose resulted in a further improvement in behavior, but a decline in academic performance. (From Sprague, R.L., & Sleator, E.K. [1977]. Hyperkinetic children: Differences in dose effects on learning and social behavior. *Science, 198,* 1274; reprinted by permission. Copyright © 1977 by the American Association for the Advancement of Science.)

used. Also, these drugs should be given only to children who have documented attention problems and/or hyperactivity and who have not responded adequately to educational and behavior modification techniques.

Pemoline (Cylert)   While amphetamines have been the primary drugs used to treat hyperactivity, another drug, pemoline, is also useful. This drug is completely different in chemical structure from amphetamines and has a longer half-life in the bloodstream. Consequently, it can be given in a single daily dose. It comes as a 37.5-milligram tablet; the child takes anywhere from 37.5 to 150 milligrams daily. Although amphetamines are usually effective right away, pemoline may need to be taken for a few weeks before it has a beneficial effect. It has few side effects other than occasional abdominal discomfort and infrequent liver dysfunction; these side effects cease when one stops taking the medication. However, it is also less effective than amphetamines. Although over 80% of ADD children respond to amphetamines, less than 50% benefit from pemoline (Knights & Viets, 1975). It is primarily used when a child has developed a tolerance to one of the amphetamines, a phenomenon that occurs in about 20% of the children (Conners & Taylor, 1980). In these children, the amphetamine stops working after 6 to 12 months of use. In some cases, switching to another type of amphetamine, for instance, Dexedrine instead of Ritalin, works. In others, pemoline may be useful.

Phenothiazines Phenothiazines are drugs that are used most often to treat psychotic disorders (Biederman & Jellinek, 1984). However, these drugs may also help in the treatment of certain types of hyperactivity. Mellaril, Thorazine, and Stelazine are all phenothiazines; they have a sedating effect and so decrease hyperactivity. However, they also reduce attention span and, thus, interfere with learning. Therefore, phenothiazines are not appropriate therapy for children with ADD-H.

The children for whom these drugs sometimes are useful are hyperactive children who have mental retardation. Sometimes, the extent of hyperactivity in these children is a very difficult problem. Since only 10%–20% of hyperactive children with retardation respond to amphetamines or pemoline, they are given phenothiazines. Half of the children show a decrease in hyperactivity when taking this type of medication (Biederman & Jellinek, 1984).

Treatment with phenothiazines must be handled with great care because they have several side effects. These drugs increase the risk of seizures in patients with epilepsy (Biederman & Jellinek, 1984) and have also been associated with liver dysfunction and excessive weight gain. Prolonged therapy with these drugs may cause a condition called tardive dyskinesia in which a person has continuous restless movements of his or her arms and legs. Most of these side effects are uncommon and disappear once the therapy is stopped. However, tardive dyskinesia may affect a number of the individuals who take phenothiazines for more than 5 years and is generally permanent (Biederman & Jellinek, 1984).

Counseling

Besides behavior modification and the use of medication, counseling both for the child and the family is a key ingredient of the treatment program. A social worker, school counselor, psychologist, or psychiatrist can provide this help and support. The child needs to know he or she is not alone, that there are other children who have similar problems. The child needs to understand what ADD is and that he or she does not have mental retardation. Counseling can provide a place for the youngster—and other family members—to discuss their anxieties, frustrations, questions, and anger. Parents and siblings may need help in understanding the implications of this disorder for their family member and for themselves. Parents may need guidance in how to set limits and how to develop realistic expectations. Everyone in the family can benefit from thoughtful support, encouragement, and information, provided not merely when a crisis hits but on a long-term basis. Just as it is important for the child to know that others have similar problems, families need to understand that they are not alone and are not to blame for their child's disorder.

Controversial Forms of Treatment

The use of other drugs and vitamins as well as the use of a restrictive diet, have been tried for the treatment of ADD. So far, these approaches have not proved effective in treating this disorder.

Other Drugs and Vitamins Other drugs besides amphetamines and pheno-thiazines have been touted for treating hyperactivity. Benadryl, an antihistamine, Tofranil, an antidepressant (Krankowski, 1965), and deanol, an antianxiety medi-cine, have all been used with little success. Caffeine once was proposed as a treatment for hyperactivity, but this, too, failed to work (Rapoport, Berg, Ismond, et al., 1984). Finally, megavitamin therapy was tried. The idea behind this approach was that a vitamin deficiency or an enzyme deficiency that could be corrected with vitamins was responsible for the hyperactivity. However, Haslam, Dalby, & Rademaker (1984) have shown that a vitamin deficiency does not exist and that megavitamin therapy, given in a controlled experiment, has no beneficial effect on hyperactivity or attention. Also, some children who received megavitamin therapy developed abnor-mal liver functioning.

Diet Another approach to the control of hyperactivity is that of changing the child's diet. Dr. Benjamin Feingold proposed that foods containing **salicylates**, sugars, food colors, and other additives led to hyperactivity (Feingold, 1975). He therefore suggested that hyperactive children refrain from eating such foods as almonds, apples, apricots, berries, cherries, cucumbers, grapes, tomatoes, and all products made from these foods (Mayer & Goldberg, 1985). He reported success in half the children he treated with this diet (Feingold, 1975). However, researchers have been unable to reproduce his results under controlled conditions. In these studies, fewer than 10% of the children responded to the Feingold diet (Conners, 1980; Varley, 1984; Wolraich, Milich, Stumbo, et al., 1985). Even though the research has not supported Feingold's results, parents report that trying the diet gives them something to do to attempt to help their child and helps to replace their feelings of helplessness and guilt (Mayer & Goldberg, 1985). It is possible that, by feeling better, parents are more able to cope with their child's problems, and that this may positively affect their child's behavior.

More recently, Egger, Carter, Graham, et al. (1985) used a highly restricted diet—called an "oligoantigenic" diet—to treat ADD-H children. This is a diet that severely limits the intake of substances that are suspected of producing allergic reactions—for example, certain artificial colors and preservatives (Weiss, 1982). About one-third of the children tried on this diet showed improvement. Further research is needed to determine if these types of diets truly hold promise for treating children with hyperactivity.

MATTHEW GROWS UP

Matthew's treatment program was a combination of the various therapies described in this chapter. In first grade, because his hyperactivity was so severe, he began to take Ritalin, 15 milligrams, before school and at lunchtime. His behavior improved. Together, Matthew's teacher and parents outlined a behavior modification program. He also received extra help in reading and mathematics. Within 6 months, Matthew changed from a withdrawn, rather somber child to one who was interested in making friends and attending school.

In physical activities, he had other problems. Since Matthew's clumsiness persisted, it was difficult for him to do well in sports, and the other children teased him. His father took him to special physical education classes to help improve his coordination. There, he met other children with similar problems. This discovery helped Matthew feel less alone and encouraged him to keep trying. He did particularly well in swimming. Even so, he continued to have "two left feet" and to be accident prone over the years.

Matthew continued to receive special resource help throughout his school years. He began to meet regularly with a social worker at school who helped him better understand and cope with his problems and frustrations. His parents frequently participated in these discussions. Some years were better than others. By 12 years of age, he no longer required Ritalin. He was much less hyperactive, but his short attention span and impulsive behavior persisted. He maintained a "C" average. Upon graduation from high school, his reading and math scores were only at the eighth grade level.

Now Matthew is entering the job market. He will make it in society but how well is uncertain. He continues to be at a disadvantage because of his disabilities. Yet he has tasted success and is willing to work hard to make a go of it. Matthew's story may well end happily.

ADD-H CHILDREN AS YOUNG ADULTS

The story of Matthew is typical of many ADD-H children. As adolescents, most of these children become more normal. They are less hyperactive, although they are still impulsive and easily distracted. They often do not attain as high an academic level as normal children do and may change jobs frequently. Some controversy exists about whether these children have a higher incidence of drug abuse, antisocial behavior, and severe psychiatric disorders as adults compared to the normal population (Hechtman, Weiss, & Perlman, 1984a; Satterfield, Hoppe, & Schell, 1982; Weiss, Hechtman, Perlman, et al., 1979). When identification and treatment are begun early, the likelihood of future success improves.

SUMMARY

Attention problems and hyperactivity are symptoms common to many disorders. The cause of the hyperactivity must be determined before effective treatment is possible. If the diagnosis is ADD-H, a program combining behavior modification techniques, special education help, possible stimulant medication, and counseling usually is effective. If the hyperactivity stems from a problem such as mental retardation, cerebral palsy, blindness, deafness, or a psychiatric disturbance, the underlying disorder will determine the kind of treatment and the prognosis. For the child with ADD who is diagnosed early, the future looks fairly positive.

REFERENCES

Abel, E.L. (1984). Prenatal effects of alcohol. *Drug and Alcohol Dependence, 14*, 1–10.

Abikoff, H., & Gittelman, R. (1985). The normalizing effects of methylphenidate on the classroom behavior of ADDH children. *Journal of Abnormal Child Psychology, 13*, 33–44.

American Psychiatric Association. (1980). *Diagnostic and statistical manual of mental disorders (DSM III)*. Washington, DC: American Psychiatric Association.

Arnold, L.E., Christopher, J., Huestis, R., et al. (1978). Methylphenidate vs. dextroamphetamine vs. caffeine in minimal brain dysfunction: Controlled comparison by placebo washout design with Bayes' analysis. *Archives of General Psychiatry, 35*, 463–473.

Barkley, R.A. (1977). A review of stimulant drug research with hyperactive children. *Journal of Child Psychology and Psychiatry, 18*, 137–165.

Bellack, A.S., & Hersen, M. (1977). *Behavior modification: An introductory textbook*. New York: Oxford University Press.

Bellinger, D.C., & Needleman, H.L. (1983). Lead and the relationship between maternal and child intelligence. *Journal of Pediatrics, 102*, 523–527.

Biederman, J., & Jellinek, M.S. (1984). Current concepts. Psychopharmacology in children. *New England Journal of Medicine, 310*, 968–972.

Camp, J.A., Bialer, J., Sverd, J., et al. (1978). Clinical usefulness of the NIMH physical and neurological examination for soft signs. *American Journal of Psychiatry, 135*, 362–364.

Caresia, L., Pugnetti, L., Besana, R., et al. (1984). EEG and clinical findings during pemoline treatment in children and adults with attention deficit disorder. An 8-week open trial. *Neuropsychobiology, 11*, 158–167.

Charles, L., Schain, R.J., & Guthrie, D. (1979). Long-term use and discontinuation of methylphenidate with hyperactive children. *Developmental Medicine and Child Neurology, 21*, 758–764.

Christensen, D.E. (1975). Effects of combining methylphenidate and a classroom token system in modifying hyperactive behavior. *American Journal of Mental Deficiency, 80*, 266–276.

Conners, C.K. (1980). *Food additives and hyperactive children*. New York: Plenum Publishing Corp.

Conners, C.K., & Taylor, E. (1980). Pemoline, methylphenidate, and placebo in children with minimal brain dysfunction. *Archives of General Psychiatry, 37*, 922–930.

Craighead, W.E., Kazdin, A.E., & Mahoney, M.J. (1981). *Behavior modification: Principles, issues and applications* (2nd ed.). Boston: Houghton Mifflin Co.

Egger, J., Carter, C.M., Graham, P.J., et al. (1985). Controlled trial of oliogoantigenic treatment in the hyperkinetic syndrome. *Lancet, 1*, 540–545.

Feingold, B.F. (1975). *Why your child is hyperactive*. New York: Random House.

Gadow, K.D. (1983). Effects of stimulant drugs on academic performance in hyperactive and learning disabled children. *Journal of Learning Disabilities, 16*, 290–299.

Gillberg, I.C. (1985). Children with minor neurodevelopmental disorders. III. Neurological and neuro-developmental problems at age 10. *Developmental Medicine and Child Neurology, 27*, 3–16.

Golinko, B.E. (1984). Side effects of dextroamphetamine and methylphenidate in hyperactive children—a brief review. *Progress in Neuro-psychopharmacology and Biological Psychiatry, 8*, 1–8.

Haslam, R.H., Dalby, J.T., & Rademaker, A.W. (1984). Effect of megavitamin therapy on children with attention deficit disorder. *Pediatrics, 74*, 103–111.

Hechtman, L., Weiss, G., & Perlman, T. (1984a). Hyperactives as young adults: Past and current substance abuse and antisocial behavior. *American Journal of Orthopsychiatry, 54*, 415–425.

Hechtman, L., Weiss, G., & Perlman, T. (1984b). Young adult outcome of hyperactive children who received long-term stimulant treatment. *Journal of the American Academy of Child Psychiatry, 23*, 261–269.

Johnson, C.F., & Prinz, R. (1976). Hyperactivity is in the eyes of the beholder. An evaluation of how teachers view the hyperactive child. *Clinical Pediatrics, 15*, 222–228.

Johnston, C., Pelham, W.E., & Murphy, H.A. (1985). Peer relationships in ADDH and normal children: A developmental analysis of peer and teacher ratings. *Journal of Abnormal Child Psychology, 13*, 89–100.

Kalachnik, J.E., Sprague, R.L., Sleator, E.K., et al. (1982). Effect of methylphenidate hydrochloride on stature of hyperactive children. *Developmental Medicine and Child Neurology, 24*, 586–595.

Kalat, J.W. (1976). Minimal brain dysfunction: Dopamine depletion? *Science, 194*, 450–451.

Knights, R.M., & Viets, C.A. (1975). Effects of pemoline on hyperactive boys. *Pharmacology, Biochemistry and Behavior, 3*, 1107–1114.

Kohler, E.M., Kohler, L., & Regefalk, C. (1979). Minimal brain dysfunction in preschool age—risk for trouble in school? *Paediatrician, 8*, 219–227.

Krager, J.M., & Safer, D.J. (1974). Type and prevalence of medication used in the treatment of hyperactive children. *New England Journal of Medicine, 291*, 1118–1120.

Krankowski, A.J. (1965). Amitriptyline in treatment of hyperkinetic children. *Psychosometics, 6*, 355–360.

Lambert, N.M., Sandoval, J., & Sassone, D. (1978). Prevalence of hyperactivity in elementary school children as a function of social system definers. *American Journal of Orthopsychiatry, 48*, 446–463.

Livingston, S. (1972). *Comprehensive management of epilepsy in infancy, childhood, and adolescence.* Springfield, IL: Charles C Thomas.

Mayer, J., & Goldberg, J. (1985). Diet and hyperactivity. *Exceptional Parent, 15*, 45–46.

Milman, D.H. (1979). Minimal brain dysfunction in childhood: Outcome in late adolescence and early adult years. *Journal of Clinical Psychiatry, 40*, 371–380.

National Institutes of Health. (1982). Defined diets and childhood hyperactivity. *Journal of the American Medical Association, 248*, 290–292.

O'Leary, S.G., & O'Leary, K.D. (1976). Behavior modification in the school. In H. Leitenberg (Ed.), *Handbook of behavior modification and behavior therapy.* Englewood Cliffs, NJ: Prentice-Hall.

Patterson, G.R. (1975). *Families: Application of social learning to family life.* Champaign, IL: Research Press.

Rapoport, J.L., Berg, C.J., Ismond, D.R., et al. (1984). Behavioral effects of caffeine in children. Relationship between dietary choice and effects of caffeine challenge. *Archives of General Psychiatry, 41*, 1073–1079.

Rapoport, J.L., & Ismond, D.R. (1984). *DSM-III training guide for diagnosis of childhood disorders.* New York: Brunner/Mazel.

Raskin, L.A., Shaywitz, S.E., Shaywitz, B.A., et al. (1984). Neurochemical correlates of attention deficit disorder. *Pediatric Clinics of North America, 31*, 387–396.

Safer, D.J. (1973). A familial factor in minimal brain dysfunction. *Behavioral Genetics, 3*, 175–186.

Safer, D.J., & Allen, R.P. (1976). *Hyperactive children: Diagnosis and management.* Baltimore: University Park Press.

Satterfield, J.H., Cantwell, D.P., Schell, A., et al. (1979). Growth of hyperactive children treated with methylphenidate. *Archives of General Psychiatry, 36*, 212–217.

Satterfield, J.H., Hoppe, C.M., & Schell, A.M. (1982). A prospective study of delinquency in 110 adolescent boys with attention deficit disorder and 88 normal adolescent boys. *American Journal of Psychiatry, 139*, 795–798.

Shaywitz, B.A., Shaywitz, S.E., Byrne, T., et al. (1983). Attention deficit disorder: Quantitative analysis of CT. *Neurology, 33*, 1500–1503.

Shaywitz, S.E., Cohen, D.J., & Shaywitz, B.A. (1978). The biochemical basis of minimal brain dysfunction. *Journal of Pediatrics, 92*, 179–187.

Shaywitz, S.E., Hunt, R.D., Jatlow, P., et al. (1982). Psychopharmacology of attention deficit disorder: Pharmacokinetic, neuroendocrine, and behavioral measures following acute and chronic treatment with methylphenidate. *Pediatrics, 69*, 688–694.

Sleator, E.K., & Von Neumann, A.W. (1974). Methylphenidate in the treatment of hyperkinetic children. *Clinical Pediatrics, 13*, 19–24.

Sprague, R.L., & Sleator, E.K. (1977). Methylphenidate in hyperkinetic children: Differences in dose effects on learning and social behavior. *Science, 198*, 1274–1276.

Stare, F.J., Whelan, E.M., & Sheridan, M. (1980). Diet and hyperactivity: Is there a relationship? *Pediatrics, 66*, 521–525.

Strauss, A.A., & Lehtinen, L.E. (1955). *Psychopathology and education of the brain-injured child* (Vol. 2). New York: Grune & Stratton.

Swanson, J.M., Sandman, C.A., Deutsch, C., et al. (1983). Methylphenidate hydrochloride given with or before breakfast. I. Behavioral, cognitive, and electrophysiologic effects. *Pediatrics, 72*, 49–55.

Varley, C.K. (1984). Diet and the behavior of children with attention deficit disorder. *Journal of the American Academy of Child Psychiatry, 23*, 182–185.

Weiss, B. (1982). Food additives and environmental chemicals as sources of childhood behavior disorders. *Journal of the American Academy of Child Psychiatry, 21*, 144–152.

Weiss, G., & Hechtman, L. (1979). The hyperactive child syndrome. *Science, 205,* 1348–1354.

Weiss, G., Hechtman, L., Perlman, T., et al. (1979). Hyperactives as young adults: A controlled prospective ten-year follow-up of 75 children. *Archives of General Psychiatry, 36,* 675–681.

Weiss, G., Kruger, E., Danielson, U., et al. (1975). Effect of long-term treatment of hyperactive children with methylphenidate. *Canadian Medical Association Journal, 112,* 159–165.

Wolraich, M., Milich, R., Stumbo, P., et al. (1985). Effects of sucrose ingestion on the behavior of hyperactive boys. *Journal of Pediatrics, 106,* 675–682.

Chapter 20

Learning Disabilities

Upon completion of this chapter, the reader will:
—know the definition of learning disability
—understand some of the ways to identify learning disabled children at a young age
—be aware of the various ways to treat learning disabled children
—be able to identify the various classroom situations used for these children

A child may have trouble learning for various reasons. As pointed out in other chapters in this book, mental retardation, cerebral palsy, epilepsy, and hearing and vision impairments may interfere with normal learning. This chapter focuses on the child who has none of these disorders but who still fails to learn effectively in school: the child with learning disabilities.

DEFINITION AND INCIDENCE OF LEARNING DISABILITIES

The term *learning disability* is difficult to define precisely. Most definitions arrive at what a learning disability is by describing what it is not. For example, a child with learning disabilities does not have mental retardation, nor does he or she have any disabling physical, emotional, or social problem. Usually, the child has had normal cultural advantages and adequate learning opportunities. Yet, despite the lack of any other developmental disability and the presence of a normal environment, the child fails to learn according to his or her abilities (Feagans, 1983).

Public Law 94-142, the Education for All Handicapped Children Act, defines learning disability as "a disorder in one or more of the basic psychological processes involved in understanding or in using language, spoken or written, which may manifest itself in an imperfect ability to listen, speak, read, write, spell or do mathematical calculations" (U.S. Office of Education, 1977). In sum, a child with learning disabilities is one who has at least average potential and yet has some problem that interferes with normal learning.

To determine the need for a special education placement for a child with learning disabilities one assesses whether there is a severe discrepancy between the child's abilities and his or her level of achievement. However, the definition of what constitutes such a discrepancy varies from state to state (Berk, 1984). In the past, the commonly used criterion was a 2-year disparity between chronological age and school achievement level. The problem with using this as a basis is that it over-estimates the existence of learning disabilities in children with IQs lower than 100 and underestimates such disabilities in children with above average intelligence. For example, a 9-year-old child with an IQ of 80 would normally be expected to function at a 7-year-old level in school. Using the past criterion, this child would be classified as learning disabled because of the 2-year discrepancy between age and achievement. On the other hand, a 9-year-old with an IQ of 130 who was functioning at a 9-year-old level in school would not be classified as learning disabled because he or she was functioning at age level. Yet, this child's level of achievement would be significantly below his or her potential. This definition, therefore, does not seem to be an accurate one because it does not take intellectual potential into account.

More recent definitions are based on significant differences between intellectual potential and school achievement. Efforts are underway to develop tools and defi-nitions to better identify children with learning disabilities before they reach school age. Using the more recent criterion, about 15% of all school children fall under this definition (Hynd & Cohen, 1983). In the United States alone, this amounts to more than 8 million children and accounts for about half of all handicapping conditions in childhood (Silverman & Metz, 1973). Included in this number are children with attention deficit disorder (ADD) who have learning disabilities as part of their disorder.

As with ADD, learning disabilities affect boys more than girls, in this case, by a ratio of 4 to 1 (Weiss & Hechtman, 1979). Reading disabilities are by far the most common form of learning disability. Poor spelling generally goes along with poor reading. Often, the child also has problems with handwriting and arithmetic. When children have difficulty in multiple areas of learning, they are thought to have a global learning disability.

SUBGROUPS OF CHILDREN WITH LEARNING DISABILITIES

In diagnosing any disorder, a practitioner may be called either a "lumper" or a "splitter." A "lumper" would put all children with a learning disability into one category. A "splitter," on the other hand, would divide a group of children with learning disabilities into various subgroups to identify them even more specifically.

In the diagnosis of learning disabilities, "splitters" have basically won the debate. However, a difficulty remains because the splitters have yet to agree on the proper subdivisions. For example, Rutter, Graham, and Yule (1970) divided children with reading problems into those with "reading retardation," commonly called dyslexics, and those with "reading backwardness," usually called slow learners. They noted that the dyslexic children basically had a language disorder and a specific reading problem. Backward readers, on the other hand, tended to have lower IQ scores, a history of birth injury, and other developmental problems. Yet, the dyslexic children had more trouble developing reading skills than the backward reading group even though they had higher IQs (Yule, 1973).

Within the dyslexic group, other researchers have proposed other divisions. For instance, Boder has suggested classifying children with reading disabilities by their type of reading errors (Boder, 1973; Boder, 1976; Fried, Tanguay, Boder, et al., 1981). Using this method of categorization, three groups are described: *dyseidetic, dysphonetic* and *mixed*. The dyseidetic group is unable to identify groupings of letters in patterns. Such children would spell and read words by their sounds (Figure 20.1); "laugh" might be "laf," and "bagel," "bagl." These children read very slowly because they must sound out each word instead of relying on a repertoire of visually recognized words. As they go along in school, these children generally remain slow readers, but they can become relatively good spellers. The dysphonetic child, on the other hand, is unable to relate symbols to sounds and thus cannot develop **phonetic** word analysis skills. This child makes bizarre spelling errors, unrelated to the sound of the word (Figure 20.2). The dysphonetic reader can identify words he or she has memorized but cannot use phonetics to sound out new words. A child with this disability may be able to approach grade level in reading but is usually a poor speller. Finally, the child with a mixed type of dyslexia has the worst of both worlds.

Wading through these categories and subdivisions can be a bit confusing. It is helpful to keep in mind that the function of the divisions is to help in selecting a treatment approach that is likely to be the most successful for a particular child.

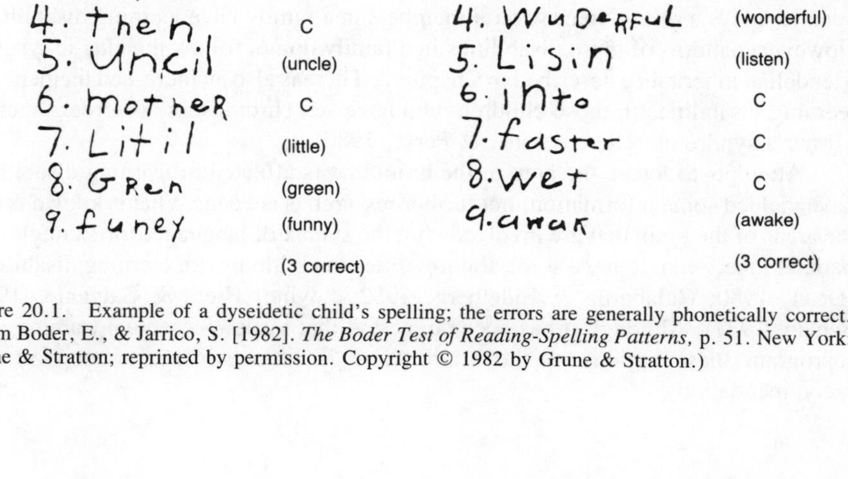

Danny   9 Yerse   GRaD - Hiy 3

KNOWN WORDS		UNKNOWN WORDS	
1. Hoss	(house)	1. Bisshis	(business)
2. Blowe	(blue)	2. PRomis	(promise)
3. aFteR	c	3 StoR	(store)
4. then	c	4. WuDaRFuL	(wonderful)
5. Uncil	(uncle)	5. Lisin	(listen)
6. motheR	c	6. into	c
7. Litil	(little)	7. faster	c
8. GRen	(green)	8. wet	c
9. funey	(funny)	9. awak	(awake)
(3 correct)		(3 correct)	

Figure 20.1. Example of a dyseidetic child's spelling; the errors are generally phonetically correct. (From Boder, E., & Jarrico, S. [1982]. *The Boder Test of Reading-Spelling Patterns*, p. 51. New York: Grune & Stratton; reprinted by permission. Copyright © 1982 by Grune & Stratton.)

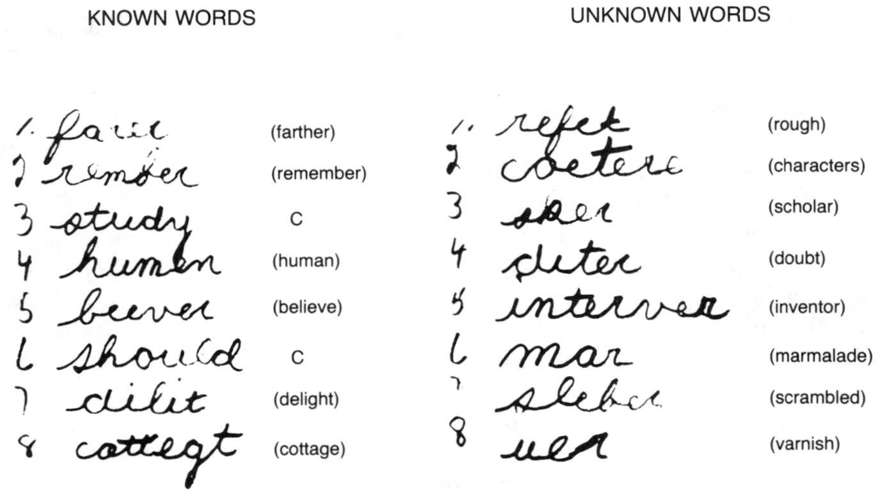

KNOWN WORDS   UNKNOWN WORDS

1. *face* (farther)   1. *refet* (rough)
2. *rember* (remember)   2. *coetere* (characters)
3. *study* c   3. *saer* (scholar)
4. *humen* (human)   4. *duter* (doubt)
5. *beever* (believe)   5. *interver* (inventor)
6. *should* c   6. *mar* (marmalade)
7. *dilit* (delight)   7. *slebc* (scrambled)
8. *cottegt* (cottage)   8. *uer* (varnish)

Figure 20.2. Example of a dysphonetic child's spelling. The spelling errors bear little resemblance to the word and are phonetically incorrect. (From Boder, E. [1973]. Developmental dyslexia: A diagnostic approach based on three atypical reading-spelling patterns. *Developmental Medicine and Child Neurology, 15,* 663–687; reprinted by permission. Copyright © 1973 by Spastics International Medical Publications.)

CAUSES OF LEARNING DISABILITIES

No one knows exactly what causes learning disabilities. Children with these disabilities do not seem to have an increased incidence of birth trauma or other environmental influences. And they tend to develop as rapidly as their siblings except in the area of language. Because of their difficulties with language, children with learning disabilities are thought to have a type of language disorder (Zuckerman & Chase, 1984).

Besides knowing that language is affected, researchers also have evidence that genetics plays a role. Often, several members in a family have learning disabilities. However, patterns of these disabilities in a family do not follow the classic types of Mendelian inheritance described in Chapter 2. There is also an increased incidence of learning disabilities in those children who have sex chromosome disorders such as Turner's syndrome (Hier, Atkins, & Perlo, 1980).

Attempts to locate the area of the brain that is affected in learning disabilities have yielded some information, but further research is needed. What is known is that the areas of the brain that are involved with the syntax of language, for example, the parietal lobe, seem to have some abnormalities in children with learning disabilities (Dean, 1980; Galaburda & Eidelberg, 1982; Levine, Hier, & Calvanio, 1981; Schain, 1977). Although it has been suggested that visual-perceptual training may reprogram these regions of the brain, there is little evidence to support this recommendation.

CHARACTERISTICS OF CHILDREN WITH LEARNING DISABILITIES

No matter what the specific form of disability, all children with learning disabilities share certain common characteristics (FCLD, 1984) (Table 20.1). They usually have difficulty from the time they enter a formal school program. In kindergarten, such a child often has trouble distinguishing various shapes and sizes. He or she finds it difficult to learn the alphabet and the different letter sounds. Handwriting is no easier. Yet, if the child has an isolated reading disability, working with numbers may be a strong point. Socially, he or she relates well to the other children, is not hyperactive, and most likely enjoys school. Since kindergarten focuses to a great extent on developing social rather than academic skills, the child with learning disabilities may fare well there.

Once he or she enters first grade, however, the situation changes. Since the youngster has not mastered the "readiness" skills necessary for reading, he or she cannot read, and spelling is equally tough. Before Christmas recess, it is usually evident that the child is having great difficulties. As the year progresses, the child falls further behind. Other symptoms develop. Because of failure in school, the child may develop behavioral and emotional problems. He or she may become depressed, develop a poor self-image, and withdraw from participating in class. Eventually, the child may either avoid going to school or become the "class clown" to get attention.

To deal effectively with these problems, the difficulties must be identified early. A program designed to meet the child's specific needs must be instituted before the emotional problems become too heavy a load.

EARLY IDENTIFICATION

In the past, learning disability was only diagnosed in children of school age. Recently, the aim has been to identify these children as early as possible. To pinpoint these

Table 20.1.   Characteristics of children with learning disabilities

Visual-perceptual problems:	Difficulty distinguishing various shapes and sizes Difficulty coloring, writing, cutting out Lack of established "handedness"—uses either right or left hand to perform a task Letter and word reversal
Attention/memory problems:	Difficulty concentrating Does not listen well Forgets easily Cannot follow instructions with many steps
Language deficits:	Delay in language development Has difficulty forming sentences and/or finding the right words
Reading problems:	Has trouble sounding out words Has difficulty understanding words or concepts Misreads letters or puts them in incorrect order

Source: Foundation for Children with Learning Disabilities (FCLD) (1984).

children before they begin a formal educational program, a profile of early language and perceptual problems was developed. However, just which items are most reliable in predicting future academic failure is still unclear (Keogh & Becker, 1973).

Disabilities in language areas are easiest to determine at an early age. Memory skills and abilities to pay attention and follow sequential commands can be evaluated. Also, the child's family history may identify other family members who had learning disabilities or delays in language development as children (Finucci, Guthrie, Childs, et al., 1976).

Although language deficits can be picked up at a fairly young age, visual-perceptual problems are more difficult to diagnose. One can look for problems in shape concepts and drawing. For example, a 3-year-old should be able to draw a circle and a cross and match colors. A 4-year-old normally can draw a "stick figure." A 6-year-old can copy a number of the pictures in the Bender-Gestalt test (Figure 20.3). A lack of these skills may indicate a learning disability, but this is not always the case.

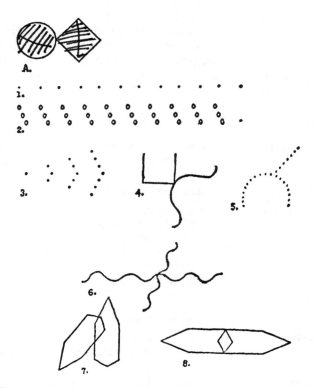

Figure 20.3. Figures used in the Bender-Gestalt test of visual-perceptual abilities. The individual is asked to copy the nine figures. (From Bender, L. [1946]. *Instructions for the use of Visual Motor Gestalt Test*, Plate I. New York: American Orthopsychiatric Association, 1946; reprinted by permission. Copyright © 1946 by Lauretta Bender and The American Orthopsychiatric Association, Inc.)

Other signs may not show up until a child is older than 7 years. For example, it is not uncommon for children under 7 years of age to reverse letters such as "b" for "d." Also, it is not until 6 years of age that a child should consistently be able to distinguish right from left. In a child older than 7, a persistence of letter reversal or an inability to discriminate right from left is characteristic of a learning disability (Accardo, 1980).

Thus, knowing how to accurately identify preschool children with learning disabilities is still in its early stages of development. One problem with too-early identification is that children who are labeled as learning disabled at 4 or 5 years of age may actually be normal. There is also the concern of creating a self-fulfilling prophecy, that of producing children with learning disabilities by tests. In one study, deHirsch, Jansky, and Langford (1966) accurately identified approximately 75% of the children in a kindergarten class who later developed learning disabilities. However, they also labeled as learning disabled a large number of the children who later had normal learning patterns.

Obviously, refinement of early identification tools should be a high priority. New tests may include auditory evoked responses and other measures of neurophysiological activity of the brain. Also, long-term follow-up studies comparing the outcomes of children who were identified and treated early versus those who were not identified until after first grade are needed.

DISTINGUISHING LEARNING DISABILITIES FROM OTHER DISORDERS

It is not surprising that the symptoms describing a child with learning disabilities sound similar to those of a child with ADD. All ADD children have learning disabilities, but not all learning disabled children have ADD. A learning disability can be an isolated phenomenon, unassociated with attention deficits, impulsiveness, clumsiness, or hyperactivity. In general, the child with an isolated learning disability has a better prognosis than a child with ADD (Levine, Brooks, & Shonkoff, 1980). If all the developmental disabilities were laid out in a spectrum, with cerebral palsy at one end and mental retardation at the other, both ADD and learning disabilities would fall somewhere in the middle (Capute, Accardo, Bender, et al., 1980). As we learn more about the workings of the brain, it may well turn out that neurochemical deficiencies exist in more than one of these disorders.

Besides those who have ADD, children with various medical and genetic diseases may also have learning problems. Girls with Turner's, or XO syndrome (see Chapter 2), have severe visual-perceptual problems (Alexander & Money, 1965). Children suffering from chronic illnesses such as diabetes, arthritis, and kidney or liver disease may have poor school performance either because of the disease itself or from psychosocial problems related to the chronic illness. Also, children with psychiatric disorders often fail in school.

The influence of a child's environment is as important as his or her physical and emotional health. For example, a child who is hungry and has poor nutrition cannot pay attention and does not learn well. Also, if the child comes from a home that does not emphasize learning, he or she will rarely achieve well in school (Bell, Abrahamson, & McRae, 1977; Bell, Aftanus, & Abrahamson, 1976). Finally, a home beset with many family problems has an impact on a child's functioning in school.

Thus, before performing a battery of psychological and educational tests on a child who is having trouble learning, a complete medical and social history should be taken. Questions to the parents might include: Is your child hyperactive? Does your child receive any medication that might affect his or her learning? Does he or she have any emotional problems? Does your child seem afraid to go to school? Does he or she avoid going to school, sometimes using sickness as an excuse? Is there any problem with vision or hearing, either now or in the past? Do you suspect that any recent changes in your home may have upset your child? Are you having problems with your child other than in school?

Once this information is obtained, the next step is to get an educational history. A child with learning disabilities can virtually always be so recognized by second grade: he or she will have a history of failure from the beginning of school. If, on the other hand, a 10-year-old child has previously done fairly well academically but suddenly starts to fail, the problem is less likely to be a specific learning disability.

EVALUATING THE LEARNING DISABLED CHILD

Treatment involves evaluation and diagnosis as well as program planning. Using a group of psychological and educational tests, one initially assesses the cognitive, visual-perceptual, and psycholinguistic strengths and weaknesses of the child as well as his or her level of achievement in different academic areas. This leads to a strategy for treatment. Most children are not tested until they have completed kindergarten. Some representative tests are discussed in the following section.

Cognitive and Other Tests

Two commonly used cognitive or IQ tests are the Wechsler Intelligence Scale for Children–Revised (WISC–R) and the Kaufman Assessment Battery for Children (K-ABC).

The WISC–R The WISC–R contains both tests of language abilities and performance tests of eye-hand skills that require minimal verbal responses (Dudley-Marling, Kaufman, & Tarver, 1981). It is divided into six verbal and six performance subtests, none of which requires reading or spelling. These subtests consist of a series of increasingly difficult questions ranging from a 6- to a 16-year-old level. On each, the child is asked to perform up to the level at which he or she consistently fails. Each subtest is then scored, with 10 being an average score. Thus, it is possible to determine a child's strengths and weaknesses by examining the results of the subtests. A variation of this test, used for children 4½ years of age and older, is called the Wechsler Preschool and Primary Scale of Intelligence (WPPSI).

The verbal subtests include: information, comprehension, arithmetic, similarities, vocabulary, and digit span. Information questions would be similar to "Who was the first President?" The comprehension test includes questions similar to "Why do we have eyes?" The arithmetic test consists of word problems rather than computation. The test of similarities examines the child's ability to categorize, asking questions similar to "How are cars and trains alike?" In the vocabulary test, the child is asked to define words. Finally, in the digit span test, an optional test, the child is asked to repeat progressively longer series of spoken numbers.

The second category, the performance subtests, includes: picture completion, picture arrangement, block design, object assembly, coding, and mazes. The picture completion test requires the child to point to missing parts in a picture. In the picture arrangement test, the child must order a series of pictures into a sequence to tell a story. The block design test has the child arrange colored blocks in a pictorial, abstract design. The object assembly test involves putting a puzzle together. In coding, the child must transpose symbols from a key on the top of a page to numbered boxes below. The final subtest, mazes, is optional and entails using a pencil to trace through progressively more complicated mazes.

Since the child with learning disabilities may have scattered abilities similar to the child with ADD (Ackerman, Peters, & Dykman, 1971), the WISC–R is useful in evaluating skills in different areas. For example, the examiner may find specific strengths in verbal areas or particular weaknesses in the visual-performance area. Such information is helpful in setting up an individualized education program (IEP).

K-ABC The Kaufman Assessment Battery for Children is a new psychometric measure designed to test children from 2½ to 12½ years of age (Kaufman & Kaufman, 1983; Wodrich, 1984). It differs from the WISC in that it minimizes the role of language and verbal skills in testing. In addition, this test is particularly useful for testing children with learning disabilities because it covers and evaluates different aspects of reading skills. Using this test, one is able to ascertain not only whether a person has a reading disability but also which type of reading disability. Thus, the dysphonetic reader can be distinguished from the dyseidetic reader.

Besides the use of cognitive tests, other tests are used to assess a child's intellectual abilities. These include tests of visual-perceptual skills, psycholinguistic abilities, and academic achievement tests (Wiig, 1984). Some of the more frequently used tests are described in Table 20.2.

Interpreting Test Results

Using these tests, a psychologist and a special educator can evaluate the child who seems to have a learning disability. The results of the tests will indicate the child's IQ, visual and perceptual problem areas, and levels of achievement in various areas of learning. From these findings, a program can be developed. Retesting at the end of the school year is important to determine the progress the child has made and the effectiveness of the program. Depending on the results of these tests, the program can be maintained or modified to better meet the child's needs for the following year.

TREATMENT APPROACHES

Right now, learning disabilities have no cure; the best approach seems to be one that teaches the child how to compensate for the disability. No single method works best

Table 20.2. Commonly used tests for evaluating the child with learning disabilities

Name of test	Consists of	Assesses	Sample items
Visual-Perceptual Tests[a]			
Bender-Gestalt Test	9 drawings the child is asked to copy	Visual-perceptual skills; eye-hand coordination	See Figure 20.3
Goodenough Draw-a-Person Test	Child is asked to draw a person; points are given for number of body parts, accuracy, and detail	Visual-perceptual skills; child's self-image	
Psycholinguistic Tests			
Illinois Test of Psycholinguistic Abilities (ITPA)	Two groups of 6 subtests	Auditory reception: visual reception; auditory/visual association; visual-motor association; verbal expression; manual expression (first 6 tests); auditory expression: grammar, **auditory sequential memory, visual sequential memory**; sound comprehension; specific language deficiencies	"Do dogs eat?" "A frog jumps, a fish _____." "Which things go together, a toothbrush and toothpaste or a bike and a cake?" "Tell me about hats." "Show me what we do with a comb."
Wepman Auditory Discrimination Test	Spoken words that sound similar	Ability to differentiate similar sounding words	"Ball, tall"
Academic Achievement Tests[b]			
The WRAT Battery (useful for determining rate of learning)	3 subtests; grade level is obtained on each subtest.	Spelling, reading, math abilities	
Woodcock-Johnson Psycho-educational Battery	Subtests in areas covering reading skills, mathematics, writing, science, social studies, humanities	General ability, academic achievement, personal interest	

Test	Description	Content/Measures
Metropolitan Readiness Test (taken during second half of kindergarten)	Screening test for entering first grade; may be first standardized measure of learning problem	Counting, number concepts, alphabet, phonetics, visual discrimination
Gates-MacGinitie Reading Tests	Vocabulary words; stories and questions about the stories	Silent comprehension and vocabulary
Durrell Reading Test		Oral reading
Word Recognition Test	List of words of varying difficulty. "Flash score": Percentage of words recognized instantly; "Untimed score: Percentage described without a time limit	Sight-reading vocabulary; word skills
Detroit Test of Learning Aptitude	19 subtests	Prerequisite skills (short-term recollection, memory, ability to follow oral directions, etc.) for reading and other school subjects; ability to understand opposites
Informal Reading Inventory (IRI)	Tests that yield 4 levels of reading ability[c]	"Independent" reading ability; "Instructional" level; "Frustration" level; "Hearing capacity" level
Key Math Diagnostic Arithmetic Test	Several subtests; yields grade equivalent	Computational skills and concepts; identifies types of errors made

Large: what, big, fun, brave." (Child picks proper definition.)

[a]Wodrich (1984).
[b]Taylor (1984), Taylor & Warren (1984), Wodrich (1984).
[c]Wilson (1981).

for all children (Hammill & Bartel, 1982; Warren & Taylor, 1984). Particular teachers prefer certain methods, and different methods are in style at different times. In general, the two main approaches attempt either to correct the underlying perceptual defect or to teach skills directly. There is no evidence that teaching prerequisite visual-perceptual skills actually improves reading.

Treatment of Perceptual Deficits

Treatment of perceptual deficits includes such methods as patterning, optometry, sensory integration, the use of an orthomolecular diet, and alpha-wave conditioning.

Patterning In 1966, Delacato proposed the theory that the development of a child patterns itself after the evolution of humans from lower primates, or as he put it, "Ontogeny recapitulates phylogeny." His approach to treating children with learning disabilities assumes that the failure to pass through a proper sequence of developmental stages in motor ability, language, visual, auditory, and other sensory areas leads to "poor neurological organization of the brain" (Delacato, 1966). To correct this, he says, the child's brain needs to be reprogrammed, and the child must pass through the proper developmental stages. This reprogramming is carried out by following a rigorous series of physical and breathing exercises as well as by restricting the intake of fluids, salt, and sugar. The diet restriction is done to increase the blood flow to the brain and to decrease the production of cerebrospinal fluid. No studies have supported the effectiveness of this approach. In fact, the American Academy of Pediatrics and other educational and medical organizations have expressed concern about the use of this method (American Academy of Pediatrics, 1982; Freeman, 1967).

Optometry Some optometrists believe that reading is essentially a visual-perceptual task that is related to the sensorimotor coordination of the child (Flax, 1973). They propose that the child use visual training exercises to overcome the perceptual problem. Yet, no research has found that eye muscle exercises have any beneficial effect on reading. Furthermore, related kinds of perceptual training that, for example, teach the child to distinguish right from left and to walk on balance boards to improve coordination have not improved reading skill (Metzger & Werner, 1984).

Sensory Integration Therapy Another method that is based on physical activity is sensory integration therapy. Ayres (1972) stated that the ability of the cortex to respond to auditory and visual stimuli depends on the organization of the stimuli in the brain stem. She observed that other abnormalities connected with the functioning of the brain stem are apparent in children with learning disabilities. These include clumsiness and poor eye muscle coordination. To deal with this, she proposed activities that involve balancing and fine motor coordination aimed at improving brain stem functioning. Since this method has not been studied in any controlled fashion, no definite conclusions can yet be drawn about its efficacy. However, initial impressions are that the method is not successful (Silver, 1975).

Orthomolecular Approach Orthomolecular diets were discussed in Chapter 9. The idea that deficiencies in vitamins or trace elements cause learning disabilities is unsubstantiated (Golden, 1984).

Alpha-Wave Conditioning An unusual alpha-wave pattern has shown up on the electroencephalograms (EEGs) of a number of children with learning disabilities. Since people can control alpha brain wave patterns with biofeedback techniques, this was tried with children who have learning disabilities. However, although 40% of children with learning disabilities display this "abnormal pattern," 25% of children without learning problems also have this pattern. Therefore, the efficacy of therapy based on this approach is highly questionable (Silver, 1975).

To summarize, little evidence supports the idea that treatment of perceptual deficits is valuable for the child with learning disabilities. Educational approaches have brought more success.

Educational Methods

So far, children with learning disabilities who have shown the greatest improvement are those who have received the most hours of specific educational intervention irrespective of the method used. Yet, long-term follow-up studies have found that only 10% of children with severe learning disabilities improved after various educational approaches were tried (Silberberg, Iversen, & Goins, 1975; Watson, Watson, & Freda, 1982). Therefore, it is difficult to advocate a single remedial program for such children. Once again, the particular reading program must meet the needs of the individual child. Commonly used approaches include teaching sight-word recognition, phonic skills, and familiar word endings. Frequently, these approaches are combined (Hewison, 1982).

The oldest educational method is the Orton-Gillingham approach, or the *visual-auditory-kinesthetic-tactile* (VAKT) technique (Orton, 1937). This is, in fact, a modification of the teaching method used by the ancient Greeks to teach reading. It is a multisensory, synthetic, alphabetic method. The child starts by learning the alphabet. He or she prints, traces, touches, and says individual letters. After he or she has mastered this, phonetics is begun. When the individual letter sounds have been learned, blends of sounds and then word phrases are introduced. Gradually, the child builds a vocabulary. However, it is a slow, painful process, as the child learns each individual sound separately. This approach is most helpful for the child who has difficulty learning whole words but who can learn phonics—the dyseidetic reader.

Another VAKT approach is the Fernald method. Here, a child begins by selecting the word he or she would like to learn. The child then checks the spelling, pronunciation, and syllabication of the word in a dictionary. Next, he or she says the word, writes it, and traces it with his or her fingers. Finally, the child writes the word from memory and places it in a file box containing new words. He or she then uses it in writing sentences and in telling stories. The child is immediately stopped and corrected if he or she makes an error, and is praised for success. Motivation plays a major role in this approach (Silberberg, Iversen, & Goins, 1975).

Still another technique is the language experience approach. Here words are introduced as part of a discussion. The teacher asks a child to tell a story and then writes on the blackboard precisely what the child says. The teacher rereads the story, and then has the child read each sentence until he or she has mastered it. The story may also be used as a basis for a field trip such as a visit to the zoo. This approach is highly motivating. It also uses the whole-word approach rather than the previously described phonetics approach. This method may be helpful for the dysphonetic reader. Its main disadvantage is the lack of a textbook from which to teach. A highly creative teacher who has much initiative is therefore required (Benton & Pearl, 1978).

A fourth approach is the color-coding method, in which letters are coupled with specific colors, and combinations of letters are learned by blending colors. Since the color scheme actually adds another level of complexity to learning, this method has not gained many advocates.

Finally, a more recent technique is the neuropsychological approach. This method emphasizes the use of the intact areas of neurological functioning to help develop remedial strategies (Hynd & Cohen, 1983). The specific strengths identified in the neuropsychological testing are utilized while the weak areas are avoided.

Because of the diversity and number of teaching methods, it is difficult to design studies to evaluate the effectiveness of the various approaches (Bell, Abrahamson, & McRae, 1977). What usually happens is that one approach is tried on a child and is continued so long as the child keeps learning. If he or she does not progress, another method is chosen. The results from the psychological and educational tests help determine which method is tried (Silberberg, Iversen, & Goins, 1975).

Classroom Situations

While the various educational approaches are quite different, they do share certain common features. First, all of them rely on a sensitive, bright, and innovative teacher. Second, they presume a small class size. Third, they involve many hours of repetition combined with a behavior modification program of positive reinforcement (see Chapter 19).

In teaching any child with learning disabilities, the main question is whether to strive to overcome the child's weaknesses or to teach to the strengths. Although one might argue either side of this question, there is little evidence to support one view over another. Therefore, the particular approach is selected according to what seems most appropriate for the specific child.

Having chosen the teaching method, the next step is to determine the educational setting. The choices range from a normal class setting to a self-contained learning disabilities class. Three types of situations are most common. The first is to have the child remain in a regular class and have a special education teacher instruct the classroom teacher on ways of handling the child's specific problems. This may be combined with after-school tutoring. Alternatively, an itinerant special education teacher could come into the class each day and give help as needed to the child with learning disabilities. The second type of situation involves a resource room. Here the child stays in a regular class for all of the subjects except the problem ones—for example, math or reading. For these, the child would go to a separate room, usually with five to eight other students and a learning disabilities teacher. The final approach is to have the child stay in a self-contained learning disabilities class for the whole day.

Each situation has advantages and disadvantages. Remaining in a regular class relieves the child of the stigma of being different and of requiring a special teacher. However, the teaching in a regular classroom may not provide enough help to the child with learning disabilities. He or she may fall further behind and become bored and inattentive. The other children may make fun of this student. Therefore, this situation is best only for those children who have a mild learning disability.

The best of both worlds would seem to be the use of a resource room. Then, the child can stay with his or her peers for the subjects that are less difficult and get special help for those that are not. Although a stigma still might be attached to being in "special education," the academic gains from a small, structured group setting tend to offset this in the long run.

Normally, only those children who have severe learning disabilities are placed in a self-contained learning disability classroom. These children have usually failed to learn in less restrictive environments. Besides their learning disabilities, they often are hyperactive and have behavior problems.

No matter what the classroom setting, any child in a special program should be reevaluated at the end of each school year, and plans should be made for the following year. Most schools have a screening committee to carry out this assessment. The parents are asked to participate in the planning, and they have the right to appeal if they do not agree with the individualized education program (IEP). In all cases, the aim is to place the child in the least restrictive setting that facilitates learning and ensures some success.

Career Education

General education teaches us about our world and provides us with basic academic skills as well as physical education, music, art, and so forth. Vocational training consists of counseling, assessment, and education for future jobs. Finally, career education focuses on the various roles, settings, and events that are important for anyone's productive work life (Brolin, Elliott, & Corcoran, 1984).

For children with learning disabilities, it is clear that career education should be an integral part of their overall educational program. This is true for a number of reasons. We know that, as adults, children with learning disabilities continue to have difficulties—such as poor retention of verbal instructions—that may interfere with their effectiveness in jobs. They may hesitate to ask questions and seek assistance. Social immaturity, clumsiness, and poor social judgments make social interactions more difficult. Also, for these individuals, colleges are often not prepared to help with their special needs (FCLD, 1984). In addition, these children are not automatically eligible for vocational training solely because they have a learning disability.

To cope with these difficulties, children with learning disabilities should receive career training beginning in elementary school (Brolin & Carver, 1982). Using this training, children can begin to understand the various roles they need to perform in society. Their self-worth is emphasized to foster an improved self-image. In middle school (grades 6–8), career and vocational assessment can help to uncover the children's interests and aptitudes. During high school, these individuals can begin to explore which careers seem best suited for them. Perhaps, they will be able to have experiences in the community that give them an opportunity to test their interests. Thus, throughout their education, career training can help these children plan for their futures. Although such training was developed for children with learning disabilities, it is appropriate and important for all children with handicaps.

Computer Technology

An adjunct to these children's educational program is the use of computer technology. The personal computer can be an effective teaching tool for the child with learning disabilities (Bender & Church, 1984). Computer programs—for example, Logo, Superpilot, and BASIC—teach logical thought processes. Typing instruction programs such as Mastertype are valuable for the child with handwriting problems. Word processing programs such as Bank Street Writer can be used to practice writing compositions. The computerized dictionary is extremely useful for those with spelling difficulties. These programs, combined with certain video games, make the computer a valuable tool for educating children with learning disabilities.

Stimulant Medication

Although treatment of children with learning disabilities has primarily focused on educational approaches, the use of stimulant medication may be helpful for some children. As was mentioned in Chapter 19, amphetamines such as Ritalin and Dexedrine are used to treat children with ADD-H. These medications are prescribed for hyperactive children to decrease their hyperactivity and to increase their attention span. Such medication may also help to improve attention in children with learning disabilities who are not physically hyperactive (Dykman, Ackerman, & McCray, 1980). If these drugs are used, their effectiveness must be carefully monitored, and they should not be a substitute for sound educational programming.

DAVID—A CASE HISTORY

David developed normally as a young child and seemed as bright and alert as his sisters. He was not hyperactive, nor did he seem particularly clumsy. However, in kindergarten, he began to have some difficulties. He got along well with the other children, but he had trouble with the work. His printing was poor, and he constantly reversed letters. Pictures drawn of his family were little more than scribbles. He had particular problems learning the alphabet and the way each letter sounded. On the Metropolitan Readiness Test, he scored below average in reading skills, although his mathematics skills were above average.

In first grade, David entered a regular class and soon began to fail. He could not learn phonetic skills, and reading remained a mystery. His spelling errors were bizarre and his printing illegible. Yet he learned how to add and subtract easily. Soon,

David underwent a battery of tests that revealed dyslexia. His full-scale IQ on the WISC–R was 120.

The school decided to keep David in a regular class for the remainder of the school year and to have an itinerant special education teacher give him extra help. This approach did not work. David fell further and further behind the other children in language skills. He misbehaved in school and began to avoid going to school, using headaches as an excuse. At the end of the first grade, his reading was more than 1 year delayed, while arithmetic skills were at an age-appropriate level. The teacher decided to give David resource help in language skills. The Orton-Gillingham approach was used.

When he entered the second grade, David was still anxious and unhappy. This time, he went to a resource room where he found only five other children. The reading specialist was kind but firm; the approach was very structured. Soon, David began to learn. It was a slow, arduous process. Besides receiving help in school, his parents worked with him at night. He remained a poor reader, but he could feel the excitement of gaining new knowledge. Friendships developed between him and the other children in the resource room. Yet, he still suffered at the hands of his less sensitive schoolmates.

At the end of the second grade, David had made 1 year's progress, still remaining a little more than a year behind in reading. He continued to attend the resource room for 30 minutes daily for 2 more years. By this time, he was an expert mathematician, which helped to offset his difficulty with reading and spelling. He still found school hard, but he stopped avoiding it. Behavior problems disappeared. With the continued support of the teachers and his parents, David has a good prognosis. He should do well because he is bright, and the early help he received has kept emotional problems from developing.

PROGNOSIS

As is true of David, the prognosis for most children with learning disabilities is good, although they frequently achieve less as adults than do normal children with similar IQs. Many go on to college and professional careers. However, most will retain some degree of learning disability as adults. In one study, 74% of the children who had reading impairment when they were 7 years old remained reading impaired years later (Watson, Watson, & Freda, 1982). The prognosis appears to depend less on the method used to help the child than on the initial severity of the learning disability, the child's IQ score, and his or her motivation to learn.

SUMMARY

A learning disability is a disorder in which a normal, healthy child fails to learn up to his or her intellectual potential in school. The underlying cause of this disorder is unknown. It may involve abnormal functioning in the parietal lobe of the brain and may have a genetic component. Whatever the cause, early detection is important because, if not helped, the child may develop emotional problems that further hinder his or her progress. An educational evaluation should be done to identify the child's strengths and weaknesses. Then, the school can develop an individualized education program for the child. Results of the program must be assessed at the end of each year and appropriate changes made. Currently, it is unclear which of the treatment methods is most helpful; a trial-and-error approach may be needed to find the most useful method for each child. Career education should be integrated into the educational program. The prognosis for the child with learning disabilities is generally good. However, despite the potential effectiveness of treatment, the child who has learning disabilities continues to have them as an adult.

REFERENCES

Accardo, P.J. (1980). *A neurodevelopmental perspective on specific learning disabilities.* Baltimore: University Park Press.

Ackerman, P.T., Peters, J.E., & Dykman, R.A. (1971). Children with specific learning disabilities: WISC profiles. *Journal of Learning Disabilities, 4,* 150–166.

Alexander, D., & Money, J. (1965). Reading abilities, object constancy and Turner's syndrome. *Perceptual and Motor Skills, 20,* 981–984.

American Academy of Pediatrics. (1982). The Doman-Delacato treatment of neurologically handicapped childen. *Pediatrics, 70,* 810–812.

American Academy of Pediatrics. (1984). Learning disabilities, dyslexia and vision. *Pediatrics, 74,* 150–151.

Ayres, A.J. (1972). Improving academic scores through sensory integration. *Journal of Learning Disabilities, 5,* 338–343.

Bell, A.E., Abrahamson, D.S., & McRae, K.N. (1977). Reading retardation: A 12 year prospective study. Implications for the pediatrician. *Journal of Pediatrics, 91,* 363–370.

Bell, A.E., Aftanas, M.S., & Abrahamson, D. (1976). Scholastic progress of childen from different socioeconomic groups matched for IQ. *Developmental Medicine and Child Neurology, 18,* 717–727.

Bender, L. (1946). *Instructions for the use of visual motor gestalt test.* New York: American Orthopsychiatric Association.

Bender, M., & Church, G. (1984). Developing a computer-applications training program for the learning disabled. *Learning Disabilities, 3,* 91–102.

Benton, A.L., & Pearl, D. (Eds). (1978). *Dyslexia: An appraisal of current knowledge.* New York: Oxford University Press.

Berk, R.A. (1984). *Screening and diagnosis of children with learning disabilities.* Springfield, IL: Charles C Thomas.

Boder, E. (1973). Developmental dyslexia: A diagnostic approach based on three typical reading-spelling patterns. *Developmental Medicine and Child Neurology, 15,* 663–687.

Boder, E. (1976). School failure—Evaluation and treatment. *Pediatrics, 58,* 394–403.

Boder, E., & Jarrico, S. (1982). *The Boder test of reading-spelling patterns.* New York: Grune & Stratton.

Brolin, D.E., & Carver, J.T. (1982). Life-centered career education for exceptional children. *Focus on Exceptional Children, 14,* 1–15.

Brolin, D.E., Elliott, T.R., & Corcoran, J.R. (1984). Career education for persons with learning disabilities. *Learning Disabilities, 3,* 1–14.

Bryan, T.H., & Bryan, J.H. (1982). *Understanding learning disabilities* (2nd ed.). Palo Alto, CA: Mayfield Publishing Co.

Capute, A.J., Accardo, P.J., Bender, M., et al. (1980). Dyslexia: Initial assessment and outcome. *Journal of Developmental and Behavioral Pediatrics, 1,* 24–28.

Clark, L. (1975). *Can't read, can't write, can't talk too good either: How to recognize and overcome dyslexia in your child.* New York: Penguin Books.

Dean, R.S. (1980). Cerebral lateralization and reading dysfunction. *Journal of School Psychology, 18,* 324–332.

deHirsch, K., Jansky, J., & Langford, W. (1966). *Predicting reading failure.* New York: Harper & Row.

Delacato, C.H. (1966). *Neurological organization and reading.* Springfield, IL: Charles C Thomas.

Dudley-Marling, C.C., Kaufman, N.J., & Tarver, S.G. (1981). WISC and WISC-R profiles of learning disabled children: A review. *Learning Disabilities Quarterly, 4,* 307–319.

Dykman, R.A., Ackerman, P.T., & McCray, D.S. (1980). Effects of methylphenidate on selective and sustained attention in hyperactive, reading-disabled, and presumably attention-disordered boys. *Journal of Nervous and Mental Disease, 168,* 745–752.

Farnham-Diggory, S. (1978). *Learning disabilities: A psychological perspective.* Cambridge, MA: Harvard University Press.

FCLD (*see* Foundation for Children with Learning Disabilities).

Feagans, L. (1983). A current view of learning disabilities. *Journal of Pediatrics, 102,* 487–493.

Finucci, J.M., Guthrie, J.T., Childs, A.L., et al. (1976). The genetics of specific reading disability. *Annals of Human Genetics, 40,* 1–23.

Flax, N. (1973). The eye and learning disabilities. *Journal of Learning Disabilities, 6,* 328–333.

Foundation for Children with Learning Disabilities (FCLD). (1984). *The FCLD guide for parents of children with learning disabilities.* New York: Education Systems.

Freeman, R.D. (1967). Controversy over "patterning" as a treatment for brain damage in children. *Journal of the American Medical Association, 202,* 83–86.

Fried, I., Tanguay, P.E., Boder, E., et al. (1981). Development of dyslexia: Electrophysiological evidence of clinical subgroups. *Brain and Language, 12,* 14–22.

Frostig, M., & Maslow, P. (1973). *Learning problems in the classroom.* New York: Grune & Stratton.

Galaburda, A.M., & Eidelberg, D. (1982). Symmetry and asymmetry in the human posterior thalamus. II. Thalamic lesions in a case of developmental dyslexia. *Archives of Neurology, 39,* 333–336.

Gearhart, B.R. (1985). *Learning disabilities: Educational strategies* (4th ed.). St. Louis: Times Mirror/ Mosby College Publications.

Geschwind, N. (1974). The development of the brain and the evolution of language. In N. Geschwind (Ed.), *Selected papers on language and the brain.* Boston: D. Reidel Publishing Co.

Golden, G.S. (1984). Symposium on learning disorders. Controversial therapies. *Pediatric Clinics of North America, 31,* 459–469.

Hammill, D.D., & Bartel, N.R. (1982). *Teaching children with learning and behavior problems* (3rd ed.). Boston: Allyn & Bacon.

Hewison, J. (1982). The current status of remedial intervention for children with reading problems. *Developmental Medicine and Child Neurology, 24,* 183–186.

Hier, D.B., Atkins, L., & Perlo, V.P. (1980). Learning disorders and sex chromosome aberrations. *Journal of Mental Deficiency Research, 24,* 17–26.

Hynd, G., & Cohen, M. (1983). *Dyslexia: Neuropsychological theory, research, and clinical differentiation.* New York: Grune & Stratton.

Kaufman, A.S., & Kaufman, N.L. (1983). *Kaufman assessment battery for children (K-ABC).* Circle Pines, MN: American Guidance Service.

Keogh, B.K., & Becker, L.D. (1973). Early detection of learning problems: Questions, cautions, and guidelines. *Exceptional Children, 40, 5–11.*

Kinsbourne, M., & Caplan, P.J. (1979). *Children's learning and attention problems.* Boston: Little, Brown & Co.

Knights, R.M., & Bakker, D.J. (Eds.). (1976). *The neuropsychology of learning disorders: Theoretical approaches.* Baltimore: University Park Press.

Levine, D.N., Hier, D.B., & Calvanio, R. (1981). Acquired learning disability for reading after left temporal lobe damage in childhood. *Neurology, 31,* 257–264.

Levine, M.D., Brooks, R., & Shonkoff, J.P. (1980). *A pediatric approach to learning disorders.* New York: John B. Wiley & Sons.

Malatesha, R.N., & Aaron, P.G. (Eds.). (1982). *Reading disorders: Varieties and treatment.* New York: Academic Press.

Metzger, R.L., & Werner, D.B. (1984). Use of visual training for reading disabilities: A review. *Pediatrics, 73,* 824–829.

Myers, P.I., & Hammill, D.D. (1969). *Methods for learning disorders.* New York: John Wiley & Sons.

Orton, S.T. (1937). *Reading, writing, and speech problems in children: A presentation of certain types of disorders in the development of the language faculty.* New York: W.W. Norton & Co.

Rutter, M., Graham, P., & Yule, W. (1970). *A neuropsychiatric study in childhood.* Philadelphia: J.B. Lippincott.

Sapir, S.G. (1985). *The clinical teaching model: Clinical insights and strategies for the learning disabled child.* New York: Brunner/Mazel.

Sapir, S., & Wilson, B. (1978). *A professional's guide to working with the learning-disabled child.* New York: Brunner/Mazel.

Schain, R.J. (1977). *Neurology of childhood learning disorders* (2nd ed.). Baltimore: Williams & Wilkins Co.

Silberberg, N.E., Iversen, I.A., & Goins, J.T. (1975). Which reading method works best? *Journal of Learning Disabilities, 6,* 547–556.

Silver, L.B. (1975). Acceptable and controversial approaches to treating the child with learning disabilities. *Pediatrics, 55,* 406–415.

Silverman, L.J., & Metz, A.S. (1973). Minimal brain dysfunction. 3. Epidemiology. Numbers of pupils with specific learning disabilities in local public schools in the United States. *Annals of the New York Academy of Sciences, 205,* 146–157.

Taylor, R.L. (1984). *Assessment of exceptional students. Educational and psychological procedures.* Englewood Cliffs, NJ: Prentice-Hall.

Taylor, R.L., & Warren, S.A. (1984). Educational and psychological assessment of children with learning disorders. *Pediatric Clinics of North America, 31,* 281–296.

U.S. Office of Education. (1977). Education of handicapped children. *Federal Register, 42,* 42478–42518.

Walker, J.E., & Shea, T.M. (1983). *Behavior managment: A practical approach for educators* (3rd ed.). St. Louis: Times Mirror/Mosby College Publications.

Warren, S.A., & Taylor, R.L. (1984). Education of children with learning problems. *Pediatric Clinics of North America, 31,* 331–343.

Watson, B.U., Watson, C.S., & Freda, R. (1982). Follow-up studies of specific reading disability. *Journal of the American Academy of Child Psychiatry, 21,* 376–382.

Weiss, G., & Hechtman, L. (1979). The hyperactive child syndrome. *Science, 205,* 1348–1354.

Wiig, E.H. (1984). Psycholinguistic aspects of learning disorders: Identification and assessment. *Pediatric Clinics of North America, 31,* 317–330.

Wilson, R.M. (1981). *Diagnostic and remedial reading for classroom and clinics* (4th ed.). Columbia: Charles E. Merrill Publishing Co.

Wodrich, D.L. (1984). *Children's psychological testing: A guide for nonpsychologists.* Baltimore: Paul H. Brookes Publishing Co.

Yule, W. (1973). Differential prognosis of reading backwardness and specific reading retardation. *British Journal of Educational Psychology, 43,* 244–248.

Yule, W. (1976). Issues and problems in remedial education. *Developmental Medicine and Child Neurology, 18,* 675–682.

Zuckerman, B.S., & Chase, C. (1984). Specific learning disability and dyslexia: A language-based model. *Advances in Pediatrics, 30,* 249–280.

Chapter 21

Cerebral Palsy

with Susan E. Harryman

Upon completion of this chapter, the reader will:
—be aware of some early clues to the diagnosis of cerebral palsy
—know the various types of cerebral palsy and their characteristics
—understand how cerebral palsy is diagnosed
—understand the role of primitive reflexes and automatic movement reactions in motor function
—be able to identify various treatment approaches to cerebral palsy, including physical therapy, medication, orthopedic surgery, neurosurgery, and biofeedback
—understand the prognoses for the different forms of cerebral palsy

---

Cerebral palsy refers not to a single disease but rather to a number of disorders of movement and posture that are due to a nonprogressive abnormality of the immature brain. The brain damage that causes cerebral palsy may also produce a number of other disorders, including mental retardation, seizures, visual and auditory deficits, and behavior problems. A child who suffers brain damage at birth because of a lack of oxygen may show signs of cerebral palsy during his or her first year of life. Another child, 4 years old, may suffer brain damage in a car accident and have symptoms of this disorder when he or she recovers from a coma. Both of these children will have cerebral palsy although the causes are quite different. In both cases, the damage occurred before the child's brain had fully matured (the age of brain maturation is usually designated as being 16 years of age). Also, the damage was not ongoing. Thus, the basic distinctions of cerebral palsy are the age of onset and the lack of progression. Consequently, neither a child with Tay-Sachs disease, a progressive central nervous system disease, nor an adult who suffered brain damage in a car accident would be diagnosed as having cerebral palsy.

Susan E. Harryman, M.S., R.P.T., is Director of Physical Therapy at The Kennedy Institute for Handicapped Children in Baltimore, Maryland.

This chapter presents an outline of the causes, types, and treatment of cerebral palsy. Also discussed are the other developmental disabilities commonly associated with cerebral palsy and the prognosis for children with this disorder.

CAUSES OF CEREBRAL PALSY

Virtually hundreds of diseases may affect the developing brain and lead to cerebral palsy. Many of these were discussed earlier in the chapters on fetal development and the birth process. Yet, only 60% of all cases of cerebral palsy have an identifiable origin (Hagberg, 1979). Events during the first trimester of pregnancy that may cause cerebral palsy include exposure to radiation or teratogenic drugs, intrauterine infections, and chromosomal abnormalities (Table 21.1). In later pregnancy, abruptio placenta and other abnormalities in the fetal-placental exchange and functioning place the child at risk. Complications during labor, delivery, and the neonatal period also result in an increased risk of developing cerebral palsy. These problems account for about 95% of the known causes of cerebral palsy. The remaining 5% of the cases result from early childhood disorders such as meningitis, head trauma, and lead intoxication (Hagberg, 1979; Hagberg, Hagberg, & Olow, 1975). Remember that in approximately 40% of the patients, no cause is identified.

TYPES OF CEREBRAL PALSY

Many classifications of cerebral palsy exist. For our purposes, three groups are used: *pyramidal, extrapyramidal,* and *mixed type.* The overall incidence of these three groups ranges from 0.6 to 2.4 per 1,000, depending on the study (Hagberg, 1979).

Table 21.1.   Causes of cerebral palsy

Causes	*Percentage of cases*
1st trimester:	7
teratogens	
chromosomal anomalies	
2nd trimester:	32
intrauterine infections	
problems in fetal/placental functioning	
Complications of labor and delivery	17
Neonatal complications:	39
sepsis	
asphyxia	
prematurity	
Childhood:	5
meningitis	
head injury	
toxins	
	100

Source: Hagberg (1979).

This means that, in the United States, about 500,000 individuals suffer from cerebral palsy. Pyramidal cerebral palsy accounts for about half of these cases, while the other two groups split the remaining half. The overall incidence of cerebral palsy fell between 1956 and 1965 but has held fairly constant at 1.5/1,000 live births since then (Kudrjavcev, Schoenberg, Kurland, et al., 1983) (Figure 21.1). Neonatal intensive care is decreasing the risk of cerebral palsy in infants who weigh about 2½ to 4 pounds at birth, but it is also enabling the survival of even smaller infants. Therefore, the improved prognoses in the 2½–4 pound infants has been offset by the higher survival rate of smaller infants who have a relatively high risk for developing cerebral palsy (Paneth, Kiely, Stein, et al., 1981).

Pyramidal (Spastic) Cerebral Palsy

Children with pyramidal cerebral palsy have suffered damage either to the motor cortex or to the pyramidal tract of the brain. As noted in Chapter 12, the motor strip of the frontal lobe passes its signals for voluntary movement to the spinal cord via the pyramidal tract. Damage to any part of this pathway leads to spasticity. Muscle tone is increased with a characteristic clasped-knife quality. When the arm or leg is moved, the initial resistance is strong, but it gives way abruptly as would a closing pocket-knife. These changes in muscle tone interfere with normal movement.

　　Depending on where the damage occurs, different parts of the body are affected. In the premature infant, a fragile area exists in the part of the brain that surrounds the lateral ventricles (see Chapter 12). The blood vessels that feed this region bleed easily, especially when the child is deprived of oxygen, which may occur in respiratory distress syndrome (Pape & Wigglesworth, 1979). Because this area includes the fibers of the pyramidal tract that primarily control movement of the legs, the legs are affected more than the arms, and the child develops *spastic diplegia* (Figure 21.2). When only the legs are affected, with no involvement of the arms, the condition is called *paraplegia* (Keats, 1965).

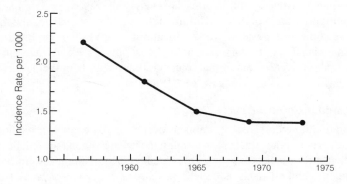

Figure 21.1.　Incidence of cerebral palsy fell between 1956 and 1965 but has remained fairly constant thereafter at about 1.5/1,000 live births. (From Kudrjavcev, T., Schoenberg, B.S., Kurland, L.T., et al. [1983]. Cerebral palsy—trends in incidence and changes in concurrent neonatal mortality: Rochester, MN, 1950–1976, *Neurology, 33,* 1433–1438; reprinted by permission.)

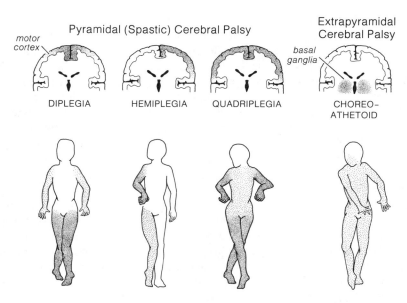

Figure 21.2.   Different regions of the brain are affected in various forms of cerebral palsy. The darker the shading, the more severe is the involvement.

If, instead, the child suffers a head injury that leads to bleeding into the area of the left pyramidal tract, the right side of the body is affected. This form of cerebral palsy is called *right spastic hemiplegia* (see Figure 21.2). In hemiplegia, the arm is usually more affected than the leg. Since the nerve fibers cross over before they enter the spinal cord, damage to one side of the brain causes abnormalities in the other side of the body.

When much of the cerebral cortex is severely damaged, *spastic quadriplegia* results (see Figure 21.2). In this condition, all four limbs are spastic, and the torso is also involved; the prognosis is worse. In this disorder, other problems, such as seizures and visual or auditory deficits, almost always exist. Overall, diplegia accounts for about 25% of pyramidal tract cerebral palsy, hemiplegia for 45%, and quadriplegia for 30% (Eiben & Crocker, 1983).

Extrapyramidal Cerebral Palsy

In extrapyramidal cerebral palsy, damage occurs to the pathways outside the pyramidal tract. These other tracts pass through the basal ganglia (see Chapter 12), and it is here that most of the damage seems to take place. The most common type of extrapyramidal cerebral palsy is called *choreoathetoid cerebral palsy* (see Figure 21.2). It involves the presence of abrupt, involuntary movements of the arms and legs. Unlike pyramidal cerebral palsy in which the problem is one of initiating movement, in choreoathetoid cerebral palsy, the difficulty is one of controlling movement and maintaining one's posture. Thus, damage affects the nerve tracts that regulate movement, not the ones that initiate it. A common cause of extrapyramidal cerebral palsy is a loss of oxygen during labor and delivery.

A child with this form of cerebral palsy has very different physical signs from one with spastic cerebral palsy. In trying to flex the child's arm, for example, one encounters a constant resistance called lead pipe rigidity, rather than the clasped-knife phenomenon of spastic cerebral palsy. Also, in extrapyramidal cerebral palsy, changes in muscle tone vary from one time to another. Sometimes the tone is increased, sometimes decreased. In addition, a physician examining the child can "shake out," or briefly reduce, the increased tone by rapidly flexing and extending the child's arm or leg (Denhoff & Robinault, 1960).

Because of the variability in tone, muscle contractures are less likely to occur in extrapyramidal cerebral palsy than in spastic cerebral palsy. On the other hand, facial muscles are more affected in choreoathetoid cerebral palsy. Consequently, the child may have more sucking, swallowing, drooling, and speaking difficulties than the child with the spastic form. Because the muscle tone fluctuates and the child experiences involuntary movements, it is more difficult for him or her to develop the stability needed for sitting and walking.

Besides choreoathetoid cerebral palsy, the other forms of extrapyramidal cerebral palsy are called *rigid* and *atonic*. Neither of these disorders has choreoathetoid movements. Instead, "lead pipe" or malleable rigidity characterizes rigid cerebral palsy, and floppy muscle tone predominates in atonic cerebral palsy. Physicians must be careful when diagnosing atonic cerebral palsy, since many forms of cerebral palsy present with symptoms of hypotonia in infancy.

Mixed-Type Cerebral Palsy

As the name implies, the mixed-type cerebral palsy includes elements of both the pyramidal and extrapyramidal forms of this disorder. For example, in a child with mixed-type cerebral palsy, the arms may be rigid while the legs are spastic. Since brain damage is often extensive, these children usually have mental retardation and other developmental disabilities.

EARLY DIAGNOSIS OF CEREBRAL PALSY

Certain groups of high risk newborns, including premature babies, twins, and small for gestational age infants, have a higher than normal incidence of cerebral palsy (Alberman, Benson, & McDonald, 1982; Hagberg, Hagberg, & Olow, 1982). Because of this increased risk, these children need to be followed closely for early signs of cerebral palsy.

Infants with cerebral palsy may behave differently from normal infants. They may sleep excessively, be irritable when awake, have a weak cry, a poor suck, and show little interest in their surroundings. Their resting position is also different. Instead of lying in a semiflexed position on the bed, they may lie in a floppy, rag doll way. Or they may have markedly increased tone and lie in an extended, arched fashion.

When examining such a child, a physician looks for abnormalities in muscle tone and reflexes. Muscle tone may be increased, decreased, or variable. It may also be asymmetrical; one side of the body may move more easily than the other side. Also, the deep tendon reflexes (DTR), such as the knee jerk, may be too quick, or the child may have tremors or *clonus* in the arms and legs.

Primitive reflexes, seen in the first 12 months of life in normal infants, usually persist in children with cerebral palsy. This persistence interferes with the normal expression of what are called *automatic movement reactions,* which are necessary for children to acquire gross motor skills. As a result, the child with cerebral palsy does not attain motor skills at the appropriate times. Although motor development is significantly delayed, cognitive and language skills may progress at a fairly normal rate. Thus, a discrepancy between the rates of motor and intellectual development is another clue to the existence of cerebral palsy.

As an affected child grows from infancy to 2 years of age, other signs of cerebral palsy become evident. Normally, infants hold their hands open after 3 months of age. In a child with cerebral palsy, the hands often remain closed in a fist. Also, a normal child does not become right- or left-handed until around 18 months of age, but a child with cerebral palsy may do so before he or she is 6 months old. This suggests that one side of the child's body is more severely involved than the other. As the child grows, this may become more obvious, because the affected limb atrophies and becomes smaller, both in circumference and in length (Keats, 1965).

Not all of these signs are found in every infant with cerebral palsy, and not all infants who have these signs develop cerebral palsy (Nelson & Ellenberg, 1982). Yet, these are indicators that can enable a physician to make a diagnosis of cerebral palsy before a child is 1 or 2 years old. With a severely affected child, the diagnosis may be clear in the first week of life (Crothers & Paine, 1959). However, in the child with mild cerebral palsy, mistakes are often made. For example, 67% of infants diagnosed as having spastic diplegia and 33% of those diagnosed as having hemiplegia or quadriplegia have been found to "outgrow" their cerebral palsy. Yet, 19% of these children who outgrew cerebral palsy were found to have mental retardation (Nelson & Ellenberg, 1982).

PRIMITIVE REFLEXES

Diagnostically, one of the chief signs of cerebral palsy is the persistence of primitive reflexes. These reflexes cause changes both in muscle tone and in movements of the limbs. They are called primitive because they are present in newborns and are controlled by the primitive regions of the nervous system: the spinal cord, the labyrinths of the inner ear, and the brain stem. As the cortex matures, these reflexes gradually are integrated into voluntary movement. During early infancy, they dominate movement; by 12 months of age, integration of the primitive reflexes is usually complete (Capute, Accardo, Vining, et al., 1977).

This is not true of a child with cerebral palsy. In such a child, primitive reflexes are stronger than normal and often last into adult life. In a previously normal child, these reflexes may reappear following a head injury or a coma. Such reflexes force the child to assume a position from which he or she has difficulty escaping (Capute, Accardo, Vining, et al., 1977).

Although there are many primitive reflexes, only three are considered in this section: the asymmetrical tonic neck reflex (ATNR), the tonic labyrinthine reflex (TL), and the positive support reflex (PS). Each of these significantly affects posture and movement, and each has a different stimulus that elicits it.

The stimulus for the *asymmetrical tonic neck reflex* is the active or passive rotation of the head. When the head is turned, the ATNR causes the arm and leg on the same side as the chin to extend more while the opposite arm and leg become more flexed (Figure 21.3). Changes in muscle tone may occur in the trunk as well. Thus, the ATNR causes an increase in muscle tone and also frequently brings about a change in position.

Infants under 3 months of age normally show the ATNR. Yet, even in infancy, a child can overcome the reflex, that is, flex and move his or her arm once it is extended. Some children with cerebral palsy cannot. They remain in the extended position until the head turns and releases the reflex. This predicament illustrates the obligatory nature of the reflex for these children.

For the *tonic labyrinthine reflex,* the stimulus is the position of the labyrinth inside the inner ear. When the neck is in an extended position or when the child is lying on his or her back, the labyrinth is tilted, and the reflex is elicited. The legs extend and the shoulders retract, or pull back (Figure 21.4). When the neck is flexed or the child is lying on his or her stomach, the hips and knees flex while the shoulders

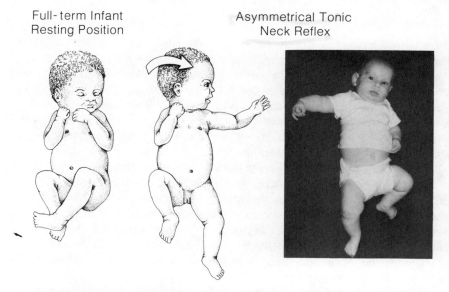

Full-term Infant
Resting Position

Asymmetrical Tonic
Neck Reflex

Figure 21.3. Asymmetrical tonic neck reflex, or fencer's response. As the head is turned, the arm and leg on the same side as the chin extend, and the other arm and leg flex.

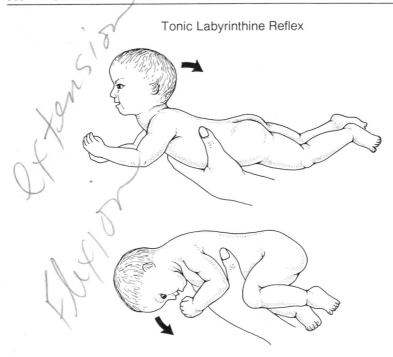

Tonic Labyrinthine Reflex

Figure 21.4. Tonic labyrinthine reflex. In the tonic labyrinthine reflex, extension of the head backward leads to retraction of the shoulders and extension of the legs. The opposite occurs if the head is flexed forward.

protract or roll forward. When the reflex is present but is not as strong, changes in muscle tone may occur without any changes in the position of the limbs.

The third primitive reflex is the *positive support reflex*. When the balls of the feet come in contact with a firm surface, the child extends the legs (Figure 21.5). This reflex enables a normal child to support his or her weight while standing. However, the increased response in a child with cerebral palsy leads to a rigid extension of the legs and feet, often accompanied by the adduction and an internal rotation of the hips. Rather than helping, this reflex then interferes with standing and walking.

Since these primitive reflexes result in changes in muscle tone and in position of the limbs, their persistence interferes with the normal development of voluntary motor activity. For example, to be able to roll over (normally accomplished at 4–5 months of age), a child must have an ATNR that is fairly well integrated with automatic movement reactions (see next section). If the ATNR lasts, the infant has difficulty beginning this movement. As he or she turns the head, the extended arm and leg hinder the start of the roll. Once the roll is begun, the flexed arm of the strong ATNR prevents its completion.

A similar problem occurs with the TL reflex and sitting. To sit independently, equilibrium reactions must be present. These reactions require constant, fine changes

Positive Support Reflex

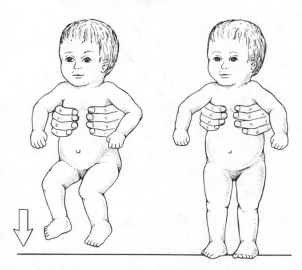

Figure 21.5. Positive support reflex. As the baby is bounced, the legs straighten to support the child's weight.

in muscle tone to maintain balance. If a strong TL reflex is present, movement of the head causes patterns of flexion and extension throughout the body. These changes are incompatible with the equilibrium reactions needed to maintain balance in a sitting position.

AUTOMATIC MOVEMENT REACTIONS

As the primitive reflexes diminish in intensity, **postural** reactions, known as automatic movement reactions, are developing (Figure 21.6). Some of the more important of these reactions include what are called righting, equilibrium, and protective reactions. These enable the child to have more complex voluntary movement and better control of posture.

Up to 2 months of age, a baby's head tilts passively in the same direction that the body is leaning. However, by 3 months of age, the baby should be able to compensate and hold his or her head upright even if the body is tilted. This is called head righting.

Before 5 months of age, if a child is placed in a sitting position and starts to fall forward, he or she will tumble over without trying to regain balance. By this age, when he or she begins to fall over, the baby will push out his or her arms to prevent the fall. This is called the *anterior protective response*. By 7 months, a similar response, the *lateral protective response,* occurs when the child starts to fall sideways (Capute, Accardo, Vining, et al., 1977). For a child to be able to sit and do other things simultaneously, balance must be refined enough so that the child can use his or her

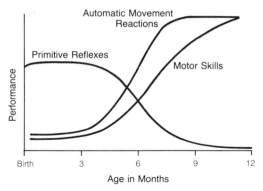

Figure 21.6.   Relationship of primitive reflexes, automatic movement reactions, and motor skills. (From Capute, A., Accardo, P., Vining, E., et al. [1977]. *Primitive reflex profile*. Baltimore: University Park Press; reprinted by permission.)

arms to reach and perform other activities as well as shift his or her weight without using arms for support. Thus, these equilibrium reactions enable the child to sit and do other things by automatically compensating when the center of gravity is shifted.

In children with cerebral palsy, not only do the primitive reflexes persist but the development of the automatic movement reactions also may lag behind or may never occur.

WALKING AND MOVEMENT

To walk, a child must be able to maintain upright posture and move forward in a smoothly coordinated manner at the same time. Even the most mildly affected child with cerebral palsy has difficulty performing the continuous changes in muscle tone that are required for normal walking. The child's walk, or gait, is affected in many ways. *Scissoring,* the most common gait disturbance, occurs because of increased tone in the muscles that control adduction and internal rotation of the hips (Figure 21.7). *Toe walking* results from an **equinus** position of the feet (see Figure 21.7) and an increased **flexor** tone in the legs.

DISABILITIES ASSOCIATED WITH CEREBRAL PALSY

Although all children with cerebral palsy have problems with movement and posture, many also have other disabilities. The most common associated disabilities are mental retardation, visual deficits, auditory disorders, and seizures (Table 21.2).

Approximately 60% of individuals with cerebral palsy have mental retardation. The particular type of cerebral palsy influences the incidence and degree of mental retardation (Robinson, 1973). Hemiplegia, the most common type of cerebral palsy, is associated with the best intellectual outcome. Most of these children have normal intelligence. Some of the children with spastic diplegia also have normal intelligence. On the other hand, fewer than 30% of individuals with spastic quadriplegia, extra-

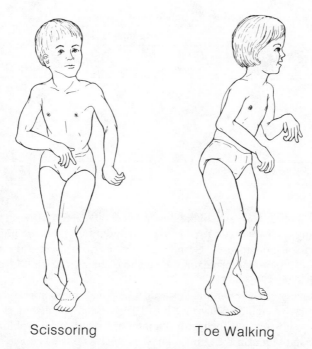

Scissoring   Toe Walking

Figure 21.7.   Scissoring results from increased tone in the muscles that control adduction and internal rotation of the hip. Toe walking is due to an equinus position of the feet and increased flexor tone in the legs.

pyramidal, and mixed-type cerebral palsy have normal intelligence. Among those children with cerebral palsy and mental retardation, 15% have mild retardation, 35% have moderate retardation, and 50% have severe to profound retardation (Robinson, 1973).

Besides mental retardation, visual problems are common and diverse in these children (Black, 1982). The premature infant may suffer retinopathy of prematurity (see Chapter 15) from excessive oxygen therapy. The child who had kernicterus may be unable to gaze in an upward direction. Individuals with hemiplegia frequently cannot see out of one part of their visual field. They also may have visual-perceptual problems that interfere with learning. About one-quarter of all children with cerebral palsy have strabismus, or squint. Overall, more than 40% of individuals with cerebral palsy also have visual or visual-perceptual deficits (Black, 1980).

Hearing, speech, and language deficits are also common and occur in about 20% of children with cerebral palsy (Platt, Andrews, & Howie, 1980; Robinson, 1973). Children with kernicterus or congenital rubella often have a high-frequency hearing loss (see Chapter 16). Extrapyramidal cerebral palsy is associated with articulation problems, and choreoathetoid movements affect tongue and vocal cord movements. Language disorders may also result from the brain damage that caused the cerebral palsy (see Chapter 17).

Table 21.2.   Deficits associated with cerebral palsy

Deficit	Percentage affected				
	Quadri-plegia	Hemi-plegia	Di-plegia	Extra-pyramidal	Mixed
Visual	55	23	38	50	64
Auditory	22	8	13	17	21
Mental retardation	67	38	56	92	79
Seizure disorder	45	12	12	45	12

Note: Study population: $N = 80$.
Source: Robinson (1973).

Roughly one-third of all children with cerebral palsy will develop seizures sometime during their lives (Keats, 1965). Pyramidal forms of cerebral palsy carry the highest incidence of seizures. Grand mal seizures occur frequently in those with hemiplegia, while minor motor seizures are common in individuals with quadriplegia and rigidity (Keats, 1965).

Finally, behavior and emotional disorders play an important role in the lives of children who have cerebral palsy (Taylor, 1959). Behavior disorders range from hyperactivity to self-injurious behavior. Numerous psychosocial problems may also develop for the individual or the family. These problems tend to become more intense during adolescence, especially in children of normal intelligence (Freeman, 1970). The ability of the family and the community to accept the child with cerebral palsy greatly affects the outcome of these problems (Barsch, 1976; Hewett, with Newson & Newson, 1970). Agencies such as the United Cerebral Palsy Association (UCP) can provide invaluable support and training for these children and their families.

TREATMENT

In developing a treatment program for a child with cerebral palsy, it is important to use an interdisciplinary approach (Taft, Matthews, & Molnar, 1983). Normally, many disciplines are involved, including occupational therapy, physical therapy, biomedical engineering, special education, speech pathology, audiology, social work, psychology, nutrition, and pediatrics (Haslam, 1973). Each discipline addresses some aspect of the child's disability. For instance, the occupational therapist evaluates the motor development of the arms, oral motor functions, visual-perceptual problems, and the activities of daily living (Finnie, 1975). The physical therapist is primarily involved in the development of posture and movement. The special educator establishes an individualized education program (IEP) for the child. The speech pathologist evaluates the child's ability to communicate. The audiologist identifies a hearing loss and recommends correction. The clinical psychologist evaluates the child's intellectual functioning, and the behavioral psychologist develops a behavior modification program, if necessary. The nutritionist recommends an appropriate diet and monitors growth. The social worker assesses family problems and coping mechanisms and offers support and counseling. The developmental pediatrician provides medical care and coordinates the various disciplines, including medical subspecialties such as orthopedics, neurology, neurosurgery, and ophthalmology.

To reiterate, the various elements of therapy may include physical therapy, occupational therapy, speech and language therapy, orthopedic surgery, and the use of medications, braces, and possibly biofeedback (Thompson, Rubin, & Bilenker, 1983). It is difficult to assess the effectiveness of these different treatment forms. Yet, in one study, treatment begun before the children were 9 months old seemed to help them walk earlier compared to those who started therapy after 1 year of age (Kanda, Yuge, Yamori, et al., 1984).

Physical Therapy

Initially, in the treatment of any child, the physical therapist evaluates posture and movement. This includes assessing tone, range of motion, primitive reflexes, and automatic movement reactions. In the United States, the principal method of physical therapy is the neurodevelopmental approach (Bobath, 1966; Thompson, 1979). This method is based on the enhancement of normal movement patterns in the child. After an evaluation, a therapy program is developed for each child. Individual techniques for positioning and handling to maintain optimal muscle tone and to facilitate equilibrium and righting reactions are established as part of each child's therapy program (Scherzer, Mike, & Ilson, 1976). Consultation with family members and others who have daily contact with the child is essential to set up a consistent program.

Patterning

Another approach to treating children with cerebral palsy is called patterning. This was discussed for the treatment of children with learning disabilities in Chapter 20. Patterning involves putting the child through a series of exercises designed to improve "neurological organization." Three to five volunteers simultaneously manipulate the child's limbs and head for hours daily in patterns that are supposed to simulate the prenatal and infantile movement of normal children. Proponents believe that if a child makes certain motions enough times, undamaged brain cells will be reprogrammed to take over the functions of the damaged cells (Zigler, 1981). The American Academy of Pediatrics is strongly opposed to this treatment. This group has found little evidence to support the theory. In addition, the regimen prescribed is so demanding and inflexible that it places considerable stress on the child and his or her family (American Academy of Pediatrics, 1982).

Physical Activity

Physical exercise is important to strengthen muscles, enhance skills, and prevent contractures (Guttman, 1976). An added benefit is that physical activity is enjoyable. The Special Olympics founded by the Joseph P. Kennedy Jr. Foundation has proven this. Each year, thousands of children with disabilities participate in running, swimming, basketball, gymnastics, and other sporting events. The rewards are invaluable for enhancing self-esteem and providing a sense of belonging. Parents and professionals should encourage all children to take part in whatever physical activity they are capable of doing.

Braces and Splints

Bracing or splinting is used along with physical therapy to maintain the range of movement, to prevent contractures at a specific joint, to provide stability, and to control involuntary movements that impair functioning (Nuzzo, 1980). Contractures develop when muscles consistently have increased tone and remain in a shortened position, severely limiting movement. The brace is usually adjusted to maintain a specific group of muscles in a lengthened or less contracted state. This improves the functioning of the joint.

One of the most commonly prescribed braces is the short leg brace. It prevents permanent shortening of the heel cords, often avoiding the need for an operation to lengthen the Achilles (ankle) tendon (see upcoming subsection on "Orthopedic Surgery"). This brace consists either of a shoe with a metal bar and leather cuff around the calf or a molded plastic splint worn inside the shoe, called an *ankle-foot* **orthosis** or AFO (Figure 21.8). Similar devices may be needed to maintain or improve range of movement and function in the wrist or hand.

Bracing devices are also used to control abnormal positions or involuntary movements that interfere with the functioning of the leg or arm. For example, an ankle splint may prevent an extended position of the foot that results from an increase in the extensor tone in the legs. Decreasing this extension at the ankle may also decrease the muscle tone in the hips and allow the child to sit in a more stable position. Also, the change in the position of the ankle allows the child to stand with his or her foot flat, improving the base of support and stability. Finally, correcting the child's abnormal foot posture may affect the position of the hips and knees when the child stands, thereby improving his or her gait. For a child with choreoathetoid cerebral palsy, a similar brace may control involuntary movements at the ankle.

To keep the hands open, a splint may be used. The thumb is held in an abducted position and the wrist in a neutral or slightly extended position (Figure 21.9). Thus, the child can make better use of his or her hand.

Most of these braces and splints are made of molded plastic. Therefore, they are custom-made and are changed as the child grows. The use of these devices may improve functioning, decrease the risk of contractures, and prevent or delay the need for corrective orthopedic surgery.

Chairs

For nonambulatory children, proper wheelchairs are essential (Schultz-Hurlburt & Tervo, 1982). The common sling-type stroller is a poor choice because it does not support the back or keep the hips properly aligned. A more supportive collapsible stroller (Pogon buggy) is indicated in Figure 21.10A. An alternative is a car seat that can be set into a stroller base (see Figure 21.10B). More appropriate for everyday use

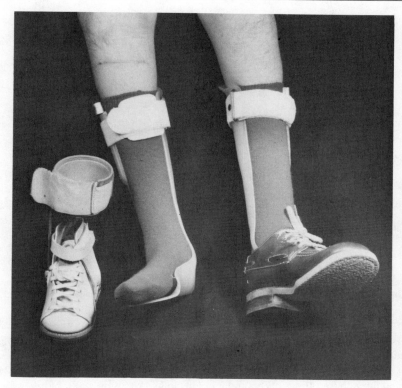

Figure 21.8. Braces. The child is wearing an ankle-foot orthosis to counter toe walking. A short leg brace used for a smaller child is shown at left.

is a high-backed straight chair (21.10c). However, some children may have difficulty using this type of chair, and modifications may be needed. For example, children with severe muscle spasms have trouble maintaining a 90° angle and an upright position. For these children, a molded insert that maintains the hips, knees, and ankles at the proper angle along with tilting the chair 10–15° will enable these children to sit comfortably and be properly supported. Children who have hypotonia may need side and head supports to keep their back and neck in position. A tray attached to the wheelchair allows the child to play with toys and to eat more independently. Motorized wheelchairs are a recent innovation that enhance the independence of those children who are able to use them. The most common type has an easily manipulated joy stick that controls both direction and speed (Breed & Ibler, 1982) (see Figure 21.10D). For children who cannot control their hand movements, other types of chairs have head switches.

Medication

Unfortunately, medications have limited usefulness in improving muscle tone in children with cerebral palsy (Young & Delwaide, 1981a,b). The medications most

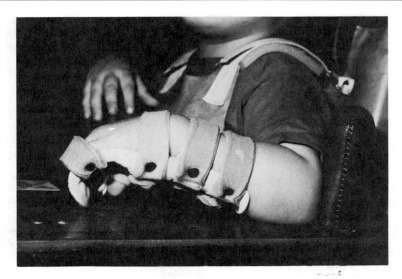

Figure 21.9. Hand splint. The thumb is held in an abducted position and the wrist in a neutral position. This may both decrease the risk of contracture and increase the use of the hand.

commonly used to control spasticity and rigidity are diazepam (Valium), baclofen (Lioresal), and dantrolene (Dantrium). No drug has been helpful for treating involuntary movement. For treating spasticity and rigidity, diazepam has proven the most useful because it decreases muscle tone (Ford, Bleck, Aptekar, et al., 1976). It is given three to four times daily, and it begins to work within 1 hour of ingestion and lasts about 4 hours. A common dose in a child with cerebral palsy is 2 milligrams three times daily. Side effects include drowsiness and excessive drooling.

Baclofen has been most effective in treating adults with multiple sclerosis and traumatic damage to the spinal cord (Young & Delwaide, 1981a,b). So far, this drug has not been used very often for treating cerebral palsy in children. The dosage in adults is 40–80 milligrams/day, divided into four doses. Drowsiness, nausea, and headache are the most common side effects.

Finally, dantrolene affects the peripheral muscles because it reduces the outflow of calcium from muscle fibers. This decreases the strength of the contraction of the muscle. About half of the children who were tested with this drug showed modest improvement (Joynt & Leonard, 1980). The dosage of dantrolene ranges from 0.5 to 3.0 milligrams/kilograms/day. It usually is given two to three times daily. Side effects include drowsiness, weakness, and increased drooling. A rare side effect of this drug is severe liver dysfunction.

Orthopedic Surgery

Because of the abnormal or asymmetrical distribution of muscle tone, children who have cerebral palsy are susceptible to the development of joint deformities. The most common of these result from permanent shortening, or contractures, of one or more

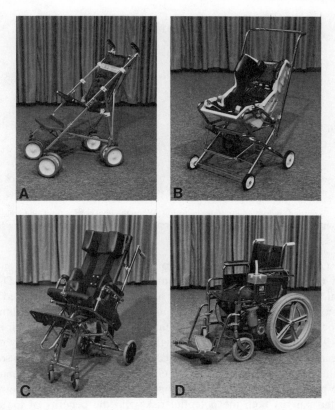

Figure 21.10. Chairs for children with cerebral palsy. A) Pogon collapsible buggy. B) Car seat/stroller. C) High-backed straight chair with inserts and head supports. D) Motorized wheelchair with joystick steering. (Photographs courtesy of William Diehl, The Kennedy Institute for Handicapped Children, Baltimore.)

groups of muscles around a joint; these limit the joint's mobility. Orthopedic surgery is done to increase the range of motion through the release, lengthening, or transfer of affected muscles. For example, a partial release or transfer of the hip adductor muscles may help to increase the range in hip abduction and improve the child's ability to sit and walk (Ferguson, 1981). A partial hamstring release, lengthening, or transfer of muscles around the knee may facilitate sitting and walking. A lengthening of the Achilles tendon at the ankle also improves walking (Figure 21.11). All of these procedures require the use of a cast or splint for 6–8 weeks after surgery and a brace at night for at least several months more (Bleck, 1979; Lee & Bleck, 1980).

A more complicated procedure is the correction of a dislocated hip that is caused by persistent, increased hip adduction over an extended period of time. If this is diagnosed when there is an incomplete or partial dislocation (**subluxation**), release of the hip adductor muscles and removal of the branch of the nerve that supplies these muscles can be effective. This operation, called an *adductor tenotomy and obturator*

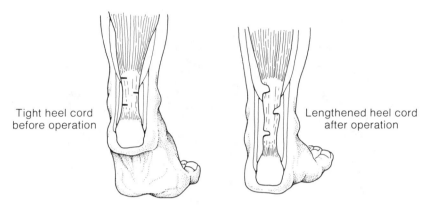

Tight heel cord
before operation

Lengthened heel cord
after operation

Figure 21.11.   Achilles tendon lengthening operation. When the heel cord is tight, the child walks on his or her toes. Surgery lengthens the heel cord and permits a more flat-footed gait.

neurectomy (ATON), usually is adequate to decrease the abnormal pull on the femur and correct the dislocation as well as improve mobility (Moreau, Drummond, Rogala, et al., 1979) (Figure 21.12). If the head of the femur is dislocated more than one-third to one-half of the way out of the hip joint socket (the acetabulum), a more complex procedure—a varus osteotomy—may be necessary (Tylkowski, Rosenthal, & Simon, 1980). In this operation, the angle of the femur is surgically changed to place the head of the femur back into the acetabulum (Figure 21.13). In some cases, the acetabulum must also be reshaped to ensure that the hip joint remains intact.

Before performing surgery, the orthopedic surgeon is careful to evaluate and explain to the parents both the potential risks and the benefits of the operation. Although surgery may both increase the mobility of the child and prevent the development of painful osteoarthritis, there is always the risk that the operation may not have the intended results or that the child may suffer complications from the surgery.

Neurosurgery

A number of neurosurgical procedures have been used to treat cerebral palsy. One of these, a *ventrolateral thalamotomy,* was discussed in Chapter 13. Besides its use in dystonia, this operation has been suggested for children with choreoathetoid cerebral palsy (Cooper, Riklan, Amin, et al., 1976; Penn, 1979). Although a number of studies have shown improvement in 10%–15% of these children following this operation, the general impression is that the procedure is not likely to help most choreoathetoid patients (Gornall, Hitchcock, & Kirkland, 1975).

Much the same conclusion is drawn regarding cerebellar and dorsal column stimulators. In these two procedures, electrodes are surgically placed either in the cerebellum or outside the coverings of the cervical spinal cord (Burton, Ray, & Nashold, 1977). The electrodes are connected to an electrical stimulator that emits a very small current. These signals are thought to block some of the abnormal impulses

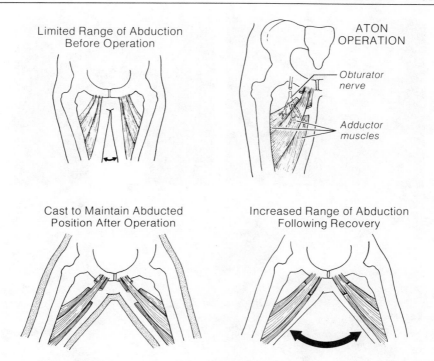

Limited Range of Abduction
Before Operation

ATON
OPERATION

Obturator
nerve

Adductor
muscles

Cast to Maintain Abducted
Position After Operation

Increased Range of Abduction
Following Recovery

Figure 21.12. Adductor tenotomy and obturator neurectomy. This operation is done to improve scissoring and to prevent hip dislocation caused by contractures of the adductor muscles in the thigh. Some of these muscles are cut, and the nerve leading to them is also severed. The child is placed in a cast to maintain a more open position. The muscles eventually grow together in a lengthened position, allowing improved sitting and/or walking.

and decrease the choreoathetosis. However, improvement is often insignificant or transient. Also, these procedures carry a risk of infection.

Biofeedback

Another approach to treatment is behavioral rather than surgical. Biofeedback involves the placement of surface electrodes over a muscle group that lacks voluntary control. The electrodes sense muscle activity and record this activity on an **electromyogram** (EMG). The patient is presented with this electrical pattern and, by trial and error, attempts to control the activity of his or her muscles to more closely resemble that of a normal pattern of muscle activity (Basmajian, 1981). When this is achieved, the individual has more coordinated movement (Bird & Cataldo, 1978; Seeger & Caudrey, 1983). This is useful if only one group of muscles is affected, and if the person has the intellectual ability to use the procedure.

Computers

In the future, computers will play an increasingly important role in the habilitation of children with cerebral palsy. Even now, computers can perform many functions to

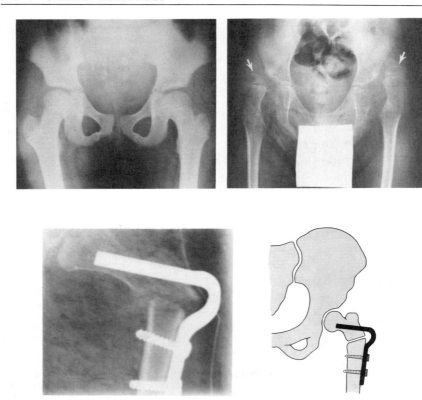

rıgure 21.13. Dislocation of the hip. The upper X rays show a normal hip to the left and a hip dislocated on both sides on the right. The arrows indicate the points of dislocation. The lower picture shows the results of a varus osteotomy to correct the left-side dislocation. The femur has been cut and realigned so that it now fits into the acetabulum. Pins, which are later removed, hold the bone in place until it heals.

help persons with disabilities live more independently. For example, computers can be used to better control the environment, to provide a lifeline with the outside world, to enable a person to work at home, and to give artificial speech, sight, and entertainment (Levy, 1983). Control of the environment can include a system that will turn the lights on and off, unlock the front door, and turn on various appliances. The telephone can also be controlled and a message automatically sent in the case of an emergency.

For individuals with severe speech deficits, the computer can provide synthesized speech. Persons with visual impairment can use the computer to receive spoken instructions and to verify letters they have written (Teja, 1983). For those who are unable to use a keyboard because of poor fine motor coordination, alternate devices to feed in information are available. Since someone with a home computer can learn how to do programming and can use a **modem** to hook up with other computers, employment at home is possible. Through such a device, a person can also do shopping and banking from home. In addition, the computer is a source of recreation, offering games and educational programs. Clearly, the uses of a computer are almost limitless and potentially may enrich the lives of many individuals with handicaps (Vanderheiden, 1982).

CASE HISTORIES OF CHILDREN WITH CEREBRAL PALSY

Tommy Tommy's birth was traumatic. His mother suffered an abruptio placenta, and she required an emergency cesarean section. She lost a great deal of blood, and the physician could not detect a fetal heartbeat during the final 3 minutes before birth. Tommy's Apgar scores were 1 at 1 minute and 2 at 5 minutes. The injection of Adrenalin into the heart and artificial ventilation were required. The doctors were able to stabilize Tommy within the first day of life, but they were afraid that significant brain damage had already occurred.

Their concern was justified. Tommy fed poorly and slept most of the time. When he was awake, he was irritable and screamed. His muscle tone remained floppy. By 3 months of age, he still held his hands in a fisted position and could not hold his head upright. He had intermittent minor-motor seizures. By 6 months of age, Tommy still made no attempt to roll over and was only beginning to make cooing sounds. When he was 12 months old, he started having choreoathetoid movements of his arms, and his muscle tone was variable (sometimes decreased and other times increased). At 2 years of age, he rolled over and reached for objects. Because of the choreoathetosis and severe mental retardation, Tommy could not actually grab objects but rather batted at them. He responded inconsistently to sounds and was later found to have a severe sensorineural hearing loss.

Emotionally, things became progressively more difficult for Tommy's parents as they realized he had severe retardation and would never be self-sufficient. However, with the support of relatives and the use of special schools and respite care, they were able to cope over the years. Now, at 21 years of age, Tommy still lives at home and attends a cerebral palsy activity center. He is happy at the center and enjoys the company of others. His cerebral palsy continues to make it impossible for him to feed or dress himself. He functions mentally at around an 18-month level. He can now sit without support but remains in a wheelchair. His parents worry about his future when they are no longer alive.

Tina Tina, a premature infant, weighed less than 2 pounds when she was born in the seventh month. She had a rocky newborn period with hypoglycemia, respiratory distress syndrome, and a patent ductus arteriosus. When finally released from the hospital at 3 months of age, she was an alert, active, and happy baby. However, her legs were definitely spastic and were held in a scissored position. She started at that age to receive regular physical therapy.

Apart from her motor development, many of her developmental milestones were normal, especially considering her prematurity. She said "mama" at 1 year of age to everyone and followed one-step commands. She could also drink from a cup. She could roll over from stomach to back, but she could not sit or stand. Her primitive reflexes persisted, and the muscle tone, especially in her legs, was increased. Her hips were noted to be partially dislocated. Although her intellectual skills fell around the 9-month level, her gross motor skills were at a 4-month level.

By 2 years of age, the scissoring of her legs became more and more troublesome, and the problem with her hips was more prominent. Dressing and sitting were difficult. An ATON operation successfully released the adductor muscles of her legs. After intensive physical therapy, she learned to roll over and sit. By 4 years of age, she was walking with short leg braces and canes. Her language development continued on course, and IQ testing using the Wechsler Intelligence Scale for Children–Revised at 6 years of age showed a verbal score of 110 and a performance score of 82. In children with cerebral palsy, such a discrepancy is common. For Tina, it was the first clue to the presence of a learning disability that became more apparent in the first grade.

Another problem, a squint, was also corrected surgically, and Tina's appearance improved. She was a vibrant, pretty, and happy child. However, her problems were not over. In the second grade, she had a number of grand mal seizures. An EEG confirmed the diagnosis of a seizure disorder, and she was placed on Dilantin. Tina is now 9 years old and has had only one seizure in the last year.

Right now, Tina is doing well in a public school setting. She is in a normal class for most of her subjects and gets help in a resource room for her reading problems. She also continues to have regular physical and occupational therapy. Both she and her parents have coped well emotionally with her disability.

PROGNOSIS

Although most children with cerebral palsy live to adulthood, their projected life expectancy is less than that of the normal population (Jones, 1975). The prognosis varies for each type of cerebral palsy. A child with a mild left hemiplegia will likely have a normal life expectancy, while a child with spastic quadriplegia may not live beyond age 40.

Although about 40% of the individuals who have cerebral palsy have normal intelligence, only a small number of these persons are able to lead normal lives (Jones, 1975). As adults, only about one-fourth are working (10% are entirely self-supporting). Another 7% work in sheltered workshop programs. An additional 39% have sufficient self-help skills to be partially independent at home. The remaining 11% who live to adulthood are in institutions (Ingram, Jameson, Errington, et al., 1964; Jones, 1975) (Table 21.3).

SUMMARY

Cerebral palsy refers to a group of disorders that cause brain damage in children. The disability is not progressive, nor does it have a cure. Certain types of cerebral palsy, such as hemiplegia and spastic diplegia, have a fairly good prognosis for independent functioning, while others, such as rigid and spastic quadriplegia, usually lead to a

Table 21.3. Living situations of adults with cerebral palsy followed over a 20-year period in the United States

| Living situation | Percentage of individuals in each living situation | | | | |
	Hemi-plegia	Choreo-athetoid	Rigid	Mixed	Total percentage
Working	39	18	0	12	26
Sheltered workshop	8	6	0	9	7
Unemployed	36	44	25	48	39
Institutionalized	8	13	19	12	11
Deceased	9	19	56	19	17

Note: Study population: $N = 336$.
Source: O'Reilly (1975).

future of dependence. In many cases, other problems besides the motor abnormalities exist, including seizures and visual, auditory, and intellectual deficits.

The most effective treatment consists of the use of an interdisciplinary approach. A number of the children with good intellectual abilities and limited handicaps can lead normal lives. Others are capable of various degrees of independence.

REFERENCES

Alberman, E., Benson, J., & McDonald, A. (1982). Cerebral palsy and severe educational subnormality in low-birthweight children: A comparison of births in 1951–53 and 1970–73. *Lancet, 1,* 606–608.
American Academy of Pediatrics. (1982). The Doman-Delacato treatment of neurologically handicapped children. *Pediatrics, 70,* 810–812.
Barsch, R.H. (1976). *The parent of the handicapped child: The study of child-rearing practices.* Springfield, IL: Charles C Thomas.
Basmajian, J.V. (1981). Biofeedback in rehabilitation: A review of principles and practices. *Archives of Physical Medicine and Rehabilitation, 62,* 469–475.
Bird, B.L., & Cataldo, M.F. (1978). Experimental analysis of EMG feedback in treating dystonia. *Annals of Neurology, 3,* 310–315.
Black, P.D. (1980). Ocular defects in children with cerebral palsy. *British Medical Journal, 281,* 487–488.
Black, P. (1982). Visual disorders associated with cerebral palsy. *British Journal of Ophthalmology, 66,* 46–52.
Bleck, E.E. (1979). *Orthopaedic management of cerebral palsy.* Philadelphia: W.B. Saunders Co.
Bobath, K. (1966). The motor deficit in patients with cerebral palsy. *Clinics in Developmental Medicine, No. 23.* London: Spastics Society Medical Educational and Information Unit, in association with William Heinemann Medical Books.
Breed, A.L., & Ibler, I. (1982). The motorized wheelchair: New freedom, new responsibility and new problems. *Developmental Medicine and Child Neurology, 24,* 366–371.
Burton, C.V., Ray, C.D., & Nashold, B.S., Jr. (Eds.) (1977). Symposium on the safety and clinical efficacy of implanted neuroaugmentive devices. *Neurosurgery, 1,* 185–232.
Capute, A.J., Accardo, P.J., Vining, E.P.G., et al. (1977). *Primitive reflex profile.* Baltimore: University Park Press.
Cooper, I.S., Riklan, M., Amin, I., et al. (1976). Chronic cerebellar stimulation in cerebral palsy. *Neurology, 26,* 744–753.
Crothers, B., & Paine, R.S. (1959). *The natural history of cerebral palsy.* Cambridge, MA: Harvard University Press.

Cruickshank, W.M. (Ed.) (1976). *Cerebral palsy: A developmental disability* (3rd ed.). Syracuse: Syracuse University Press.

Denhoff, E., & Robinault, I.P. (1960). *Cerebral palsy and related disorders: A developmental approach to dysfunction.* New York: McGraw-Hill Book Co.

Eiben, R.M., & Crocker, A.C. (1983). Cerebral palsy within the spectrum of developmental disabilities. In G.H. Thompson, I.L. Rubin, & R.M. Bilenker (Eds.), *Comprehensive management of cerebral palsy.* New York: Grune & Stratton.

Ferguson, A.B. (1981). *Orthopaedic surgery in infancy and childhood* (5th ed.). Baltimore: Williams & Wilkins Co.

Finnie, N.R. (1975). *Handling the young cerebral palsied child at home.* New York: E.P. Dutton & Co.

Ford, F., Bleck, E.E., Aptekar, R.G., et al. (1976). Efficacy of dantrolene sodium in the treatment of spastic cerebral palsy. *Developmental Medicine and Child Neurology 18,* 770–783.

Freeman, R.D. (1970). Psychiatric problems in adolescents with cerebral palsy. *Developmental Medicine and Child Neurology, 12,* 64–70.

Gornall, P., Hitchcock, E., & Kirkland, I.S. (1975). Stereotaxic neurosurgery in the management of cerebral palsy. *Developmental Medicine and Child Neurology, 17,* 279–286.

Guttman, L. (1976). *Textbook of sport for the disabled.* Aylesbury, England: H.M. & M. Publishers.

Hagberg, B. (1979). Epidemiological and preventive aspects of cerebral palsy and severe mental retardation in Sweden. *European Journal of Pediatrics, 130,* 71–78.

Hagberg, B., Hagberg, G., & Olow, I. (1975). The changing panorama of cerebral palsy in Sweden, 1954–1970: I. Analysis of the general changes. *Acta Paediatrica Scandinavica, 64,* 187–192.

Hagberg, B., Hagberg, G., & Olow, I. (1982). Gains and hazards of intensive neonatal care: An analysis from Swedish cerebral palsy epidemiology. *Developmental Medicine and Child Neurology, 24,* 13–19.

Haslam, R.H.A. (Ed.). (1973). Habilitation of the handicapped child. *Pediatric Clinics of North America, 20,* 1–268.

Hewett, S., with Newson, J., & Newson, E. (1970). *The family and the handicapped child: A study of cerebral palsied children in their homes.* Chicago: Aldine Publishing Co.

Hreidarsson, S.J., Shapiro, B.K., & Capute, A.J. (1983). Age of walking in the cognitively impaired. *Clinical Pediatrics, 22,* 248–250.

Illingworth, R.S. (1983). *The development of the infant and young child: Normal and abnormal* (8th ed.). New York: Churchill Livingstone, Inc.

Ingram, T.T.S., Jameson, S., Errington, J., et al. (1964). *Living with cerebral palsy: A study of school leavers suffering from cerebral palsy in Eastern Scotland.* London: Spastics Society Medical Educational and Information Unit in association with William Heinemann Medical Books.

Jones, M.H. (1975). Differential diagnosis and natural history of the cerebral palsied child. In R.L. Samilson (Ed.), *Orthopaedic aspects of cerebral palsy.* Philadelphia: J.B. Lippincott Co.

Joynt, R.L. & Leonard, J.A., Jr. (1980). Dantrolene sodium suspension in treatment of spastic cerebral palsy. *Developmental Medicine and Child Neurology, 22,* 755–767.

Kanda, T., Yuge, M., Yamori, Y., et al. (1984). Early physiotherapy in the treatment of spastic diplegia. *Developmental Medicine and Child Neurology, 26,* 438–444.

Keats, S. (1965). *Cerebral palsy.* Springfield, IL: Charles C Thomas.

Kudrjavcev, T., Schoenberg, B.S., Kurland, L.T., et al. (1983). Cerebral palsy—trends in incidence and changes in concurrent neonatal mortality: Rochester, MN, 1950–1976. *Neurology, 33,* 1433–1438.

Lee, C.L., & Bleck, E.E. (1980). Surgical correction of equinus deformity in cerebral palsy. *Developmental Medicine and Child Neurology, 22,* 287–292.

Levy, R. (1983). Interface modalities of technical aids used by people with disability. *American Journal of Occupational Therapy, 37,* 761–765.

Low, N.L. (1980). A hypothesis why "early intervention" in cerebral palsy might be useful. *Brain Development, 2,* 133–135.

Molnar, G.E. (1982). Intervention for physically handicapped children. In M. Lewis & L.T. Taft (Eds.), *Developmental disabilities: Theory, assessment and intervention.* New York: SP Medical and Scientific Books.

Moreau, M., Drummond, D.S., Rogala, E., et al. (1979). Natural history of the dislocated hip in spastic cerebral palsy. *Developmental Medicine and Child Neurology, 21,* 749–753.

Nelson, K.B., & Ellenberg, J.M. (1982). Children who "outgrew" cerebral palsy. *Pediatrics, 69,* 529–536.

Nuzzo, R.M. (1980). Dynamic bracing: Elastics for patients with cerebral palsy, muscular dystrophy and myelodysplasia. *Clinical Orthopedics, 148,* 263–273.

O'Reilly, D.E. (1975). Care of the cerebral palsied: Outcome of the past and needs for the future. *Developmental Medicine and Child Neurology, 17,* 141–149.

Paneth, N., Kiely, J.L., Stein, Z., et al. (1981). Cerebral palsy and newborn care. III. Estimated prevalence rates of cerebral palsy under differing rates of mortality and impairment of low birth-weight infants. *Developmental Medicine and Child Neurology, 23,* 801–806.

Pape, K.E., & Wigglesworth, J.S. (1979). Haemorrhage, ischaemia and the perinatal brain. *Clinics in Developmental Medicine, Nos. 69 & 70.* Philadelphia: J.B. Lippincott Co.

Penn, R.D. (1979). The neurosurgical treatment of cerebral palsy. *Pediatric Annals, 8,* 614–619.

Platt, L.J., Andrews, G., & Howie, P.M. (1980). Dysarthria of adult cerebral palsy. II. Phonemic analysis of articulation errors. *Journal of Speech and Hearing Research, 23,* 41–55.

Robinson, R.O. (1973). The frequency of other handicaps in children with cerebral palsy. *Developmental Medicine and Child Neurology, 15,* 305–312.

Scherzer, A.L., Mike, V., & Ilson, J. (1976). Physical therapy as a determinant of change in the cerebral palsied infant. *Pediatrics, 58,* 47–52.

Schlesinger, E.R., Allaway, N.C., & Peltin, S. (1959). Survivorship in cerebral palsy. *American Journal of Public Health, 49,* 343–349.

Schultz-Hurlburt, B., & Tervo, R.C. (1982). Wheelchair users at a children's rehabilitation center: Attributes and management. *Developmental Medicine and Child Neurology, 24,* 54–60.

Schwejdap, P., & Vanderheiden, G. (1982). Adaptive firmware card for the Apple II. *Byte,* 276–314.

Seeger, B.R., & Caudrey, D.J. (1983). Biofeedback therapy to achieve symmetrical gait in children with hemiplegic cerebral palsy: Long-term efficacy. *Archives of Physical Medicine and Rehabilitation, 64,* 160–162.

Taft, L.T., Matthews, W.S., & Molnar, G.E. (1983). Pediatric management of the physically handicapped child. *Advances in Pediatrics, 30,* 13–60.

Taudorf, K., Melchior, J.C., & Pedersen, H. (1984). CT findings in spastic cerebral palsy. Clinical, aetiological and prognostic aspects. *Neuropediatrics, 15,* 120–124.

Taylor, E.M. (1959). *Psychological appraisal of children with cerebral defects.* Cambridge, MA: Harvard University Press.

Teja, E. (1983). Ears for your computer. *Computers and Electronics,* 35–39.

Thompson, G.H., Rubin, I.L., & Bilenker, R.M. (1983). *Comprehensive management of cerebral palsy.* New York: Grune & Stratton.

Thompson, S. (1979). *The role of physical therapeutic measures in the management of the cerebral palsy child: Introduction and background.* Paper presented at 33rd Annual Meeting of the American Academy for Cerebral Palsy and Developmental Medicine in San Francisco.

Tylkowski, C.M., Rosenthal, R.K., & Simon, S.R. (1980). Proximal femoral osteotomy in cerebral palsy. *Clinical Orthopaedics and Related Research, 151,* 183–192.

Vanderheiden, G. (1982). Computers can play a dual role for disabled individuals. *Byte,* 136–162.

Vanderheiden, G., & Grilley, K. (Eds.). (1976). *Non-vocal communication techniques and aids for the severely physically handicapped: Based upon transcriptions of the 1975 Trace Center national workshop series on non-vocal communication techniques and aids.* Baltimore: University Park Press.

Young, R.R., & Delwaide, P.J. (1981a). Drug therapy: Spasticity (first of two parts). *New England Journal of Medicine, 304,* 28–33.

Young, R.R., & Delwaide, P.J. (1981b). Drug therapy: Spasticity (second of two parts). *New England Journal of Medicine. 304,* 96–99.

Zigler, E. (1981). A plea to end the use of the patterning treatment for retarded children. *American Journal of Orthopsychiatry, 51,* 388–390.

Chapter 22

Epilepsy

Upon completion of this chapter, the reader will:
—understand what constitutes a seizure and how it happens
—know the various types of seizures
—be able to identify the various drugs used to treat seizures and know for which seizures they are effective
—realize what to do in case of a seizure
—be aware of the prognosis for people with seizure disorders

At some time during their lives, about 6% of the population in the United States will have a seizure (Goldman, 1985a; Rose, Penry, Markush, et al., 1973). Over half of these seizures occur in early childhood, associated with either a high fever or head trauma (Nelson & Ellenberg, 1981). Usually, these are single episodes that never recur and do not require medication. The electroencephalogram (EEG), or brain wave test, remains normal (Figure 22.1). These children do not have epilepsy.

Individuals with repeated seizures have epilepsy, also called a seizure disorder. About 50% of all the children with epilepsy have normal intelligence. Those who do have normal intelligence also have a higher incidence of learning disabilities (Bourgeois, Prensky, Palkes, et al., 1983). Their seizures are generally well controlled with anticonvulsant medication, and these drugs can usually be stopped if the child has no seizures for several years. Of those with mental retardation, some children have seizures as part of a multihandicapping condition that may include cerebral palsy and sensory deficits. These children often have more complex seizure patterns that are harder to control, and they require lifelong medication.

This chapter defines seizures and describes various types of seizures, diagnostic tests, anticonvulsant medications, and other forms of treatment, as well as the prognosis for epilepsy.

WHAT IS A SEIZURE?

A seizure, or convulsion, starts in an area of the cortex containing nerve cells (neurons) that are more apt to discharge than normal cells. This discharge spreads and

325

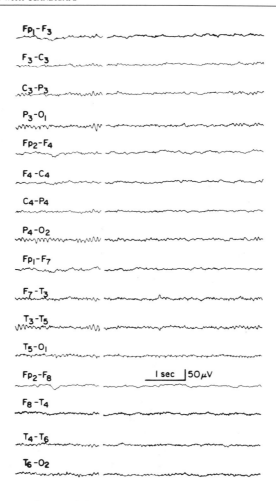

Figure 22.1. Appearance of a normal electroencephalogram (EEG). Note the relatively regular, undulating brain wave pattern. (From Niedermeyer, E., & Lopes da Silva, F. [1981]. *Electroencephalography: Basic principles, clinical applications, and related fields.* Baltimore: Urban & Schwarzenberg; reprinted by permission.)

recruits the neurons that surround the center of the seizure, causing them to discharge electrically. If the spread is limited to a small area, only an arm or leg may twitch. If it involves the entire cortex, a grand mal seizure results, and the entire body is affected. It is this excessive and periodic discharge that constitutes a seizure. Such a discharge, depending on its location, may lead to loss of consciousness, involuntary movements, or abnormal sensory phenomena.

Common causes of seizures include anoxia, hypoglycemia, trauma, and infections. What appears to happen is this: All nerve cells are enclosed by a membrane containing a pump that maintains a high level of the mineral sodium outside the cell and a high concentration of potassium inside the cell. When the cell is stabilized in this way, a nerve impulse is not generated. However, if there is a breakdown in this membrane so that sodium flows in and potassium flows out of the cell (a process called **depolarization**), a neural impulse is generated and travels down the nerve fiber. Conditions such as anoxia and hypoglycemia create an increased susceptibility to depolarization and, therefore, a greater risk of seizures. Structural damage to the nerve cell from trauma or infection has a similar effect.

TYPES OF SEIZURES

Generally, seizures are classified according to whether the entire cortex or only a part of it is affected (Commission on Classification, 1981). Thus, they are either generalized or partial seizures. Individuals who have a seizure disorder have one or more of these types of seizures. Generalized seizures include grand mal, petit mal or absence, Lennox-Gastaut, atonic seizures, and infantile spasms. Partial seizures are either simple or complex. Besides this classification, some seizures that exist in early childhood, that is, neonatal seizures and febrile convulsions, are somewhat unique and are considered separately.

Neonatal Seizures

Seizures in a newborn appear to be different from those seen in an older child (Freeman, 1983). Rarely do they involve all four extremities. Instead, one limb may jerk, or the eyes might move rhythmically or stare. The reason the seizure does not spread very much is because the newborn's immature cortex has a sparse network of neurons (Figure 22.2). Since the spread of the seizure relies on the recruitment of nearby cells, the fewer the number of cells surrounding the abnormal area, the more localized the seizure.

In the newborn, the most common causes of seizures are anoxia, intracerebral hemorrhages, brain malformations, hypocalcemia, sepsis, and hypoglycemia (see Chapter 6). The prognosis depends more on the underlying cause than on the severity of the seizure (Matsumoto, Watanabe, Sugiura, et al., 1983). In some instances, the seizures are easily controlled and never recur. In other cases, the seizures are precursors of a severe handicapping condition.

The two causes of seizures associated with good prognoses are hypocalcemia, or low blood calcium, and hypoglycemia (Lombroso, 1983). Hypocalcemia, a cause of seizures in full-term babies, is rare in premature infants. It is reversed by giving a calcium supplement. Seldom are there any complications, and the children normally are sent home from the hospital without any anticonvulsant medication. The same is true for children who have seizures caused by transient hypoglycemia, or low blood sugar. This type of seizure is more frequent in premature and small for gestational age infants. The hypoglycemia is treated by administering glucose. Rarely do these children require anticonvulsant medication (Freeman, 1983).

On the other hand, infants who have seizures caused by anoxia, intracerebral hemorrhages, brain malformations, or sepsis have a poorer prognosis. Severe

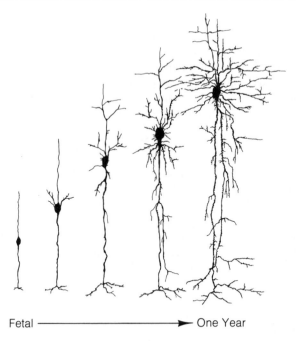

Fetal ————————————→ One Year

Figure 22.2.   Progressive development of neurons during fetal life and the first year of life. Because of the few interconnections, the newborn rarely has a full-fledged grand mal seizure; it may well involve only one or two limbs. By 1 year, the increased interconnections lead to a typical grand mal seizure in a susceptible child.

hypoxia and/or intracerebral hemorrhages lead to lethargy, poor feeding, and abnormal changes in muscle tone as well as seizures. These children have a greater chance of also having developmental disabilities. Brain malformations are usually associated with mental retardation and cerebral palsy. In all of these cases, seizures generally persist through childhood, and anticonvulsant treatment is required.

Febrile Convulsions

Although it is rare for a child between 1 and 6 months of age to have a seizure, between 6 months and 5 years of age, about 1 in 200 children will have at least one convulsion associated with a high fever (Nelson & Ellenberg, 1981) (Figure 22.3). The peak age for having this type of seizure is 18 months. Upper respiratory illnesses, stomach flu, and rashes (roseola) are common antecedents of such seizures. Occasionally, children have febrile convulsions after they have received a diphtheria-pertussis-tetanus (DPT), polio, or measles shot (Hirtz, Ellenberg, & Nelson, 1984).

Why some children are more likely to have febrile convulsions than others is unclear. However, many families have more than one member who has suffered a febrile convulsion in childhood. Thus, this suggests a possible genetic factor.

The most likely time for a febrile convulsion to occur is when a fever is on the rise, usually above 102°F (39°C). The seizure is grand mal in type, with **tonic-clonic**

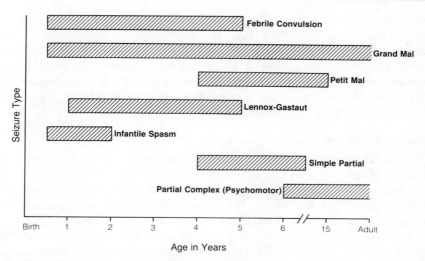

Figure 22.3.   Ages of occurrence of various types of seizures.

movements of all extremities. It generally lasts less than 5 minutes, although this may seem an eternity to the parents. By the time the child is brought to the emergency room, the seizure usually has stopped, and the child is lethargic or sleeping. On examination, the physician will find no problems other than the infection that led to the seizure. A spinal tap, or **lumbar puncture**, is often done the first time such a seizure occurs to make sure the child does not have meningitis (Gerber & Berliner, 1981). The child is not hospitalized, nor does he or she need anticonvulsant medication. If an EEG is taken a few weeks after the episode, its results are usually normal. There is no evidence that these seizures affect intellectual development (Smith & Wallace, 1982).

A child who has already had one febrile convulsion runs about a 30%–40% risk of having another before 4 years of age. If the child has a second convulsion, the risk is 50% for having additional febrile seizures (Nelson & Ellenberg, 1981). About 10% of children who have febrile convulsions go on to have recurrent seizures and, therefore, epilepsy (Nelson & Ellenberg, 1976). Children who have a family history of epilepsy, abnormal neurological development before their first febrile convulsion, or an atypical febrile convulsion that lasts longer than 15 minutes are more likely to develop epilepsy.

After a child has two febrile convulsions, prophylactic treatment with anti-convulsants is often begun and is continued until he or she is about 30 months old, when the recurrence risk becomes low (Consensus Development Conference, 1980). The most commonly used drug is phenobarbital (Antony & Hawke, 1983). For this drug to be effective, it must be taken once daily. Studies have shown that it reduces the risk of recurrence of febrile convulsions to 2% (Pearce, Sharman, & Forster, 1977). Possible side effects include hyperactivity, other behavioral problems, and sleepiness (Wolf, Forsythe, Stunden, et al., 1981). Valproic acid, or Depakene, is at least as effective as phenobarbital. However, it must be taken three times a day and may, although rarely, cause liver failure (Mamelle, Mamelle, Plasse, et al., 1984). Recently, researchers have suggested giving Valium as a suppository at the onset of a fever to prevent the occurrence of a febrile convulsion in susceptible children (Knudsen, 1985). Physicians have suggested using tepid baths and acetaminophen to control a fever. Whether such treatment is effective in preventing febrile convulsions is unclear (Camfield, Camfield, Shapiro, et al., 1980).

Grand Mal Seizures

Of the generalized seizures, grand mal is the most common and is the prototype when one thinks of epilepsy. This type of seizure can occur at any age (see Figure 22.3). When a person has a grand mal seizure, he or she sometimes has an aura, or sensation, that the seizure is about to begin. The seizure starts with the person losing consciousness and falling to the floor. He or she initially becomes rigid during what is called the tonic stage. During this period, the individual may stop breathing, turn blue (cyanotic), or bite the tongue. Next is a clonic phase with rhythmic jerking of the body, sweating, and **incontinence** (Figure 22.4). The entire seizure usually lasts less than 5 minutes and is followed by a deep sleep. Upon recovery, the person has no memory of the seizure itself.

These seizures can occur as often as three to five times a day or as seldom as once a year. A child with grand mal seizures is normally treated with anticonvulsants until he or she has been free of seizures for 2–3 years. Stopping the medication after this time is successful in about 80% of children with this type of seizure (Emerson, D'Souza, Vining, et al., 1981).

While grand mal seizures are not usually dangerous, they may become life-threatening in the case of *status epilepticus*. This is defined as a seizure or group of seizures that lasts more than 30 minutes, during which the child never regains consciousness (Rothner & Erenberg, 1980). Status epilepticus occurs most often during the first 3 years of life. The danger comes because the brain requires a constant flow of glucose and other energy compounds. During a prolonged seizure, the small reserves of these compounds in the brain are rapidly depleted, and blood circulation to the brain is impaired. The effect of this combination of events is possible injury to or death of brain tissue.

Therefore, status epilepticus is a medical emergency requiring rapid and effective treatment. For anyone working with a young child with epilepsy, this means that the child must get to a hospital if a seizure lasts more than 15 minutes. At the emergency room, the child is usually given a shot of the drug, Valium. This medication usually stops the seizure within 2–3 minutes. With treatment, the child should not suffer any adverse effects.

Petit Mal or Absence Seizures

Petit mal or absence seizures are much less common than grand mal seizures and account for less than 5% of all seizure disorders. These occur most often in individuals who are between 4 and 15 years old (Dodson, Prensky, DeVivo, et al.,

Grand Mal

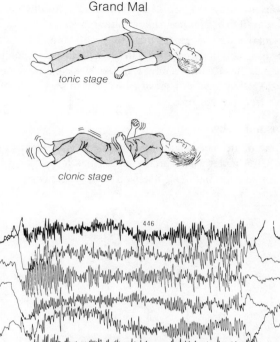

tonic stage

clonic stage

Figure 22.4. EEG pattern of a child with grand mal seizures. There is a burst of spike activity over the entire cortex during the course of the seizure. (EEG from Niedermeyer, E., & Lopes da Silva, F. [1981]. *Electroencephalography: Basic principles, clinical application, and related fields*. Baltimore: Urban & Schwarzenberg; reprinted by permission.)

1976). In this type of seizure, a person suddenly stares vacantly into space, blinks, and loses consciousness (Figure 22.5). The child's muscle tone remains normal, and he or she does not fall. Neither tonic-clonic movement nor drowsiness takes place. The child is unaware of the episode and may well continue a conversation begun just prior to the seizure. This type of seizure usually lasts less than 10 seconds and may occur as often as 20–40 times a day. If the seizures remain undetected and untreated, a child may do poorly at school because he or she misses much of the instruction while having these frequent seizures.

Lennox-Gastaut Seizures

A variant form of absence seizure is called Lennox-Gastaut. It fits into this category because the EEG pattern has certain similarities to that seen in petit mal seizures. However, this seizure manifests itself differently and carries a much more ominous

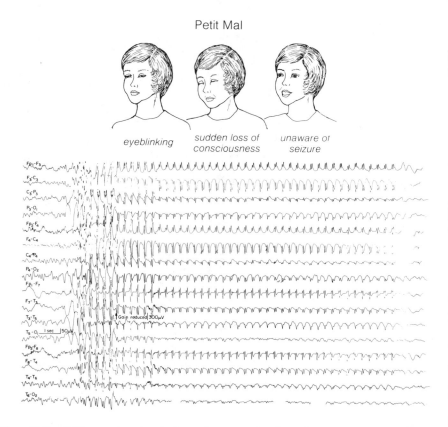

Figure 22.5.   EEG pattern in petit mal seizures shows a regular, slow spike and wave pattern that lasts less than 30 seconds. (EEG from Niedermeyer, E., & Lopes da Silva, F. [1981]. *Electroencephalography: Basic principles, clinical applications, and related fields*. Baltimore: Urban & Schwarzenberg; reprinted by permission.)

prognosis. A person with Lennox-Gastaut experiences a variety of different types of seizures; some are similar to petit mal seizures, some are tonic, and others are **myoclonic** in nature. This mixed pattern is commonly seen in children who previously had infantile spasms (see following subsection) (Kurokawa, Goya, Fukuyuma, et al., 1980). These seizures are difficult to control with medications and are usually associated with other developmental disabilities such as mental retardation and cerebral palsy.

Atonic Seizures

Atonic seizures, a form of generalized seizure, are characterized by an involuntary, sudden change in muscle tone. During these seizures, the individual either loses tone and crumbles to the floor like a rag doll (**akinetic**) or seems to be thrown down suddenly (kinetic). No tonic-clonic movements occur, and the person recovers in a matter of seconds. Drugs that are effective in treating atonic seizures include Depakene, Ativan (lorazepam), and Clonopin (clonazepam).

Infantile Spasms

Infantile spasms, the final type of generalized seizure to be discussed, start at around 6 months of age and disappear by 24 months (Lacy & Penry, 1976). However, their usual aftermath is the development of a Lennox-Gastaut EEG pattern, myoclonic and/or grand mal seizures, and severe mental retardation. The infantile spasm takes the form of a sudden jackknifing forward of the body 5 to 10 times in a row for about 30 seconds; this recurs as often as every 10 minutes. A specific EEG pattern called hypsarrhythmia is found (Figure 22.6). A number of diseases including Tay-Sachs disease, phenylketonuria, and Down syndrome are connected with an increased risk of infantile spasms (Lacy & Penry, 1976). Yet, in about half of the cases, the cause of the seizure is unknown. In these children, early treatment with adrenocorticotropic hormone (ACTH) or other steroid medications usually stops the spasms (Hrachovy, Frost, Kellaway, et al., 1983; Snead, Benton, & Myers, 1983). Even with treatment, over 90% of these children have mental retardation (Matsumoto, Watanabe, Negoro, et al., 1981; Singer, Rabe, & Haller, 1980).

Partial Seizures

Partial seizures, a new medical term, covers seizures that are localized to one specific area of the brain. These seizures may be either simple partial or partial complex seizures.

Simple Partial Seizures A common example of a simple partial seizure is one that only affects a single arm or leg. This is called a focal-motor seizure. The seizure may start in one limb and then move upward to gradually involve other parts of the body. When this happens, the seizure is called a jacksonian seizure (Livingston, 1972).

Partial Complex Seizures Partial complex seizures are also called psychomotor or temporal lobe seizures. Clinically it is important to distinguish these seizures from petit mal seizures, which they resemble. Before a person experiences a partial complex seizure, he or she often has a premonition about it. The individual may feel

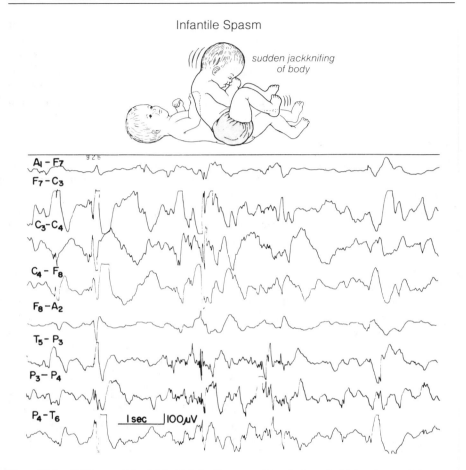

Figure 22.6.   EEG pattern of a child with infantile spasms. Note the irregular high-voltage activity. This pattern is called hypsarrhythmia. (EEG from Niedermeyer, E., & Lopes da Silva, F. [1981]. *Electroencephalography: Basic principles, clinical applications, and related fields*. Baltimore: Urban & Schwarzenberg; reprinted by permission.)

ill at ease or have a headache. This warning may come as much as a day before the actual seizure.

Because the temporal lobe controls such senses as smell, sound, and taste as well as some emotions, the individual may experience a variety of sensations during a seizure. He or she might smell acrid or sweet odors, have a funny taste in the mouth, hallucinate, undergo a feeling of "deja vu," or feel fearful or angry (Figure 22.7).

The seizure often includes blinking, lip smacking, chewing, or other automatic actions including unbuttoning and buttoning one's clothing. Unlike petit mal seizures, which last about 10 seconds, partial complex seizures continue from 30 seconds to 5 minutes. The EEG shows seizure activity restricted to the area of the

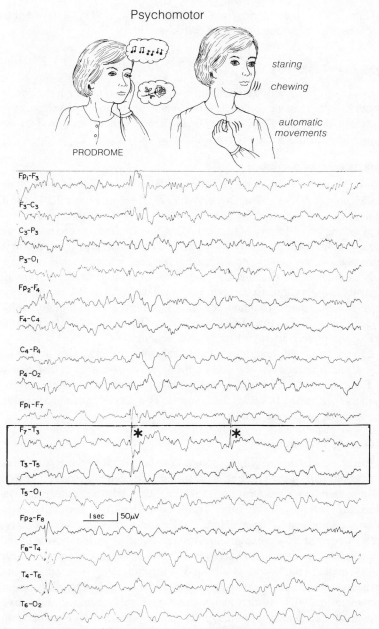

Figure 22.7.   In partial complex or temporal lobe seizures, the abnormal spike discharges (noted by the asterisks) are confined to the temporal lobe of the brain, leads F₇-T₃ and T₃-T₅. The remainder of the EEG record appears normal. (EEG from Niedermeyer, E., & Lopes da Silva, F. [1981]. *Electroencephalography: Basic principles, clinical applications, and related fields*. Baltimore: Urban & Schwarzenberg; reprinted by permission.)

temporal lobe. About half of the individuals with this type of seizure have a grand mal seizure at one time or another (Gomez & Klass, 1983).

DIAGNOSIS OF EPILEPSY

The diagnosis of epilepsy is based on a history of recurrent seizures. The EEG is helpful both in localizing the area in the brain where the focus of the seizure exists and in determining the type of epilepsy (Figure 22.8). Other tools used to evaluate epilepsy include various kinds of brain imaging techniques.

The Electroencephalogram

Approximately 80% of all children with epilepsy have abnormal EEG patterns (Ajmone-Marsan & Zivin, 1970). In grand mal seizures (see Figure 22.4), the normal EEG pattern may be interrupted by bursts of seizure activity throughout the brain. When a person is on anticonvulsant medication, the EEG returns to normal because the drug suppresses the seizure activity. In petit mal seizures, the wave pattern is more discrete and has slower spikes and waves that last only a few seconds but may occur repeatedly throughout the time the EEG is recorded (see Figure 22.5). As mentioned earlier, partial complex seizures are typified by seizure activity that occurs only in the temporal lobe rather than throughout the brain (see Figure 22.7). Finally, in infantile spasms (see Figure 22.6), the EEG shows chaotic bursts of activity throughout the brain unlike the pattern in any other kind of seizure.

In some cases, even though a child has seizures, the EEG may appear normal. Under these circumstances, a few other approaches can be used to discover seizure activity. For example, a child might wear a monitor that records an EEG continuously over 24 hours (Bachman, 1982; Mizrahi, 1984). This record can then be analyzed for more subtle signs of seizure activity.

Brain Imaging Techniques

Besides EEGs, new brain imaging techniques can help identify discrete areas of brain damage in about half of the children with epilepsy (Bachman, Hodges, & Freeman, 1976). These techniques are most useful with children who have more than one type of seizure and for those with other handicaps. One such technique is the CT (computerized tomography) scan. Here a series of X rays of cross-sections of the brain are synthesized by a computer to form an image of various levels of the brain (Figure 22.9). The most common abnormality seen is cortical atrophy, or shrinkage of the gray matter (Bachman, Hodges, & Freeman, 1976). A similar image is obtained using an even newer method called nuclear magnetic resonance, or magnetic resonance imaging (MRI). Rather than using X rays, this technique makes use of the natural magnetic characteristics of the molecules in the brain. It is even better than the CT scan for differentiating gray and white matter (see Figure 22.9). Lastly, PET (positron emission tomography) scans highlight the metabolic activity of the brain rather than its physical structure (Engel, 1984). For example, the focus of a seizure might "light up," as it uses up much more glucose than a normal area. This tool can

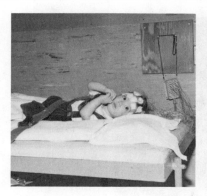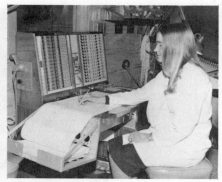

Figure 22.8. The taking of an electroencephalogram.

also be used to examine the pattern of neurotransmitters in various areas of the brain (Figure 22.10). Doing a PET scan requires the injection of small amounts of radioactive material.

TREATMENT OF EPILEPSY

Usually, epilepsy is treated with anticonvulsant medication. Other treatment approaches include a special diet, called a ketogenic diet, and surgery.

Anticonvulsant Drugs

Once a seizure disorder is diagnosed, appropriate medications are started to control the seizures (Table 22.1). The most commonly used anticonvulsants, their dosage,

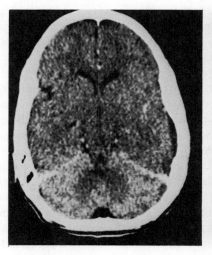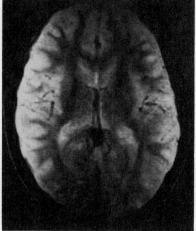

Figure 22.9. Brain imaging techniques. A normal CT scan is shown on the left and an MRI scan of the same patient on the right. The MRI scan gives a clearer image of brain structure than the CT scan.

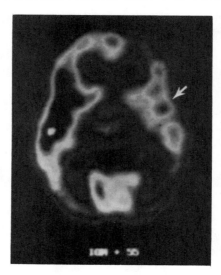

Figure 22.10. Position emission tomography (PET). The PET scan outlines area of decreased metabolic activity in the right temporal lobe of a patient with partial complex seizures. (From Theodore, W.H., Newmark, M.E., Sato, S., et al. [1983]. [18]F Fluorodeoxyglucose positron emission tomography in refractory complex partial seizures. *Annals of Neurology, 14,* 429–437; reprinted by permission. Copyright ©1983 by Little, Brown & Company, Boston.)

and side effects are listed in Table 22.2. A single anticonvulsant is chosen, and the dosage is adjusted so that seizures are controlled and side effects are minimized (Johnston & Freeman, 1981; Schmidt, 1983). Ordinarily, drug levels in the blood are monitored a few times a year. However, if a person has side effects, a blood level is taken immediately to make sure the dosage is not toxic. Once an individual is stabilized on a medication, the physician may order another EEG to see if the pattern has improved. Also, the person may keep a record of his or her seizures to document the frequency and to determine the effectiveness of the medication.

For about half of the children with epilepsy, one drug is sufficient to control the seizures (Elwes, Johnson, Shorvon, et al., 1984). For the other half, two drugs are required. It is extremely uncommon for a child to require more than two anticonvulsants. The child who has mixed-type seizures or infantile spasms is the most likely to need more than one medication. Some of the frequently used anticonvulsants are discussed in the following subsections.

Dilantin (Phenytoin) Dilantin, the trademark name for phenytoin, is one of the two most commonly used anticonvulsants; the other is phenobarbital. Dilantin probably controls a seizure by preventing the recruitment of nerve cells that surround the focus of the seizure, thereby stopping the seizure's progress (Freeman & Lietman, 1973). It accomplishes this by increasing the activity of the membrane pump in the surrounding nerve cells so that the concentration of sodium outside the cells and the potassium inside the cells is maintained. The surrounding cells, then, are less likely to depolarize and become part of the spreading seizure. Thus, Dilantin controls the

Table 22.1. Types of seizures and the medication/diet commonly used to treat them

Type of seizure	Pheno-barbital	Dilantin	Tegretol	Depakene	Clonopin	Mysoline	Zarontin	ACTH	Ketogenic diet
Grand mal	X	X	X	X	X	X			X
Petit mal				X	X		X		
Infantile spasms				X	X			X	X
Lennox-Gastaut				X	X				X
Simple partial/partial complex	X	X	X	X	X	X			

Table 22.2.   Anticonvulsant medications

Drug	How supplied (mg)	Tablet/ capsule/liquid (T/C/L)	Dosage (mg/kg/day)	Frequency of dosage per day	Side effects
Dilantin	50, 100	T/C/L	3–8	2	Ataxia; lethargy; gum swelling; rash; hairiness
Pheno-barbital	15–60	T/L	3–10	1–2	Lethargy; rash; hyperactivity
Mysoline	50, 200	T/L	12–25	2	Lethargy; ataxia
Zarontin	250	T/L	20–40	2	Vomiting; sedation; dizziness; liver damage
Tegretol	200	T	20–40	2	Lethargy; ataxia; rash; aplastic anemia
Clonopin	0.5, 2.0	T	0.03–0.1	3	Ataxia; sedation; salivation; personality disturbances
Depakene	250, 500	C/L	20–60	3	Lethargy; hair loss; anorexia; liver damage
ACTH	40, 80 units	Injection	20–80 units/day	1	Cataracts; brittle bones; diabetes; hypertension

Source: Physician's Desk Reference (1985).

spread rather than prevents the initiation of a seizure. The person may have an aura, but a full-fledged seizure should not occur.

Dilantin is primarily used to control grand mal and partial complex seizures. Young children usually take it twice a day, while older children can receive it in a single daily dose. Among the common side effects are swelling of the gums, excessive hairiness, and skin rash. Individuals with severe handicaps run a risk of developing rickets (Morijiri & Sato, 1981). Signs of toxicity include vomiting, lethargy, and an unsteady gait (ataxia) (Livanainen & Savolainen, 1983). All of these symptoms disappear when the drug is stopped or is restarted at a lower dose. Generally, Dilantin is considered to be safe and effective, but it does have a relatively high incidence of bothersome side effects. Also, it may cause malformations in the developing fetus of a pregnant woman with epilepsy (see Chapter 4) (Nakane, Okuma, Takahasi, et al., 1980).

Phenobarbital   Similar to Dilantin, phenobarbtial is used to treat grand mal and partial complex seizures. Yet, phenobarbital works quite differently from

Dilantin. It prevents the onset of a seizure by raising the intensity of the stimulus needed to trigger the seizure. However, once this threshold is exceeded, the seizure begins. Thus, a person using this drug tends either not to have an aura of a seizure at all or to have a complete seizure. Side effects of phenobarbital include drowsiness, irritability, and skin rash. Also, about 30%–40% of the children who are begun on phenobarbital become hyperactive and experience other behavioral and learning problems; eventually, they have to stop taking the medication (Ferrari, Barabas, & Matthews, 1983). An overdose leads to severe drowsiness that generally improves within 24 hours of stopping the medication (Brill & Mitchell, 1981).

Mysoline (Primidone) Mysoline, a trade name for primidone, is similar in chemical structure to phenobarbital. It is primarily used to treat grand mal seizures, but it is also useful in treating partial complex seizures. Drowsiness and ataxia are the most common side effects. These side effects disappear when the drug is discontinued (Delgado-Escueta, Treiman, & Walsh, 1983).

Zarontin (Ethosuximide) Unlike the other drugs mentioned so far, Zarontin is used exclusively for treating petit mal seizures. Common side effects are drowsiness and dizziness.

Tegretol (Carbamazepine) Similar to Mysoline, Tegretol is used principally to treat grand mal and partial complex seizures. Side effects are generally milder and less frequent than those of either Dilantin or phenobarbital. They include ataxia, double vision, drowsiness, and nausea. On rare occasions, a person may develop a bone marrow problem that leads to anemia (*Physician's Desk Reference,* 1985). Because of its few side effects, Tegretol is being used increasingly as a drug of first choice in treating grand mal seizures.

Clonopin (Clonazepam) Clonopin is similar in structure to Valium, but it is more effective than Valium for the long-term management of seizures. Clonopin has been used to treat all the different types of seizures. However, it is most often used for infantile spasms and myoclonic seizures. Drowsiness is common after the medication is started but usually subsides after a few weeks. In children with cerebral palsy, other side effects include decreased muscle tone, drooling, and swallowing difficulties (Eadie, 1984). A similar drug, Ativan (lorazepam), has recently become available and is also used to treat these types of seizures (Walker, Homan, Crawford, et al., 1984).

Depakene (Valproic Acid) Depakene is the newest anticonvulsant. Like Clonopin, it has been used to treat all forms of seizures. However, it is most effective as a second drug to treat grand mal seizures and as a primary drug to treat petit mal and myoclonic seizures. It works by increasing the level of the neurotransmitter gamma-aminobutyric acid (GABA), which suppresses seizure activity. Side effects, present in about 20% of the cases, include nausea, drowsiness, and hair loss (Eadie, 1984). These problems usually improve over time and stop if the drug is discontinued. A more severe but very rare complication is liver damage. Fewer than 1 in 100,000 individuals who take this drug develop severe, irreversible liver failure (Sherard, Steiman, & Couri, 1980). Depakene is considered to be a safe and effective drug.

ACTH (Adrenocorticotropic Hormone) ACTH, a steroid releasing hormone, is used only to treat infantile spasms. This drug must be injected into muscle tissue. If successful, it may be replaced in a month or so by oral steroid medication such as prednisone. Treatment is sometimes stopped after a few months or may be continued on a long-term basis; it is effective in stopping about 80% of infantile spasms if it is started within 1 month of the onset of the seizures (Singer, Rabe, & Haller, 1980). The problem with this form of therapy is that steroids have significant side effects, including weakening of the bone structure, high blood pressure, cataracts, and an increased risk of infection. Thus, they must be used with extreme care.

When to Stop Anticonvulsants

In the past, once an individual was placed on anticonvulsants, it was assumed he or she required them for life, similar to the diabetic's need for insulin. However, in most cases, this does not seem to be true. Recently, a number of studies have been published that report the effects of stopping anticonvulsant therapy in children who have been seizure free for 2–4 years (Emerson, D'Souza, Vining, et al., 1981; Shinnar, Vining, Mellits, et al., 1985; Thurston, Thurston, Hixon, et al., 1982). Thurston et al. (1982) followed children for 15–23 years after they stopped treatment and found that overall 72% of them remained free of seizures (Figure 22.11). If they did have seizures, usually these occurred within a year after stopping therapy. The risk of recurrence was higher in children with mental retardation, in children who started having seizures before they were 2 years old, in individuals who had experienced more than 30 seizures, and in those who had an abnormal EEG pattern when they stopped treatment (Emerson, D'Souza, Vining, et al., 1981) (Figure 22.12).

The Ketogenic Diet

Besides anticonvulsants, another approach to treating difficult-to-manage seizures is the ketogenic diet. This diet is high in fats and low in carbohydrates. To compensate for the deficiency in carbohydrates, the body breaks down the fats, leading to a condition called **ketosis**. This causes a decrease in seizure activity in about half of the children treated (Livingston, 1972). However, this diet is difficult to follow, especially for older children who will steal candy and other carbohydrate treats. Also, it is incompatible with a normal rate of growth. In addition, if the ketosis is not maintained, the seizures recur.

Surgery

Although used infrequently, surgery is another treatment for epilepsy. For at least one disorder, psychomotor or partial complex seizures, surgery has proved to be effective in individuals for whom medication has not worked. The surgery involves the removal of the abnormal region of the temporal lobe. This region is identified with the use of an EEG. Once this area is removed, over 50% of previously uncontrollable psychomotor seizures come under control (Davidson & Falconer, 1975; Lindsay, Ounsted, & Richards, 1984). However, this approach should only be used after anticonvulsants have failed. Well over 80% of partial complex seizures respond to Dilantin, Mysoline, Depakene, or Tegretol (Lindsay, Ounsted, & Richards, 1984).

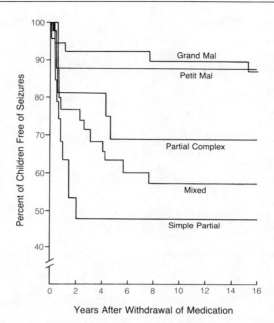

Figure 22.11.   Percentage of children who remained free of seizures after withdrawal of anticonvulsants. Over 80% of children with grand mal and petit mal seizures remain seizure-free compared to 50% to 70% of children with other types of seizures. All children had been free of seizures for at least 4 years before stopping medication. (From Thurston, J.H., Thurston, D.L., Hixon, B.B., et al. [1982]. Prognosis in childhood epilepsy. Additional follow-up of 148 children 15 to 23 years after withdrawal of anticonvulsant therapy. *New England Journal of Medicine, 306,* 831–836; reprinted by permission of *The New England Journal of Medicine.*)

WHAT TO DO IN THE EVENT OF A SEIZURE

Even though anticonvulsant medication generally improves seizures, many individuals with epilepsy continue to have convulsions. Seizures may be as infrequent as once a year or as often as 50 a day. The role of a professional or a parent who has to deal with the seizure depends on its type and duration. Repeated petit mal seizures require no immediate action, provided they stop within 15 minutes. An increased frequency, however, should alert one to the possible need for a change in medication.

A more difficult problem is a grand mal seizure. With this seizure, the child may fall and injure him- or herself, or he or she may choke, stop breathing, or turn blue. All these complications are unusual, but they do occur. The appropriate first aid procedure is as follows: The child should be laid on the floor or on a bed to avoid injury and turned on one side to prevent choking or aspiration if he or she vomits. One should not insert a spoon or finger between the person's teeth to prevent swallowing of the tongue. A person is physically unable to swallow the tongue. The main result of trying to insert a spoon would be a bitten finger or a broken tooth. The person helping the child should listen to the chest for breath sounds. If no breath sounds are heard for a minute, artificial ventilation should be started (see Appendix D). Rarely is this

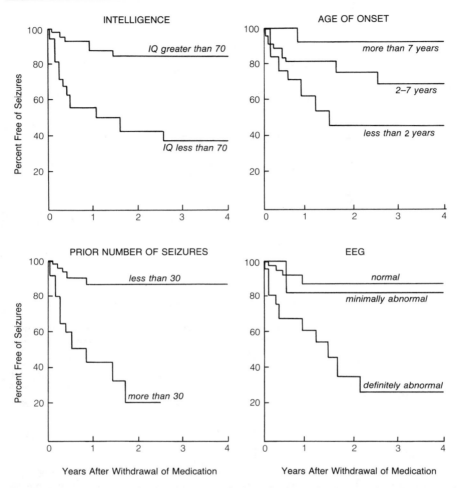

Figure 22.12. Percentage of children who remain free of seizures for 4 years after withdrawal of anticonvulsants. The risk of recurrence of seizures was higher in children with mental retardation, in those with onset of seizures before 2 years of age, in those with a history of many seizures, and in those who continued to have abnormal EEGs. All children had been free of seizures for 4 years before stopping medication. (From Emerson, R.D., D'Souza, B.J., Vining, E.P., et al. [1981]. Stopping medication in children with epilepsy: Predictors of outcome. *New England Journal of Medicine, 304*, 1125–1129; reprinted by permission of *The New England Journal of Medicine*.)

needed, since most children stop breathing for less than 30 seconds. If the seizure lasts more than 15 minutes, someone should call an ambulance, and the child should be taken to an emergency room to receive treatment. Otherwise, the seizure may turn into status epilepticus.

Another important aspect in the treatment of a seizure is the psychological impact it may have on the child. Many children who have grand mal seizures are incontinent during a seizure. When this happens, having a change of clothing on hand and explaining the seizure to those around the child may help relieve some of the anxiety and embarrassment associated with epilepsy.

CASE HISTORIES OF CHILDREN WITH EPILEPSY

The stories of Judy, Jamie, and Billy help illustrate some of the variety in epilepsy and its treatment.

Judy Judy was 2 years old when she had her first seizure during a high fever. Her mother was giving her a sponge bath, trying to bring down her fever, when she began having tonic-clonic movements. Her parents rushed her to a nearby hospital. When she arrived there 15 minutes later, she was still convulsing. A shot of Valium stopped the convulsion within 5 minutes. Later that night, although lethargic, Judy responded to her name and to simple questions. Blood tests were done, and she underwent a spinal tap. Neither meningitis nor a chemical imbalance was found. The physician told Judy's parents that she had a febrile convulsion. He indicated that this was not dangerous but might recur before she was 4 years old. He reassured Judy's parents that she was fine and had not suffered brain damage. The parents were also instructed that the best prevention of future seizures was to keep her fever from going above 102°F by using acetaminophen plus sponge baths.

By the next day, Judy was quite normal. She did have another convulsion several months later, but this time her parents were better prepared, and it was not as traumatic for them. After this seizure, she was placed on phenobarbital prophylactically. She took one tablet (60 milligrams) daily for 2 years, until, at the age of 4, she stopped taking the drug. She has been well since then and is now an "A" student in the sixth grade.

Jamie Jamie, the second child to be highlighted here, was more seriously affected with epilepsy. Like Judy, Jamie's first seizure was a grand mal type. However, it was not associated with fever and occurred when she was 5 years old. There was no infection or injury to explain the seizure. Unlike Judy's normal EEG, Jamie's showed a grand mal seizure pattern. She was placed on Dilantin to control the seizures. Despite the medication, Jamie's seizures continued. The family had difficulty coping with the illness, and they found it hard to give her the support and encouragement they knew she needed. Jamie felt ostracized in school; she was self-conscious about her disability, and she developed few friendships. Jamie was very sad and forlorn. Phenobarbital was soon added to the Dilantin, and her seizures became less frequent. However, the physician had difficulty reaching an appropriate dose for Jamie. Sometimes it was too high, and she was lethargic and irritable. At other times, it was too low, and she had a seizure. Finally, the right dose was determined, and her seizures came under good control. At 10 years of age, after being seizure-free for 2 years, medications were stopped. She has remained free of seizures for the past 3 years.

Unfortunately, the emotional problems for Jamie and her family persisted. Eventually, they were referred to a social worker for counseling. Jamie began to feel better and to gain self-esteem. Her parents developed ways to handle her situation more effectively. Now, at 14 years of age, Jamie is doing well in class and is making more friends. Though still hesitant, Jamie has made progress. Her prognosis depends, to a great extent, on those around her and how much support and encouragement she receives from them.

Billy The least encouraging of the cases is that of Billy. For him, seizures are but one part of a more complicated and serious condition. Billy was born prematurely and had sepsis as a newborn. He developed infantile spasms when he was 2 months old; he also was microcephalic. By 6 months, it was clear Billy had spastic cerebral palsy and severe mental retardation. His seizures were poorly controlled, even though he took Depakene. By 16 months of age, he averaged 20 to 30 seizures a day. His mother preferred not to put him on additional medication, because she found doing so made him lethargic and uninterested in his environment.

His parents know Billy has profound retardation, and they worry about his future. He is now in a cerebral palsy preschool program, and his parents are strengthened by the support of the occupational and physical therapists who work with Billy. For now, both Billy and his family are coping. Yet, his seizures continue.

PROGNOSIS

Many people with epilepsy live normal lives. Some are able to stop their medications after they have been free of seizures for at least 2 years. Driving a car is allowed if a person has had no seizures for some time, laws pertaining to which vary from state to state. The most troublesome side effects are the long-term psychological ones (Holdsworth & Whitmore, 1974). Social acceptance is a major problem for individuals who continue to have seizures as adults (Hermann, 1982). This may be the reason why individuals with epilepsy who continue to have seizures have a lower educational and occupational level of achievement than those who no longer have seizures (Harrison & Taylor, 1976; Holowach, Thurston, & O'Leary, 1972; Voeller & Rothenberg, 1973).

The lives of children with epilepsy who have multiple handicaps are even more affected. For them, epilepsy is often merely a part of a condition that includes cerebral palsy and mental retardation. The prognosis for these children is generally determined more by the degree of cerebral palsy and mental retardation than by the presence of seizures.

SUMMARY

Epilepsy refers to a condition in which there are normally functioning neurons that discharge at the least provocation and cause a convulsion. Generalized seizures include grand mal, petit mal, atonic, and infantile spasms. Partial seizures include simple and complex. Seizures may occur singly or in combination and may start in the newborn period, in infancy, or in later childhood. For many individuals, the seizures are an isolated disability and can be controlled with medication. Many children are successfully withdrawn from medication after they are free of seizures for 2–4 years. These children lead basically normal lives. However, for the child with multiple handicaps, the prognosis is far worse.

Even with adequate control of the seizures, the problem of the stigma attached to epilepsy persists. To combat this stereotyping, improved education enabling the public to accept this illness as no different from any other chronic disorder is needed.

REFERENCES

Ajmone-Marsan, C., & Zivin, L.S. (1970). Factors related to the occurrence of typical paroxysmal abnormalities in the EEG records of epileptic patients. *Epilepsia, 11,* 361–381.

Antony, J.H., & Hawke, S.H.B. (1983). Phenobarbital compared with carbamazepine in prevention of recurrent febrile convulsions. A double-blind study. *American Journal of Diseases in Children, 137,* 892–895.

Bachman, D.S. (1982). Twenty-four-hour ambulatory electroencephalographic monitoring in pediatrics. (Abstract). *Annals of Neurology, 12,* 207.

Bachman, D.S., Hodges, F.J., & Freeman, J.M. (1976). Computerized axial tomography in chronic seizure disorders of childhood. *Pediatrics, 58,* 828–832.

Bourgeois, B.F., Prensky, A.L., Palkes, H.S., et al. (1983). Intelligence in epilepsy: A prospective study in children. *Annals of Neurology, 14,* 438–444.

Brill, C.B., & Mitchell, M.H. (1981). Seizures and other paroxysmal disorders. *Advances in Pediatrics, 28,* 441–489.

Camfield, P.R., Camfield, C.S., Shapiro, S.H., et al. (1980). The first febrile seizure-antipyretic instruction plus either phenobarbital or placebo to prevent recurrence. *Journal of Pediatrics, 97,* 16–21.

Chevrie, J.J., & Aicardi, J. (1978). Convulsive disorders in the first year of life: Neurological and mental outcome and mortality. *Epilepsia, 19,* 67–74.

Commission on Classification and Terminology of the International League Against Epilepsy. (1981). Proposal for revised clinical and electroencephalographic classification of epileptic seizures. *Epilepsia, 22,* 489–501.

Committee on Drugs. (1985). Behavioral and cognitive effects of anticonvulsant therapy. *Pediatrics, 76,* 644–647.

Consensus Development Conference. (1980). Febrile seizures: Long term management of children with fever-associated seizures. *Pediatrics, 66,* 1009–1012.

Davidson, S., & Falconer, M.A. (1975). Outcome of surgery in 40 children with temporal lobe epilepsy. *Lancet, 1,* 1260–1263.

Davis, A.G., Mutchie, K.D., Thompson, J.A., et al. (1981). Once-daily dosing with phenobarbital in children with seizure disorders. *Pediatrics, 68,* 824–827.

Delgado-Escueta, A.V., Treiman, D.M., & Walsh, G.O. (1983). The treatable epilepsies. *New England Journal of Medicine, 308,* 1508–1514, 1576–1584.

Dodson, W.E., Prensky, A.L., DeVivo, D.C., et al. (1976). Management of seizure disorders: Selected aspects. *Journal of Pediatrics, 89,* 527–540, 695–703.

Eadie, M.J. (1984). Anticonvulsant drugs. An update. *Drugs, 27,* 328–363.

Elwes, R.D., Johnson, A.L., Shorvon, S.D., et al. (1984). The prognosis for seizure control in newly diagnosed epileptics. *New England Journal of Medicine, 311,* 944–947.

Emerson, R., D'Souza, B.J., Vining, E.P., et al. (1981). Stopping medication in children with epilepsy: Predictors of outcome. *New England Journal of Medicine, 304,* 1125–1129.

Engel, J., Jr. (1984). The use of positron emission tomographic scanning in epilepsy. *Annals of Neurology, 15 (Suppl.),* S180–S191.

Engel, J., Jr., Troupin, A.S., Crandall, P.H., et al. (1982). Recent developments in the diagnosis and therapy of epilepsy. *Annals of Internal Medicine, 97,* 584–598.

Ferrari, M., Barabas, G., & Matthews, W.S. (1983). Psychologic and behavioral disturbances among epileptic children treated with barbiturate anticonvulsants. *American Journal of Psychiatry, 140,* 112–113.

Freeman, J.M. (1983). Neonatal seizures. In F.E. Dreifuss (Ed.), *Pediatric epileptology: Classification and management of seizures in the child.* Boston: John Wright, PSG.

Freeman, J.M., & Lietman, P.S. (1973). A basic approach to the understanding of seizures and the mechanism of action and metabolism of anti-convulsants. *Advances in Pediatrics, 20,* 291–321.

Gerber, M.A., & Berliner, B.C. (1981). The child with a "simple" febrile seizure: Appropriate diagnostic evaluation. *American Journal of Diseases in Children, 135,* 431–433.

Goldman, J. (1985a). Let's talk about seizures, part I. Questions and answers for children. *Exceptional Parent, 15,* 24–28.

Goldman, J. (1985b). Let's talk about seizures, part II. Questions and answers for children. *Exceptional Parent, 15,* 54–57.

Gomez, M.R., & Klass, D.W. (1983). Epilepsies of infancy and childhood. *Annals of Neurology, 13,* 113–124.

Harrison, R.M., & Taylor, D.C. (1976). Childhood seizures: A 25-year follow-up. *Lancet, 1,* 948–951.

Hauser, W.A., Anderson, V.E., Loewenson, R.B., et al. (1982). Seizure recurrence after a first unprovoked seizure. *New England Journal of Medicine, 307,* 522–528.

Hermann, B.P. (1982). Neuropsychological functioning and psychopathology in children with epilepsy. *Epilepsia, 23,* 545–554.

Hirtz, D.G., Ellenberg, J.H., & Nelson, K.B. (1984). The risk of recurrence of non febrile seizures in children. *Neurology, 34,* 637–641.

Holdsworth, L., & Whitmore, K. (1974). A study of children with epilepsy attending ordinary schools. I. Their seizure patterns, progress and behavior in school. *Developmental Medicine and Child Neurology, 16,* 746–758.

Holowach, J., Thurston, D.L., & O'Leary, J. (1972). Prognosis in childhood epilepsy. *New England Journal of Medicine, 286,* 169–174.

Hrachovy, R.A., Frost, J.D., Kellaway, P., et al. (1983). Double-blind study of ACTH vs. prednisone therapy in infantile spasms. *Journal of Pediatrics, 103,* 641–645.

Johnston, M.V., & Freeman, J.M. (1981). Pharmacologic advances in seizure control. *Pediatric Clinics of North America, 28,* 179–194.

Knudsen, F.U. (1985). Effective short-term diazepam prophylaxis in febrile convulsions. *Journal of Pediatrics, 106,* 487–490.

Kurokawa, T., Goya, N., Fukuyuma, Y., et al. (1980). West syndrome and Lennox-Gastaut syndrome: A survey of natural history. *Pediatrics, 65,* 81–88.

Lacy, J.R., & Penry, J.K. (1976). *Infantile spasms.* New York: Raven Press.

Lindsay, J., Ounsted, C., & Richards, P. (1984). Long-term outcome in children with temporal lobe seizures. V. Indications and contra-indications for neuro-surgery. *Developmental Medicine and Child Neurology, 26,* 25–32.

Livanainen, M., & Savolainen, H. (1983). Side effects of phenobarbital and phenytoin during long-term treatment of epilepsy. *Acta Neurologica Scandinavica, 68 (Suppl. 97),* 49–67.

Livingston, S. (1972). *Comprehensive management of epilepsy in infancy, childhood, and adolescence.* Springfield, IL: Charles C Thomas.

Lombroso, C.T. (1983). Prognosis in neonatal seizures. *Advances in Neurology, 34,* 101–113.

Mamelle, N., Mamelle, J.C., Plasse, J.C., et al. (1984). Prevention of recurrent febrile convulsions—a randomized therapeutic assay: sodium valproate, phenobarbital and placebo. *Neuropediatrics, 15,* 37–42.

Matsumoto, A., Watanabe, K., Negoro, T., et al. (1981). Infantile spasms: Etiologic factors, clinical aspects and long term prognosis in 200 cases. *European Journal of Pediatrics, 135,* 239–244.

Matsumoto, A., Watanabe, K., Sugiura, M., et al. (1983). Long-term prognosis of convulsive disorders in the first year of life: Mental and physical development and seizure persistence. *Epilepsia, 24,* 321–329.

Mazziotta, J.C., & Engel, J. (1984). The use and impact of positron computed tomography scanning in epilepsy. *Epilepsia (Suppl. 2), 25,* S86–S104.

Mizrahi, E.M. (1984). Electroencephalographic/polygraphic/video monitoring in childhood epilepsy. *Journal of Pediatrics, 105,* 1–9.

Morijiri, Y., & Sato, T. (1981). Factors causing rickets in institutionalized handicapped children on anticonvulsant therapy. *Archives of Disease in Childhood, 56,* 446–449.

Nakane, Y., Okuma, T., Takahasi, R., et al. (1980). Multi-institutional study on the teratogenicity and fetal toxicity of antiepileptic drugs: A report of a collaborative study in Japan. *Epilepsia, 21,* 663–680.

Nelson, K.B., & Ellenberg, J.H. (1976). Predictors of epilepsy in children who have experienced febrile seizures. *New England Journal of Medicine, 295,* 1029–1033.

Nelson, K.B., & Ellenberg, J.H. (Eds.). (1981). *Febrile seizures.* New York: Raven Press.

Niedermeyer, E., & Lopes da Silva, F. (1981). *Electroencephalography: Basic principles, clinical applications, and related fields.* Baltimore: Urban & Schwarzenberg.

Pearce, J.L., Sharman, J.R., & Forster, R.M. (1977). Phenobarbital in the acute management of febrile convulsions. *Pediatrics, 60,* 569–572.

Physician's desk reference (39th ed.). (1985). Oradell, NJ: Medical Economics Co.

Riikonen, R. (1984). Infantile spasms: Modern practical aspects. *Acta Paediatrica Scandinavica, 73,* 1–12.

Rose, S.W., Penry, J.K., Markush, R.E., et al. (1973). Prevalence of epilepsy in children. *Epilepsia, 14,* 133–152.

Rothner, A.D., & Erenberg, G. (1980). Status epilepticus. *Pediatric Clinics of North America, 27,* 593–602.

Schmidt, D. (1983). Single drug therapy for intractable seizures. *Journal of Neurology, 29,* 221–226.

Sherard, E.S., Steiman, G.S., & Couri, D. (1980). Treatment of childhood epilepsy with valproic acid: Results of the first 100 patients in a 6-month trial. *Neurology, 30,* 31–35.

Shinnar, S., Vining, E.P.G., Mellits, E.D., et al. (1985). Discontinuing anti-epileptic medication in children with epilepsy after two years without seizures: A prospective study. *New England Journal of Medicine, 313,* 976–980.

Singer, W.D., Rabe, E.F., & Haller, J.S. (1980). The effect of ACTH therapy upon infantile spasms. *Journal of Pediatrics, 96,* 485–489.

Smith, J.A., & Wallace, S.J. (1982). Febrile convulsions: Intellectual progress in relation to anti-convulsant therapy and to recurrence of fits. *Archives of Disease in Childhood, 57,* 104–107.

Snead, O.C., Benton, J.W., & Myers, G.J. (1983). ACTH and prednisone in childhood seizure disorders. *Neurology, 33,* 966–970.

Theodore, W.H., Newmark, M.E., Sato, S., et al. (1983). ^{18}F Fluorodeoxyglucose position emission tomography in refractory complex partial seizures. *Annals of Neurology, 14,* 429–437.

Thompson, P.J., & Trimble, M.R. (1982). Anticonvulsant drugs and cognitive functions. *Epilepsia, 23,* 531–544.

Thurston, J.H., Thurston, D.L., Hixon, B.B., et al. (1982). Prognosis in childhood epilepsy. Additional follow-up of 148 children 15 to 23 years after withdrawal of anticonvulsant therapy. *New England Journal of Medicine, 306,* 831–836.

Voeller, K.K.S., & Rothenberg, M.B. (1973). Psychosocial aspects of the management of seizures in children. *Pediatrics, 51,* 1072–1082.

Volpe, J. (1973). Neonatal seizures. *New England Journal of Medicine, 289,* 413–416.

Walker, J.E., Homan, R.W., Crawford, I.L., et al. (1984). Lorazepam: A controlled trial in patients with intractable partial complex seizures. *Epilepsia, 25,* 464–466.

Wolf, S.M., Forsythe, A., Stunden, A.D., et al. (1981). Long-term effect of phenobarbital on cognitive function in children with febrile convulsions. *Pediatrics, 68,* 820–823.

Wright, F.S. (1984). Epilepsy in childhood. *Pediatric Clinics of North America, 31,* 177–188.

Chapter 23

Caring and Coping
The Family of a
Child with Handicaps

Upon completion of this chapter, the reader will:
—Understand the various stages of the development of the family over the life cycle
—Be aware of the impact a child's disability has on the parents, the child him- or herself, the siblings, and the grandparents
—Be alert to how societal attitudes and reactions influence the outcome for these children and their families
—Recognize some of the ways in which professionals can best help these families

Up to now, this book has focused on the medical information and physical aspects of various kinds of disabilities. Equally important is the emotional impact that these disabilities have on the different family members. How the family handles the day-to-day stresses, concerns, and needs of its members determines, to a great extent, the outcome for these individuals (Cobb & Hancock, 1984). Besides giving sound medical advice, professionals must be attuned to the emotional needs of the families they serve. This means seeing the entire family as the "patient" and not simply addressing the physical aspects of the child's situation.

This chapter examines the life cycle of families and looks at how having a child with a disability affects family members throughout this life cycle. The impact on the parents, the child him- or herself, siblings, and grandparents is reviewed. Also discussed is how professionals might best serve these families and the role that society plays in the outcome for these individuals.

THE LIFE CYCLE OF THE FAMILY

The stages that families go through as they progress through life together are analogous to the developmental stages of an individual. In each stage, the family must fulfill certain emotional tasks (Carter & McGoldrick, 1980). Events that happen in most families trigger the progression of the family from one stage to another. For example, the birth of a child ushers in a new stage for the family. When this event occurs, each member must adjust to and accommodate the presence of this new member (Terkelsen, 1980).

For our purposes, the six-stage life cycle model is used (Carter & McGoldrick, 1980). In the first stage, the unattached adult is separating from his or her original family. The adult is becoming established in work and is developing intimate relationships with peers. The adult is, in effect, becoming his or her own separate person. During the second stage, two families are joined with the marriage of their offspring. The newly married couple becomes committed to their new family, and old relationships are realigned to accommodate the inclusion of these new members. The family with young children is the focus of the third stage, when still newer members are accepted into the family. The marital relationship adjusts to make space, both emotional and physical, for the children. The adults become parents, and the relationships with the families of origin are realigned once again to adjust to new and expanded roles.

In the fourth stage, the children are adolescents and are beginning to test out the waters of independence. The relationships between parents and children need to shift to allow the children to broaden their horizons and to branch out more into the world. In the fifth stage, the children usually move out of the home. The marital relationship has to readjust once again to having only two people in the home. Relationships with the children adjust from that of child-adult to adult-adult. During this stage, parents are often dealing with ill health or the deaths of their parents and are accommodating new members into the family as daughters-in-law and sons-in-law. Finally, in the sixth stage the family in later life again has to handle a shifting of roles. Often, elderly parents become more dependent on their sons and daughters. Parents may engage in some sort of review of their own lives and may work at integrating their failures and successes.

For all families, the adjustments and realignments each member must make during the various times of change are often stressful. When a family has a child with a disability, the stressful times are compounded, and the adjustments are multiplied. For example, the individual with a handicap may remain in one stage, that of the dependent child, for the rest of his or her life. Thus, on each occasion when a life change should occur, the difference between the family with a child who has a handicap and one with a normal child is further accentuated. Each family member is affected differently during various times of the life cycle.

EFFECTS ON PARENTS

When a couple is expecting a child, they fantasize about their "dream child," what the child will be and how he or she will look (McCollum, 1984). If the child is born with a handicap, the fantasied child is lost (McCollum, 1984; Solnit & Stark, 1961). The parents experience tremendous pressure and stress in trying to adjust to their loss

(Mori, 1983; Powell & Ogle, 1985), and a grieving process takes place. The stages of grieving described in the literature are useful for understanding this process (Kubler-Ross, 1969). However, it is important to keep in mind that these stages are neither time-bound nor orderly in their progression (Blacher, 1984b; Cobb & Hancock, 1984). Each stage can recur, and some elements of the various stages may be combined.

Initially, in their grief, parents may feel shock and disbelief and may deny the truth (Blacher, 1984b). Along with these feelings may be physical manifestations such as frequent sighing, insomnia, an empty feeling in the stomach, loss of appetite, restlessness, and irritability (McCollum, 1984). Next, parents tend to feel angry, resentful, or bitter. "Why us?" is a frequent question. They may have feelings of lowered self-esteem as well, believing that somehow something they did contributed to or even caused the situation. The anger may be directed toward themselves, their child, God, the hospital staff, or others (Blacher, 1984b). When they feel angry with their child, they often then feel guilty because they don't think it is right to be angry with the child. Often, feelings are jumbled and difficult to sort out. On the other hand, for some parents who, after the birth, suspect that their child has a handicap, being told that a handicap does in fact exist provides them with a sense of relief. Their doubts have received a name, something with which to work.

Some parents then experience a "bargaining" stage, during which they might go from doctor to doctor, trying to find a better prognosis or a not so serious diagnosis. It is also a time when parents may turn to unconventional forms of treatment in hopes of finding a cure for their child. This stage is often filled with frustration and a sense of failure.

After a period of time, parents may feel more adjusted to their family's situation (Blacher, 1984b). They then are better able to redirect their energies toward handling the problems of their child and those of other family members. Yet, even at this point, feelings of anger, denial, and guilt may recur (Butler, 1983), especially if parents find out their child has more problems than they first were told or anticipated. As Helen Featherstone, the mother of a child with severe handicaps, states, "Few parents, even though they are coping effectively, ever reach an 'emotional promised land'" (Featherstone, 1980).

In addition, some parents continue to live in a state of "chronic sorrow" (Kennedy, 1970; Olshansky, 1962). In these situations, not only are the parents burdened by what seems to them to be never-ending sadness, but they also have to contend with the feeling that something is wrong with them for feeling this way. However, even in this state, parents are able to experience some sense of accomplishment and take pleasure in what their child can achieve. Still, the chronic sorrow touches all aspects of their lives, and the underlying sadness colors their feelings and responses to the world.

For all parents, the coping process continues somewhat unpredictably. Although many parents experience these feelings in the sequence just described, many do not. Also, mothers and fathers tend to experience this period of grief and adjustment differently. For instance, mothers usually assume the majority of the care of the children. Therefore, their personal lives are affected most by having children and even more so by the birth of a child with a handicap (Glendinning, 1983). The relationship between the mother and the child is affected by the infant's temperament and needs as well as by the mother's mood (Affleck, Allen, McGrade, et al., 1982b). Often, children with disabilities are less responsive to their mother's attention and efforts (Harper, 1984; Wasserman, Seidman, & Allen, 1984). Because of this, the mother may find it difficult to play with and encourage the child. This may result in her emotional withdrawal from the child (Wasserman, Seidman, & Allen, 1984). Also, if the mother feels depressed, it is more difficult for her to respond to her child (Affleck, Allen, McGrade, et al., 1982b). Some relief from her daily duties and understanding for her feelings expressed by others help the mother to continue her efforts to assist her child.

For fathers, there seems to be a greater tendency to deny the reality of their child's disability and its emotional impact (Cobb & Hancock, 1984). Fathers tend to focus more on long-term problems, especially financial ones, than do mothers, and respond less emotionally. Mothers, on the other hand, are usually most concerned with their ability to handle the day-to-day care of the child. Also, while mothers seem to gain a great deal of satisfaction and relief from talking about their difficulties, fathers, largely because of social taboos related to males expressing grief, generally react by keeping their feelings inside (Glendinning, 1983). In addition, fathers tend to be more concerned about their child's behavior outside the home, his or her social status, and the child's likelihood for future occupational success (Seligman, 1983).

As time passes and the parents settle into the routine of caring for their child, they often identify special difficulties. One parent said, "There's a real 'daily grind' of care that only those who experience it can really understand" (Glendinning, 1983). These day-to-day special problems include additional laundry, special diets and treatment, social restrictions and isolation, extra financial costs, added anxiety about the future and the child's health, and continued loss of sleep (Glendinning, 1983; Mori, 1983; Tavormina, Boll, Dunn, et al., 1981).

These added stresses may also place a great deal of strain on a marriage (Seligman, 1983). Sometimes, the parents find it difficult to accept each other's styles of coping—for example, the silent versus the needing-to-talk style. If these issues remain unresolved, they may eventually lead to divorce (Abrams, 1970). Yet, the effect on a marriage is not always negative. Some couples have mentioned that they felt drawn closer together because of their child with disabilities (Glendinning, 1983).

Child Abuse and Neglect

When families have no relief from the exceedingly taxing care of a child with disabilities, and the parents are feeling overwhelmed, the potential for child abuse increases dramatically (Solomons, 1979). This risk is even higher in single-parent families. Several child abuse studies indicate that children with developmental disabilities make up a high proportion of the population of abused and neglected children, anywhere from 29%–70% (Blacher, 1984a; Diamond & Jaudes, 1983; Solomons, 1979).

The incidence of sexual abuse also tends to be relatively high among children with disabilities (Watson, 1984). Other factors besides stress that may contribute to this high incidence are the emotional and social isolation of the parents (Solomons, 1979). Sometimes, these factors are compounded by the child's unresponsiveness to the parents' attention and perhaps his or her hypersensitivity to any stimulation, including gentle touching (Friedrich & Boriskin, 1976).

In some situations, the child is not abused but is neglected. In these homes, the child does not receive some part of care that he or she needs. For example, he or she may not attend school, may miss medical appointments, or may not be given required medication. Continued neglect may threaten the child's development and eventual outcome. Although some of these situations end up in the child's removal from the home, in many others, the family and the child protective worker, a social worker, are able to determine ways to improve the situation.

In all cases, the best treatment is prevention. To help reduce the risk of abuse and neglect, professionals must be open to discussing the parents' feelings of overwhelming burden and their frustrations at handling their child. Nonjudgmental responses are necessary to help these families. In addition, practical measures such as respite care, parent support groups, hotlines, and financial relief help to break the isolation of these families and ease their burdens.

EFFECTS ON THE CHILD WITH A DISABILITY

Although children with handicaps deal with difficulties the rest of us do not have to face, no conclusive evidence shows that they have more adjustment difficulties than other children (Cobb & Hancock, 1984). Yet, to grow up feeling worthwhile, it is important for these children to see themselves as persons *with handicaps* rather than as handicapped persons (Roth, 1981). In this way, the emphasis is on the individual rather than on the handicap.

One area that is more significant for children with physical disabilities than for normal children is their attitude toward their bodies. Whether the child was born with the disability or acquired it later on seems to affect how he or she feels toward his or her body (Kessler, 1979; Rousso, 1984; Vargo, 1978). For instance, children with congenital disabilities may feel whole and intact since the disability has always been a part of them (Rousso, 1984). From the beginning, then, such children have a different perspective from their parents. For them, there has been no loss. Yet, the manner in which parents react to their child's disability greatly determines how the child will think of himself or herself (Harvey & Greenway, 1982). On the other hand, when a person becomes disabled later in childhood, he or she experiences the same grief that parents do when they learn their child has a handicap (Vargo, 1978). This shared experience can either enhance understanding or add to the child's and parents' sorrow.

Because of the limitations of their disability and the attitudes and reactions of those around them, children with handicaps are often socially isolated (Fraser, 1980). This means the child is likely to have less well-developed social skills and, thus, is more awkward in social interactions. The child remains uncomfortable around other people and they around him or her. One adaptive strategy may be for children with disabilities to acknowledge their disability and its implications for them (Cobb & Hancock, 1984). In this way, they might reduce others' discomfort and increase their opportunities for social exchanges. The advantage for children with disabilities would be the refinement of their social skills and greater comfort and flexibility in interactions with others.

Adolescence is a particularly difficult time for all of us and our families, but for adolescents with disabilities, the frustrations and uncertainties of this stage are magnified (Cobb & Hancock, 1984; Winter & DeSimone, 1983). It is a time when youngsters with disabilities are most likely to accept society's image of the ideal body and to reject themselves and the way they look (Strax, 1976). It is also a time when peer acceptance is crucial, and when such acceptance is less likely for the teenager with disabilities (Cobb & Hancock, 1984). As a woman in her mid-20s who has spina bifida eloquently described her adolescence: "You take all the questions of who am I and what am I going to do, and you multiply that by 10 and you have me. . . . Everybody was in twos, except me . . . and the body beautiful was a terrible image to have to keep up with" (Y. Perret, personal interview with Joan R., August 1, 1984).

Thus, adolescence is a time of special struggle for the teenager who has a disability. Besides difficulties with being accepted by others, such an adolescent also has more trouble achieving a balance between dependence and independence (Abramson, Ash, & Nash, 1979). This is because many of these individuals have to live for a longer time, perhaps for a lifetime, being dependent—at least to some extent—on others. Acknowledging and accepting this dependency in a realistic fashion is important for the adjustment of these persons. Yet, it is also vital for them to be able to be as independent as possible and to have hope and dreams for the future (Cobb & Hancock, 1984).

In addition, performance in academic and social areas becomes more important during this time. If the adolescent with disabilities finds he or she cannot succeed at a particular task, he or she may be less motivated to try. Others, especially parents and teachers, may expect either too much or too little of this person. In either case, he or she winds up failing or not performing what is possible (Abramson, Ash, & Nash, 1979). Therefore, it is crucial for parents and teachers to help the teenager recognize what is attainable and encourage him or her to try.

During this time, as in other times, open communication with parents is critical. For example, the adolescent needs to be able to talk about his or her sexuality and to be seen as a sexual person (Rousso, 1985). This is often difficult for parents to recognize, but is extremely valuable. It is also important for the adolescent to be able to explore ways to meet his or her needs for intimate contact with other people. The teenager needs help in sorting out and expressing concerns and feelings in this area (Winter & DeSimone, 1983). An acceptance by themselves and others of these concerns and feelings helps teenagers to continue to develop a better sense of who they are and a recognition of their self-worth. In this way, they will be better able to engage in positive social interactions and to accomplish their goals (Morgan & Leung, 1980; Starr & Heiserman, 1977).

When the adolescent becomes a young adult, the individual and the family are normally dealing with issues of separation. Also, the young adult is beginning to set up his or her direction in terms of employment and other interests (Carter & McGoldrick, 1980). This, then, is another difficult time for individuals with disabilities, since they may be limited in their employment choices, and they may not be able to leave home. Yet, many persons with disabilities can be independent and self-supporting. Thus, it remains important for family members and others who are involved with these individuals to encourage them to try, to find resources that may assist in their independence, and to look for alternatives if one path does not work out for them.

EFFECTS ON SIBLINGS

Not only are the children with disabilities and their parents affected, but also the brothers and sisters of the children. These siblings have special needs and concerns. They may, for example, wonder about the cause of their sibling's handicap and worry about that child's future. They might fear that they will "catch" their brother or sister's disability or will pass it on to their children. Some siblings question whether they were somehow responsible for the handicap. Sometimes, they feel relieved that they do not have a disability and then feel guilty about this. They may wonder why they seem to have mixed feelings toward their sibling. For instance, they may resent the attention their sibling receives, but then feel guilty about their resentment (Ellifritt, 1984). Or they may question whether their parents love them as much as their sibling with a disability, because that child often receives so much of the parents' attention and time. They may also wonder how they can help their parents (Powell & Ogle, 1985).

At some time or another, all children who have a sibling with a handicap need to ask questions, to sort out their feelings, and to have time alone with their parents (Breslau, Weitzman, & Messenger, 1981; Mori, 1983). Parents should try to answer their questions honestly and fully. Also, it is very helpful if parents can recognize and accept that these children often feel torn between protecting their brother or sister, whom they love, and being accepted by children outside the family, who often tease them and their sibling (Featherstone, 1980).

Although some of the literature has emphasized the negative effects on the siblings of a child with handicaps, recent findings point to a number of positive effects as well (Cobb & Hancock, 1984; Glendinning, 1983). For instance, Simeonsson & McHale (1981) found that these siblings were more altruistic, idealistic, expressed greater humanitarian interests, and were more tolerant toward others. In addition, most of these siblings had healthy relationships with their parents, felt comfortable having their friends meet their sibling with a disability, and also were willing to explain their sibling's disability if asked. These brothers and sisters generally helped at home in some way with their sibling with a disability and did not feel burdened by this responsibility.

EFFECTS ON GRANDPARENTS

The last group of family members to be considered is grandparents, who are often influential and important to both the parents and their children. For grandparents, grandchildren are often a source of joy, comfort, and satisfaction. Having grandchildren may renew their purpose in life and revive some feelings of importance (Mori, 1983). When a child is born with a handicap, grandparents as well as parents may mourn. Sometimes, the grandparents' denial of the disability lasts longer than that of the parents and may actually interfere with the parents' adaptation to the disability. Grandparents may discourage the parents from participating in programs for the child because they believe the "special" help is not necessary (Gabel & Kotsch, 1981). In some instances, the grandparents may blame their son- or daughter-in-law for bringing the "bad blood" into the family that caused the disability (Mori, 1983). Yet, often, after a difficult period of time, grandparents can prove to be sources of support and assistance to the parents. It is important for both parents and grandparents to recognize the value of grandparents to the family. They can help with practical needs such as babysitting and can sometimes offer a perspective that provides answers to what may seem insurmountable problems (Mori, 1983).

SOCIETY AND COMMUNITY REACTIONS

So far, this chapter has concentrated on the internal dynamics and workings of the family and its members. The social context of the family is equally important in determining the outcome for its members. Attitudes of those outside the family affect reactions and relationships within the family. Especially significant to the family with a child who has a disability is the reaction of others to this child. For example, families often find they must deal with the reactions of their neighbors to their child. These reactions may range from helpful and kind to fearful or even obnoxious. Some may seem to view the child's disability as contagious, that he or she will somehow infect the neighborhood. Others accept the family and the child as ordinary people who perhaps need some extra help. Families may find that they must establish some guidelines for handling their relationships with their neighbors. If parents are able to briefly explain the child's disability, they often find this removes the mystery and makes the situation feel more normal.

Neighbors' reactions are often typical of the kinds of reactions the family encounters in the rest of society. One important factor in others' reactions is the significance that is placed on the disability itself. For example, if society defines a child who has a handicap as a sick person, then expectations of that child will be different from those of a society that regards those with physical disabilities as normal (Fraser, 1980).

In the United States, society has tended to stigmatize those with physical disabilities (Goffman, 1963; Vargo, 1978). That is, we tend to view persons with disabilities as somehow having less value. This sets these individuals apart and makes their adaptational tasks that much more difficult (Cobb & Hancock, 1984; O'Moore, 1980). This attitude creates, in a sense, a radically different world for those who have physical disabilities. It may also mean that these children face different developmental tasks; thus, traditional developmental theory may not apply accurately to them (Gliedman & Roth, 1980). These children may be at a double disadvantage: they may need to be exceptional in personal and interpersonal characteristics to be appealing to peers, and yet it is difficult for them to develop interpersonal skills because they are isolated and rejected as part of a stigmatized minority (Cobb & Hancock, 1984), a kind of "Catch-22." This may result in children with disabilities accepting this negative view of themselves, with a resultant loss in self-worth and self-esteem (Mauer, 1976). Or they may try to somehow "pass" as normal, trying to hide their disability so that others will accept them and will not view them as unequal. Deciding how to present oneself to a world that often views a disability in this fashion is very difficult.

The entire family is affected by these reactions to the child with a disability. Attitudinal changes come slowly, but certainly are necessary if these families' already-difficult jobs are not to be made harder by societal pressures and prejudices.

ROLE OF THE PROFESSIONAL

Professionals can do much to lighten the burden that families with a child who has disabilities carry. In beginning to work with these families, we must all examine and come to terms with our own attitudes toward individuals with disabilities (Cobb & Hancock, 1984). As members of a society that stigmatizes these persons, we are not immune to adopting some of these attitudes ourselves. Thus, this is an important first step in our work. We must also recognize that in working with these families, we will experience times of frustration and feelings of helplessness because we cannot do as much for them as we would like. Knowing that this will happen may help us handle these feelings when they occur.

Another important consideration is the nature of the relationship that we have with families. The key is to recognize that this relationship is not really an equal one; that is, the parent is unfortunately not often viewed as being on an equal footing with the professional (Glendinning, 1983). Unless we are sensitive to this, clients may be reluctant to express their feelings or to make suggestions. It is necessary, therefore, for us to recognize the "expertise and experience" of the parents (Glendinning, 1983).

As we maintain some awareness of our own reactions and recognize the type of relationship we have with parents, we can proceed to help them through the problematic times of the life cycle. There are particular transitional times when what we do can make a great deal of difference to these families.

This is especially true at the time of diagnosis of the child. The response the family receives at this time may set a tone and have a much greater impact on these families than will their future contacts with the same professionals (Cobb & Hancock, 1984). When information is given, it should be in clear, concrete language rather than obscure jargon (Luterman, 1979). Adequate time needs to be allowed for counseling and for questions (Barsch, 1968; Cobb & Hancock, 1984; Glendinning, 1983). Parents must be given time to come to grips with the shock of the diagnosis. Often, it is necessary to repeat the information for the parents, as this time of heightened emotion makes it difficult for them to absorb what is being said.

During times of crisis, professionals, especially social workers, may find that much progress can be accomplished with families. Although we all resist making major changes and adaptations in our lives, during crisis, we are more open to suggestions because we are so anxious to resolve our feelings of stress. By being aware of this, professionals can help families to examine not only the symptoms of the crisis but also any underlying causes and to look at ways to alleviate these problems.

As professionals and parents work together to develop a treatment plan for the child, it is important to keep in mind the time, energy, and resources that the family has so that the plan is realistic and manageable (Wolfensberger, 1967). Such plans should be reviewed as frequently as every 3 months for a young child and at 6–12 month intervals for an older child. Sometimes, parents are resistant to professionals' suggestions. Rather than label parents as noncompliant, it is crucial to look at the reason(s) for their resistance. Perhaps what the professional is suggesting goes against some value the parents have or does not fit into their cultural perspective. Taking a closer look can often provide valuable information. Also, demands are often placed on parents that are nearly impossible. For instance, they are expected to care for the needs of the child but not overprotect him or her, and to find a way to grieve over, yet not reject, the child. They also are asked to treat the child as normal but not deny the disability. We must be sensitive to these expectations and work to enhance the family's efforts, not focus on their weaknesses (Glendinning, 1983).

Finally, parents often say that they need more help in the practical, day-to-day care of a child who has a disability (Featherstone, 1980; Glendinning, 1983; Wolfensberger, 1967). When we work with a family, we can ask about their daily routine and try to determine how we might lighten the load of that routine and what community services might be most helpful to them. We need, therefore, to be aware of what services are available in their communities. For example, is there a parent support group that might help to break the isolation of these parents? Is there respite care? If so, what does it cost? What are the eligibility requirements, if any? Are homemaker services available? Is this family eligible for some sort of financial help, especially with their medical bills? (See Chapter 25.)

These are some of the ways in which we might better serve these families. Certainly, the role the professional plays with these families helps to determine the prognosis for the child and the outcome for the entire family. It also can aid in making their rocky road to the future a little smoother.

CASE STUDY

Jimmy had always been slower in his development than his brother David. He did not walk until 20 months and was not talking until 3 years of age. Throughout this time, Jimmy's parents would ask their pediatrician how Jimmy was doing. They were comforted by his reassurances that their son would catch up, but some of their doubts continued to linger.

By the time Jimmy was 4 years old and had made little additional progress, his parents could no longer believe he was doing fine. They began to look for an answer, a reason for his delay in development. They located a developmental pediatrician who spent time with them and Jimmy. In meetings with her and the multidisciplinary team at the center where she worked, Jimmy's parents learned that Jimmy had mental retardation. Even though they had suspected this, they still felt numb and shocked. The members of the team advised them on ways to help Jimmy. They reassured them that Jimmy's retardation was not their fault.

Gradually, with the support and assistance of this professional team and the encouragement of their own parents, Jimmy's parents began to adjust to the reality of Jimmy's condition. They became involved with a group of parents of children with retardation and learned they were not alone in experiencing ambivalent feelings about their child. This helped them a great deal.

When Jimmy was 5 years old, his parents entered him in a special education program. He was happy there and made progress. Jimmy's mother became active in his school, volunteering her services there once a week. Jimmy's achievements pleased her.

For Jimmy's father, however, the situation was more difficult. He was not involved in Jimmy's schooling and found Jimmy's slow progress to be disconcerting. In the support group, Jimmy's father was able to express these feelings. This helped him and provided his wife with a better understanding of these feelings.

The family remained in contact with the treatment center. Through the center, they found out about respite care, and the parents were able to go on some weekend vacations. This was rejuvenating for them. They also learned about special community programs that were available to children with retardation and their families.

Jimmy is now 8 years old and remains in a special education program. He continues to make slow but steady progress. Although his parents continue to have their ups and downs, the bad times are less frequent and are weathered more easily. Jimmy's brother has also been getting more attention from his parents and feels better about himself and his brother.

Through the help and guidance of people who cared for them and through their own hard work, this family has survived and is functioning well.

SUMMARY

As the family progresses through its life cycle, its members face various changes and adjustments. These are magnified for the family with a child who has a disability. Parents, siblings, and extended family members are all affected. The child with a disability has a particularly difficult time during adolescence, when acceptance by peers and one's body image become critical factors. Negative attitudes about disabilities that are apparent in society also affect the family's adjustment. Professionals, too, may play a significant role in the outcome for the family. Even though the family has to cope with extra burdens, most families develop positive relationships among their members and manage to cope effectively with their extra cares.

REFERENCES

Abrams, R.C. (1970). The impact of cerebral palsy on the patient and his family. In M. Debuskey (Ed.), *The chronically ill child and his family*. Springfield, IL: Charles C Thomas.

Abramson, M., Ash, M.J., & Nash, W.R. (1979). Handicapped adolescents—a time for reflection. *Adolescence, 55*, 557–565.

Affleck, G., Allen. D.A., McGrade, B.J., et al. (1982a). Maternal caretaking perceptions and reported mood disturbance at hospital discharge of a high risk infant and nine months later. *Mental Retardation, 20*, 220–225.

Affleck, G., Allen, D., McGrade, B.J., et al. (1982b). Home environments of developmentally disabled infants as a function of parent and infant characteristics. *American Journal of Mental Deficiency, 86*, 445–453.

Affleck, G., McGrade, B.J., McQueeney, M., et al. (1982). Relationship-focused early intervention in developmental disabilities. *Exceptional Children, 49*, 259–261.

Babington, C.H. (1981). *Parenting and the retarded child*. Springfield, IL: Charles C Thomas.

Banta, E.M. (1984). Perceptions of parent-child relations by parents and siblings of deaf-blind children. *Dissertation Abstracts International, 45*, 806A.

Barsch, R.H. (1968). *The parent of the handicapped child: The study of child-rearing practices*. Springfield, IL: Charles C Thomas.

Blacher, J. (Ed.). (1984a). *Severely handicapped young children and their families: Research in review*. New York: Academic Press.

Blacher, J. (1984b). Sequential stages of parental adjustment to the birth of a child with handicaps: Fact or artifact? *Mental Retardation, 22*, 55–68.

Boston Women's Health Book Collective, Inc. (1978). *Ourselves and our children: A book by and for parents*. New York: Random House.

Breslau, N., Weitzman, M., & Messenger, K. (1981). Psychologic functioning of siblings of disabled children. *Pediatrics, 67*, 344–353.

Burden, R.L. (1980). Measuring the effects of stress on the mothers of handicapped infants: Must depression always follow? *Child Care, Health and Development, 6*, 111–125.

Buscaglia, L. (1983). *The disabled and their parents: A counseling challenge* (rev. ed.). Thorofare, NJ: SLACK.

Butler, A.B. (1983). There's something wrong with Michael: A pediatrician-mother's perspective. *Pediatrics, 71*, 446–448.

Carter, E.A., & McGoldrick, M. (Eds.). (1980). *The family life cycle: A framework for family therapy*. New York: Gardner Press.

Cobb, L.S., & Hancock, K.A. (1984). Development of the child with a physical disability. *Advances in Developmental and Behavioral Pediatrics, 5*, 75–107.

Cruikshank, W.M. (Ed.). (1980). *Psychology of exceptional children and youth*. Englewood Cliffs, NJ: Prentice-Hall.

Darling, R., & Darling, J. (1982). *Children who are different*. St. Louis: C.V. Mosby Co.

Diamond, L.J., & Jaudes, P.K. (1983). Child abuse in a cerebral-palsied population. *Developmental Medicine and Child Neurology, 25*, 169–174.

Dickman, I.R., & Gordon, S. (1983). *Getting help for a disabled child—advice from parents*. Public Affairs Pamphlet No. 615. New York: Public Affairs Committee.

Donaldson, J. (1980). Changing attitudes toward handicapped persons: A review and analysis of research. *Exceptional Children, 46*, 504–514.

Dorner, S. (1975). The relationship of physical handicap to stress in families with an adolescent with spina bifida. *Developmental Medicine and Child Neurology, 17*, 765–776.

Ellifritt, J. (1984). Life with my sister—guilty no more. *Exceptional Parent, 14*, 16–21.

Fairfield, B. (1983). Parents coping with genetically handicapped children: Use of early recollections. *Exceptional Children, 49*, 411–415.

Featherstone, H. (1980). *A difference in the family: Life with a disabled child*. New York: Basic Books.

Field, T., Roopnarine, J.L., & Segal, M.M. (Eds.). (1984). *Friendships in normal and handicapped children*. Norwood, NJ: Ablex Publishing Corp.

Fraser, B.C. (1980). The meaning of handicap in children. *Child Care, Health and Development, 6,* 83–91.

Friedrich, W.N., & Boriskin, J.A. (1976). The role of the child in abuse: A review of the literature. *American Journal of Orthopsychiatry, 46,* 580–590.

Gabel, H., & Kotsch, L. (1981). Extended families and young handicapped children. *Topics in Early Childhood Special Education, 1,* 29–35.

Gamble, M. (1984). Helping our children accept themselves. *Exceptional Parent, 14,* 48–51.

Glendinning, C. (1983). *Unshared care: Parents and their disabled children*. London: Routledge & Kegan Paul.

Gliedman, J., & Roth, W. (1980). *The unexpected minority: Handicapped children in America*. New York: Harcourt Brace Jovanovich.

Goffman, E. (1963). *Stigma*. Englewood Cliffs, NJ: Prentice-Hall.

Greenfeld, J. (1972). *A child called Noah*. New York: Holt, Rinehart & Winston.

Harper, D.C. (1984). Child behavior toward the parent: A factor analysis of mothers' reports of disabled children. *Journal of Autism and Developmental Disorders, 14,* 165–182.

Harte, T.J.F. (1981). The relationship between self-concept, empathy training, and attitudes toward the physically handicapped in ten to eleven year old boys and girls. *Dissertation Abstracts International, 41,* 4741B.

Harvey, D., & Greenway, P. (1982). How parent attitudes and emotional reactions affect their handicapped child's self-concept. *Psychological Medicine, 12,* 357–370.

Hewett, S. (1976). Research on families with handicapped children—an aid or an impediment to understanding? *Birth Defects, The Original Article Series, 12,* 35–46.

Kennedy, J.F. (1970). Maternal reactions to the birth of a defective baby. *Social Casework, 51,* 410–416.

Kessler, M.S. (1979). Age of disability onset as a psychological factor in anxiety and self-esteem of wheelchair-bound individuals. *Dissertation Abstracts International, 39,* 6547A.

Kubler-Ross, E. (1969). *On death and dying*. New York: Macmillan Co.

Lear, R. (1980). *Play helps: Toys and activities for handicapped children*. London: William Heinemann Medical Books.

Linkowsi, D.C., & Dunn, M.A. (1974). Self-concept and acceptance of disability. *Rehabilitation Counseling Bulletin, 17,* 28–32.

Lonsdale, G. (1978). Family life with a handicapped child: The parents speak. *Child Care, Health and Development, 4,* 99–120.

Luterman, D. (1979). *Counseling parents of hearing-impaired children*. Boston: Little, Brown & Co.

McCollum, A.T. (1984). Grieving over the lost dream. *Exceptional Parent, 14,* 9–12.

Mauer, R.A. (1976). Young children's affective responses to a physically disabled story book hero. *Dissertation Abstracts International, 37,* 918–919.

Moran, M.A. (1984). Families of developmentally disabled infants in early intervention. *Dissertation Abstracts International, 44,* 2916B.

Morgan, B., & Leung, P. (1980). Effects of assertion training on acceptance of disability by physically disabled university students. *Journal of Counseling Psychology, 27,* 209–212.

Mori, A.A. (1983). *Families of children with special needs: Early intervention techniques for the practitioner*. Rockville, MD: Aspen Systems Corp.

Murray, R.F. (1976). Psychosocial aspects of genetic counseling. *Social Work in Health Care, 2,* 13–23.

Newson, E., & Hipgrave, T. (1983). *Getting through to your handicapped child*. New York: Cambridge University Press.

O'Hara, D.M., & Levy, J.M. (1984). Family adaptation to learning disability: A framework for understanding and treatment. *Learning Disabilities, 3,* 63–76.

Olshansky, S. (1962). Chronic sorrow: A response to having a mentally defective child. *Social Casework, 43,* 190–193.

O'Moore, M. (1980). Social acceptance of the physically handicapped child in the ordinary school. *Child Care, Health and Development, 6,* 317–318.

Paterson, G.W. (1975). *Helping your handicapped child*. Minneapolis: Augsburg Publishing House.

Powell, T.H., & Ogle, P.A. (1985). *Brothers & sisters—a special part of exceptional families*. Baltimore: Paul H. Brookes Publishing Co.

Prensky, A.L., & Palkes, H.S. (1982). *Care of the neurologically handicapped child: A book for parents and professionals*. New York: Oxford University Press.

Rhodes, S.L. (1977). A developmental approach to the life cycle of the family. *Social Casework, 58,* 301–311.

Ringe, L.B. (1981). Body attitudes, self-esteem, and physical disability. *Dissertation Abstracts International, 41,* 3586B.

Roth, W. (1981). *The handicapped speak.* Jefferson, NC: McFarland & Co, Inc.

Rousso, H. (1984). Fostering healthy self esteem. Part One. *Exceptional Parent, 14,* 9–14.

Rousso, H. (1985). Fostering self-esteem. Part Two. What parents and professionals can do. *Exceptional Parent, 15,* 9–12.

Schild, S. (1976). Counseling with parents of retarded children. In F.J. Turner (Ed.), *Differential diagnosis and treatment in social work.* New York: Free Press.

Schloss, P.J. (1984). *Social development of handicapped children and adolescents.* Rockville, MD: Aspen Systems Corp.

Seligman, M. (Ed.). (1983). *The family with a handicapped child: Understanding and treatment.* New York: Grune & Stratton.

Simeonsson, R.J., & McHale, S.M. (1981). Review. Research on handicapped children: sibling relationships. *Child Care, Health and Development, 7,* 153–171.

Solnit, A.J. & Stark, M.H. (1961). Mourning the birth of a defective child. *Psychoanalytic Study of the Child, 16,* 523–537.

Solomons, G. (1979). Child abuse and developmental disabilities. *Developmental Medicine and Child Neurology, 21,* 101–108.

Starr, P., & Heiserman, K. (1977). Acceptance of disability by teenagers with oral-facial clefts. *Rehabilitation Counseling Bulletin, 20,* 198–201.

Strax, T.E. (1976). Adolescence—a period of stress, the search for an identity. *Birth Defects, The Original Article Series, 12,* 63–70.

Tavormina, J.B., Boll, T.J., Dunn, N.J., et al. (1981). Psychosocial effects on parents of raising a physically handicapped child. *Journal of Abnormal Child Psychology, 9,* 121–131.

Terkelsen, K.G. (1980). Toward a theory of the family life cycle. In E.A. Carter & M. McGoldrick (Eds.). *The family life cycle: A framework for family therapy.* New York: Gardner Press.

Vargo, J.W. (1978). Some psychological effects of physical disability. *American Journal of Occupational Therapy, 32,* 31–34.

Vernon, M. (1979). Counseling the parents of birth-defective children. *Postgraduate Medicine, 65,* 197–200.

Wasserman, G.A., & Allen, R. (1985). Maternal withdrawal from handicapped toddlers. *Journal of Child Psychology and Psychiatry, 26,* 381–387.

Wasserman, G.A., Seidman, S., & Allen, R. (1984). Toddlers with congenital anomalies and their mothers: The research of the Child Development Program at the New York State Psychiatric Institute. *Rehabilitation Literature, 45,* 202–205.

Watson, J.D. (1984). Talking about the best kept secret: Sexual abuse and children with disabilities. *Exceptional Parent, 14,* 15–20.

Webster, E.J. (1977). *Counseling with parents of handicapped children: Guidelines for improving communication.* New York: Grune & Stratton.

Wikler, L., Wasow, M., & Hatfield, E. (1981). Chronic sorrow revisited: Parents' vs. professional depiction of the adjustment of parents of mentally retarded children. *American Journal of Orthopsychiatry, 51,* 63–70.

Winter, M., & DeSimone, D. (1983). I'm a person, not a wheelchair! Problems of disabled adolescents. In R.L. Jones (Ed.), *Reflections on growing up disabled.* Reston, VA: Council for Exceptional Children.

Wishart, M.C., Bidder, R.T., & Gray, O.P. (1980). Parental responses to their developmentally delayed children and the South Glamorgan Home Advisory Service. *Child Care, Health and Development, 6,* 361–376.

Wolfensberger, W. (1967). Counseling the parents of the retarded. In A.A. Baumeister (Ed.), *Mental retardation: Appraisal, education, and rehabilitation.* Chicago: Aldine Publishing Co.

Zimmerman, J.L.W. (1982). Social interaction patterns between blind multi-impaired infants and their mothers: An analysis of the process. *Dissertation Abstracts International, 42,* 3113A.

Zola, I.K. (1982). *Missing pieces: A chronicle of living with a disability.* Philadelphia: Temple University Press.

Chapter 24

Some Ethical Dilemmas

Upon completion of this chapter, the reader will:
—Understand a number of ethical issues concerning persons with handicaps, including genetic screening, prenatal diagnosis, abortion, treatment issues, human experimentation, sterilization, institutionalization, and rights to education

---

Recent medical advances have led to improved care for children both before and after birth. In the last 10 years, the death rate for all infants has been cut in half. For premature infants, the decline has been equally dramatic (Dunea, 1983). Neonatal intensive care units now exist in some 600 hospitals across the country (Dunea, 1983). Yet children with severe developmental disabilities continue to be born. In some ways, the same technology that has contributed to the saving of tiny premature infants may also add to the incidence of developmental disabilities, since these babies are at greater risk for these disorders than full-term infants.

Because of the complex technology and the choices available for the care of children with developmental disabilities, numerous difficult ethical questions are raised. For example: Should prenatal diagnosis be performed on women who are at risk genetically for having a child with a severely disabling disease? If yes, should affected fetuses be aborted? Are there instances in which medical care should be withheld from a newborn infant with disabilities? Is it ethical to perform experimental research on children with handicaps? Should young adults with mental retardation be sterilized? Where should children with handicaps live—at home or in institutions? What does society owe children with handicaps in terms of an education?

In this chapter, these ethical questions are examined from various perspectives.

GENETIC SCREENING

Both Ann and her husband, Danny, have learned through a genetic screening program that they are carriers of Tay-Sachs disease. If Ann becomes pregnant, her chances of carrying a child with Tay-Sachs disease are 1 in 4. Such a child would have little future because there is no treatment for Tay-Sachs, and all children with this disease die at a young age. Neither Ann nor Danny is willing to consider abortion of an affected fetus. They are faced with a dilemma. Should Ann risk becoming pregnant and simply hope for a well-born child, or do she and Danny have an obligation to society—and to themselves—not to take that risk?

If Ann does become pregnant and carries the fetus to term, she runs a significant risk of having a child with Tay-Sachs disease. Medical or institutional care for this child would be costly, and the state would be likely to bear most of the burden. If Ann accepted the possibility of therapeutic abortion, she could ensure that no child of hers would be born with Tay-Sachs disease. Therefore, does the state have a right to prevent the birth of her affected child (Reilly, 1977)?

Even more basic is the question of whether the state has a right or a duty to perform genetic screening. Right now, genetic screening is available for carriers of Tay-Sachs disease and sickle cell anemia. In the future, genetic screening is likely to be available for other severe diseases. Will we eventually decide that these screening programs should be legislated and that, if a test is positive, an individual should be required to undergo a particular treatment? Is it possible that individuals like Ann and Danny would not be allowed to marry because of their "bad genes"? At the heart of this issue is whether or not the individual's freedom of choice is more important than society's preferences. Right now, our society favors respecting the individual's choice.

A similar question emerges in considering newborn screening tests. One example is the test for phenylketonuria (PKU). Virtually all newborns have blood drawn before they are discharged from the hospital to test for PKU and other inborn errors of metabolism (see Chapter 8). The rationale is that early identification of PKU permits treatment that prevents mental retardation. If therapy is delayed, brain damage invariably occurs. As a result, most states have passed laws requiring this test on all newborns. Even considering its worthwhile nature, is it ethical to mandate this test? Some parents may object to the requirement, saying that it violates their right to give informed consent.

A way around this problem is to remove the compulsory nature of the test. In Maryland, for instance, the law requiring this test was repealed, and parents instead are offered the test on a voluntary basis (Culliton, 1976). Over 95% of parents agree to have the test performed. The end result, therefore, is close to what had been previously legislated. However, using this approach, the rights of both the state and the family are protected.

PRENATAL DIAGNOSIS, THERAPEUTIC ABORTION, AND FETAL THERAPY

Closely linked to the question of genetic screening are the issues surrounding prenatal diagnosis and therapeutic abortion.

Susan is 38 years old and is pregnant for the first time. There is no family history of genetic disease. However, her obstetrician has advised her to have prenatal diagnosis performed because of her age. Susan is unsure. She knows the procedure carries only a slight risk to her and her fetus (Fletcher, 1981). Nonetheless, she is hesitant, primarily because she wants to avoid the possible decision about abortion should the fetus be found to have Down syndrome. After much thought and a few contacts with a genetic counselor, Susan decides not to have the prenatal diagnosis.

In recognition of some of the concerns individuals have about prenatal diagnosis and the difficulties they face in deciding whether or not to have such diagnosis performed, the Hastings Center has suggested certain criteria that prenatal diagnostic programs should follow. These include: 1) A woman at risk should not be denied prenatal diagnosis simply because she has decided against having an abortion; 2) Counseling must be noncoercive and respectful of the various different opinions about abortion; 3) Physicians must inform parents about possible postnatal treatment, if it exists; 4) All results of the prenatal diagnosis should be shared with parents. In addition, these guidelines express opposition to the use of amniocentesis for sex choice alone, but also oppose any restrictions on this option, to protect parents' right to choose (Fletcher, 1981; Powledge & Fletcher, 1979). While the use of prenatal diagnosis often does lead to the therapeutic abortion of an affected fetus, parents who are opposed to abortion might use this information to prepare themselves and their families for the birth of a child with a disability and for the care of that child. Thus, the use of prenatal diagnosis should not be offered only to those who would consider an abortion.

When making her decision, Susan's opposition to abortion was the key factor, and many other individuals who oppose prenatal diagnosis share her view. It is not the prenatal diagnostic techniques that are the problem, they would argue, but rather that these techniques often lead to abortion (Fletcher, 1981). There is a wide range of positions on whether or not abortion is morally justifiable (Weber, 1976). At one extreme are those who believe that abortion is never acceptable. They say the unborn fetus is a human being from the moment of conception and that its life must be protected under all circumstances (Churchill & Siman, 1982; Drinan, 1970). And, they would say, once abortion is allowed, this may lead to infanticide and then genocide. They would argue that once one takes the first step on the "slippery slope" of allowing some destruction of life, it is difficult, if not impossible, to control the rest of the steps (Horan & Delahoyde, 1982).

A slightly less extreme viewpoint is that abortion is acceptable only if the mother's life is in danger. Those who advocate this position also believe that the fetus is a human being from the time of conception. Nevertheless, they argue that the life of the mother must be considered before that of the fetus.

Those in the middle might argue that abortion is morally acceptable in certain defined situations, but not in others. For example, members of this group would allow abortion following rape or incest, or when the fetus is malformed or has a severe genetic disorder. The difficulty with this position is drawing the line as to which conditions are serious enough to justify abortion (Veatch, 1977). Those who reject this position fear that as prenatal diagnosis becomes more widespread, women will be

368 / CHILDREN WITH HANDICAPS

pressured to undergo abortion of any damaged or potentially damaged fetus. Combined with this pressure may be society's unwillingness to continue to pay for care of persons with disabilities (Kolata, 1980).

Finally, at the other extreme are those who believe that abortion is acceptable whenever a woman wants it. Those who advocate this position argue that a woman has a right to privacy and that part of exercising that right means being able to choose to have an abortion and having access to a safe abortion if she determines it is needed (Churchill & Siman, 1982). Such advocates believe that the fetus is not human until it is able to live independently outside the mother's womb, generally considered to be after the 24th week of gestation. Prior to that time, a woman should have the right to make a choice as she sees fit.

Recently, the possibility of fetal therapy adds further dimensions to the abortion debate. As the treatment of the fetus for certain disorders becomes more and more possible, important questions are raised about the rights of the mother as a patient and the rights of the fetus as a patient. How to weigh the risks and benefits to the fetus and the mother is difficult to determine (Ruddick & Wilcox, 1982). Over the past few years, some court cases have granted certain rights to the fetus. In one case, a mother was ordered to undergo treatment to protect the fetus (Bainbridge, 1983). As the fetus is assigned more rights, one of the results may be an impact on the availability of, legality of, and access to abortion.

In the future, the resolution of the abortion issue will depend on defining the moral and legal status of the fetus. What is likely to happen is that the U.S. Supreme Court will decide much of this essentially ethical question as it considers and reviews future challenges to *Roe v. Wade* (the landmark 1973 abortion case) and other related cases.

WITHHOLDING TREATMENT

Judy is 3 days old and has Down syndrome. She also has an intestinal blockage that requires surgery. Her parents are young, ages 18 and 20, and Judy is their first child. Their financial resources are limited. They are concerned about how severe Judy's retardation will be and whether or not they can emotionally handle having a child with retardation. They are counseled that most Down syndrome children have moderate retardation and often are very happy children. They hesitate to give permission to perform surgery. Perhaps it would be better to allow Judy to die. Yet, do they have the right to refuse surgery for their child?

Another newborn, Tommy, has spina bifida. He is likely to have normal intelligence, but the location of the opening in the spine is in the upper back region. Thus, he will be paralyzed below this level and most likely will be unable to walk or to control his bowel and bladder functions. He also runs a risk of becoming hydrocephalic. Immediate surgery is needed to cover the spinal opening and prevent infection. He will also require a great deal of expensive medical care in the future because he will probably develop orthopedic, neurosurgical, and kidney problems. However, without surgery as a newborn, he is likely to develop meningitis and die. Tommy's parents are in their mid-twenties and have two normal children at home.

They are torn between their obligation to their other children and to Tommy. Should they permit surgery?

Similar to Judy and Tommy, many children with handicaps are born with medical problems that are life-threatening in the newborn period. For example, approximately 10% of the children with Down syndrome have a narrowing of the small intestine called duodenal atresia (Penrose & Smith, 1966). This condition leads to vomiting and dehydration. If untreated, these infants starve to death during the first weeks of life. Approximately 1 in 1,000 infants are born with spina bifida (Gallo, 1984). The opening in the spine that is part of this condition places these infants at great risk for developing meningitis, an infection that carries a mortality rate of over 50% (Freeman, 1973; Lorber, 1974).

For both of these defects, surgical correction is not difficult. The damaged portion of the small intestine can be removed surgically, and the child can then eat and drink normally. Likewise, the spinal opening in spina bifida can be closed. The catch is that these children often have remaining disabilities for their entire lives. The ethical question raised is whether or not parents or someone else has the right to withhold treatment from these infants.

Right now, these decisions are made by parents through communication with their child's physician. Roughly 10 years ago, a landmark study showed that of 299 deaths in an intensive care nursery, 43 (14%) were related to the withholding of treatment (Duff & Campbell, 1973). Whether the frequency of these decisions remains this high is uncertain, but such painful decisions do continue to be made. To examine the question of withholding treatment, one must consider the related issues of informed consent, the definition of a human being, and the quality of life versus the sanctity of life.

Who should decide whether or not surgery takes place? Traditionally, the patient himself, if able, or his or her parents have made the decision. For parents to be able to give informed consent, they must receive information from the physician as to the risks of the procedure, the possible benefits, and the long-term prognosis for their child. In giving information, physicians may be affected by their own biases concerning whether a particular infant's life is worth continuing (Bridge & Bridge, 1981). When the physician describes an operation, he or she, consciously or unconsciously, may accentuate certain risks or benefits (Duff & Campbell, 1973; Shaw, 1973) and influence the parents' decision. An awareness of these factors is important in the decision-making process.

Once the parents have received the information, the question is whether they can really give informed consent. Some argue that parents faced with the birth of a child with defects are in a state of shock, overwhelmed by fear, guilt, and horror (Johnson, 1980; Shaw, 1973). These feelings, then, may keep them from making a reasonable decision (Ellis, 1982). The parents may feel they have no alternative but surgery. Others argue that even though parents have these feelings, it does not mean that their right to decide and their wishes should be overridden (Strong, 1984). Generally, studies have found that parents' decisions in these situations are thoughtful, reasonable, and responsible (Strong, 1984).

And the question arises that if parents are not able to decide, who is and who should? Does the physician or the state have the right? In the past, the courts have supported parents' right to make this decision. However, two recent, highly publicized cases suggest that the state may be more ready to intervene now than in the past.

Baby Doe and Baby Jane Doe

The first case is that of Baby Doe, which, because of its significance, is discussed here in some detail. Baby Doe was born in Indiana with Down syndrome and a tracheoesophageal fistula, a condition in which the esophagus is not connected to the stomach. Thus, he could not eat normally. His parents decided not to give permission for him to have corrective surgery. He was then denied food and water, and he died at 6 days of age. The Indiana courts let the parents' decision stand (Fost, 1982). However, that was not the end of the situation. Shortly after his death, there ensued a public outcry.

In June 1982, the federal government notified all hospitals that it was unlawful to withhold treatment from a baby with handicaps. Nine months later, in March 1983, the government, through the U.S. Department of Health and Human Services (DHHS), issued another order, which required the placement of a sign in public areas in nurseries and delivery rooms stating that discrimination against children with handicaps was prohibited. The notice also warned that federal funds would be withdrawn from hospitals that violated this order. In addition, the order announced the establishment of an agency in Washington, D.C., that would investigate any violation of this order at a moment's notice. A toll-free number was given. (On four occasions, investigative squads went to hospitals to check into complaints; no violations were found [Dunea, 1983].) Following the publication of these regulations, there was much criticism of them. The American Academy of Pediatrics and others filed a suit against the government (Holder, 1983). In April 1983, a federal court judge struck down the rule, calling it "arbitrary, capricious, and intrusive" (Culliton, 1983; Dunea, 1983; U.S. District Court, 1983). The government said it would appeal the case.

In April 1984, the American Academy of Pediatrics released their "Guidelines for Infant Bioethics Committees" and urged hospitals to establish such committees to help decide these difficult situations (Annas, 1984). Later, in October 1984, the U.S. Congress passed some important amendments to the Child Abuse Prevention and Treatment Act. These amendments expanded the definition of "medical neglect" to include "withholding of medically indicated treatment from a disabled infant" (Krauthammer, 1985). To implement these amendments, the Department of Health and Human Services issued its final rule (U.S. DHHS, 1985). This rule defined further what was meant by withholding treatment and medical neglect (Murray, 1985). It supported the trend toward aggressive treatment of life-threatening medical problems in infants who had other physical or mental disabilities. Interestingly, violation of the rule carried fairly minor penalties. The maximum sanction was a loss of a limited amount of federal money. Neither criminal nor civil actions were authorized or threatened. In some ways, then, this final rule may have a minimal impact on what has been practiced in these situations in nurseries across the country. However, the final word is not yet in. The issue is still being reviewed in the courts, and it is there that increasing numbers of these decisions may be made in the future.

Another relevant and important case is that of Baby Jane Doe who was born in October 1983 in New York with spina bifida and hydrocephaly. Her prognosis, according to her doctors, was severe retardation, epilepsy, paralysis, and constant urinary tract infections. She was transferred to Stony Brook Hospital where surgery was to be performed. After further consultation with physicians, nurses, religious counselors, and a social worker, her parents decided not to consent to surgery. Instead, they chose to treat her with antibiotics to protect her against an infection of her spinal column (Steinbock, 1984).

At this point, a local lawyer heard of the case through a confidential tip. He filed a suit seeking the appointment of a guardian for the child and additional treatment for the child. The judge appointed a guardian, ruled that the infant was in need of immediate surgery, and authorized the guardian's consent to surgery. The case was appealed, and the appellate court reversed the judge's order, saying that the parents' decision was in the best interests of the infant and that the courts had no basis for intervention. The highest court in New York upheld this later decision. However, the federal government sued, saying it had a right to see the hospital records on this child. This request was turned down, but the government has appealed the case (Steinbock, 1984). The Supreme Court, at the request of the Reagan administration, agreed to consider in its session that began in October 1985 whether it is illegal for hospitals to grant parents' wishes to withhold nourishment or medically indicated treatment from a child with handicaps (Denniston, 1985). As of March 1986 the court had not ruled on this case. Thus, the final outcome in this case is uncertain. As of the summer of 1985, Baby Jane Doe was still alive but had severe handicaps (Schmeck, 1985).

In instances where the courts have overruled the parents, the issue that then arises is whether it remains the parents' responsibility to care for the child with handicaps whom they did not want to keep alive. One might argue that if the state decides to save a child's life, then it and not the parents should be responsible for the future care of the child (Shaw, 1973). There is some irony in the government's arguing for the treatment and saving of these infants' lives at the same time that funding for programs to help care for and educate children with handicaps is being cut (Murray, 1985).

EXPERIMENTAL TREATMENT OF AND RESEARCH ON CHILDREN WITH HANDICAPS

On October 26, 1984, physicians at Loma Linda University Medical Center in California implanted a heart from a 7-month-old baboon named Goobers into the body of an infant who was born with a serious heart condition. This infant, later known as Baby Fae, lived for 20 days with this new heart but died of kidney and heart failure that resulted from a reaction to the foreign tissue in her body (Joseph & Rose Kennedy Institute of Ethics, 1985).

The case of Baby Fae was not the first of its kind. In the 1960s, xenografts, or transplants between different species, were tried. A chimpanzee's heart and another chimpanzee's kidneys were transplanted into the bodies of two poor, dying, black men. These men did not survive (Annas, 1985). In these cases, there were many questions raised about whether the men had given informed consent or whether they were simply taken advantage of for research purposes (Annas, 1985). In the case of Baby Fae, too, consent questions have been raised (Annas, 1985; Capron, 1985). Was the consent in her case an informed, voluntary one? How does one ensure that, in these cases, a request for consent is balanced and fair?

Besides the consent question, other issues have been raised. Much discussion has centered on the experimental nature of the transplant. Some would argue that there was not enough evidence to support trying this form of treatment, since similar transplants in the past have not worked (Reemtsma, 1985). Another related concern is that other treatment options may not have been explored thoroughly. For instance, some critics point out that it does not seem that the doctors looked for a human heart for Baby Fae (Gore, 1985). Given this possibility, could it mean that the prime focus of this treatment was the experimental nature of it, or was it done in the belief that it would provide Baby Fae with the best chances for survival (Joseph & Rose Kennedy Institute of Ethics, 1985)? If this was truly an experiment, was it justified (McCormick, 1985)?

In addition to these concerns, others have pointed out that experimental treatment such as that used in this case must be advanced with extreme care. For some time, hospitals and treatment centers have had institutional review boards (IRBs) that pass judgment on the potential risks and benefits of various research proposals. Some say that the review process in the case of Baby Fae was deliberate and careful, and the patient's well-being was of the utmost concern (Sheldon, 1985). Others question whether this was so because of the experimental nature of the procedure and the seriousness of the situation (Joseph & Rose Kennedy Institute of Ethics, 1985).

Finally, some individuals have expressed concern about the use of animals in the treatment of humans. They argue that animals should not be viewed as merely a resource for humans to use as they see fit. Rather, they should be accorded certain rights and treated with respect and consideration for their well-being (Regan, 1985). This is an issue that may be raised more and more frequently as this type of experimental treatment is further developed.

Besides organ transplantation, another novel treatment is gene therapy. In this treatment, a gene, either made synthetically or obtained from another organism (see Chapter 8), is inserted in the place of a defective or missing gene. Because this form of therapy tampers with, to some extent, the essence of who we are, many scientists argue for adherence to strict criteria before this form of therapy is tried. For example, they say that this form of therapy should only be tried on individuals who have limited alternatives. Also, the therapy should have potential to help the patient, and its risks and benefits must be explained carefully. In addition, before any gene is administered to a person, animal studies must show that this treatment has a reasonable chance of success, and that the researchers expect the treatment will not harm the person

(Anderson & Fletcher, 1980; Mercola & Cline, 1980). These criteria apply to the use of gene therapy in the nonsex cells. The use of this therapy in the sex cells (the sperm and the egg) is considered taboo because of the implications of this type of manipulation for future generations (Motulsky, 1983).

As is illustrated by the above examples, experimental treatment of children revolves around two central points: informed consent and benefit to the individual.

Some persons argue that research that does not directly benefit a child or person with retardation is unethical (Plamondon, 1979). Thus, a parent or guardian should have no legal right to consent to such studies (Jonsen, 1978). While an adult may choose for altruistic reasons to engage in research that would benefit society, a child or person with retardation is neither given that choice nor is he or she rationally able to make that decision. Others have argued that even children and individuals with retardation have an obligation to benefit society and that their consent may be presumed (so long as their parents give their consent) in experiments of minimal risk to them (Capron, 1985).

Of additional concern is research that may benefit the individual but may also involve significant risks (Gaylin, 1982). In these instances, the risks versus the benefits must be weighed, and both the consent of the participant, if possible, and that of the parent should be obtained.

Unfortunately, procedures to safeguard children and persons with retardation from nonbeneficial research have not always been followed. In the early 1950s and 1960s, research was done on healthy children with mental retardation in a state institution in New York. These children were infected with mild hepatitis to study the natural course of this disease (Jonsen, 1978). When this information became public, there was a great uproar. Subsequently, the National Commission for the Protection of Human Subjects formulated guidelines for research on children and individuals with retardation (Jonsen, 1978). These guidelines stated, first, that research must be scientifically sound and significant. Second, if at all possible, the research should first be done on animals, followed by adults and older children before using young children. Third, informed consent must be obtained from at least one parent and the participant, if the latter is able to give consent. Finally, the risks must be minimized. Once these criteria are met, research may be performed so long as the risk does not exceed that encountered normally in the children's daily lives. If the risk is more than that, the research may be done only if the expected benefits to the individual subject outweigh the possible risks. When there is no direct benefit to the participant, the research is acceptable only if the risk is minimal and the research is likely to yield knowledge that is vital to the understanding and treatment of the individual's disease (Jonsen, 1978).

STERILIZATION

Another issue involving consent is the involuntary sterilization of persons with mental retardation. The most common methods of sterilization are tubal ligation, hysterectomy, and vasectomy.

In the United States, the use of voluntary sterilization is growing, and research on reversible forms of sterilization has a greater likelihood of success now than in the past because of advances in microsurgery and reconstructive techniques. The possibility of having a reversible form of sterilization adds new dimensions to the debate over involuntary sterilization of individuals with mental retardation (Blank, 1984). In reviewing this debate, one must keep in mind that what is appropriate birth control for a person with mild retardation may not be for a person with severe retardation. Thus, the extent of retardation is a critical factor.

Proponents of sterilization state that it potentially has a number of benefits. First, as a form of genetic engineering, some would argue that it may decrease the incidence of mental retardation. It is clear that the risks of having children with mental retardation are higher among individuals with mental retardation (Blank, 1984). Yet, at least 80% of children with mental retardation are born to parents of normal intelligence (Macklin & Gaylin, 1981; Rosenberg, 1980). Thus, critics of this perspective would say that this is not sufficient reason to involuntarily sterilize people.

A second reason given for sterilization is that it avoids the stress of parenthood for individuals unable to cope with the normal pressures of living independently. However, little empirical data exist that support the assumption that persons with mental retardation, especially those with mild retardation, are unable to care for their children (Blank, 1984; Rosenberg, 1980). The issue is less clear for persons with more severe mental retardation. Those with IQs less than 50 function at a mental age below 8 years. Without help, caring for and raising a child is likely to be beyond these individuals' capabilities. In addition, the burden of childrearing may tax their coping skills too much.

An additional point that is raised on this parenting issue is that the risk of child abuse is increased in individuals with mental retardation because they can deal less effectively with stress. Opponents of this view contend that singling out persons with mental retardation is discriminatory. For such selection to be just, all normally intelligent individuals with a history of child abuse, abandonment, drug abuse, and alcoholism would also need to be considered for sterilization (Blank, 1984).

A third argument for sterilization says that it may improve personal hygiene. Hysterectomy, one form of sterilization, not only prevents conception but also stops menstruation (Chamberlain, Rauh, Passer, et al., 1984). For some females with retardation, menstruation may be frightening and difficult. Some families find it extremely hard to cope with an adolescent with severe retardation who has begun to menstruate. The advantages of a hysterectomy are that it improves personal hygiene and makes the care of the woman easier. Opponents retort that the benefit to the family does not outweigh the loss of freedom for the individual (Rosenberg, 1980). They suggest that other forms of contraception such as birth control pills or an intrauterine device (IUD) are more appropriate measures.

Even if all were to agree that it is wise to sterilize individuals with severe retardation, the question of consent must be addressed. A major stumbling block is the definition of consent: It must be voluntary and informed, and the person involved must be capable of making a decision (Haavik & Menninger, 1981). This may be a "Catch-22" situation. If we believe that an individual is capable of giving consent, might not that individual also be competent to raise children? In other words, if an individual is competent in some areas, doesn't that imply competence in other areas of that person's life? If a person is unfit to raise children, isn't that person also unable to give consent (Derouin, 1982)?

To deal with the sterilization question, some have suggested letting the parent or guardian of the individual with mental retardation make the decision. However, this raises an additional issue because the interests of the parent may conflict with those of the child.

Some individuals argue that only the courts can order involuntary sterilization if a person is unable to give consent (Bayles, 1981). Some courts have found that judges can order sterilization under *parens patriae,* that is, in providing for society's best interests (Haavik & Menninger, 1981). Other cases have held that having children is a basic civil right of any individual in this country regardless of the level of intelligence (Vining & Freeman, 1978).

Recently, the states have stepped into the controversy, and, since 1980, an increasing number of state legislatures have passed sterilization statutes. Some states have tried to pass legislation that authorizes coercive sterilization, especially on poor women, but none has passed so far (Blank, 1984). Approximately 20 states now have some law permitting a review of requests for sterilization (Passer, Rauh, Chamberlain, et al., 1984).

Similarly, the courts have experienced a dramatic change in their attitude toward sterilization. As recently as the 1970s, courts were reluctant to order sterilization and generally ruled that they had no authorization to do so (Blank, 1984). Now, it appears that courts are carefully and cautiously authorizing some sterilizations to be performed. In an attempt to develop a more balanced approach to making these decisions, one court set certain standards and procedures to follow (Annas, 1981). These include: 1) The court must appoint a guardian to protect the individual's interests in the case; 2) The court should receive independent medical and psychological evaluations of the individual by qualified professionals; 3) The judge must meet personally with the individual before deciding whether the person is incompetent to decide; 4) Clear and convincing evidence must prove the person is incompetent; 5) Sterilization must be in the individual's best interests. To determine this, the court must consider the possibility of pregnancy occurring, the potential physical and mental harm from pregnancy and from sterilization, the feasibility of other forms of contraception, and the ability of the individual to care for a child in the future (Annas, 1981). This model of decision making seems to be a balanced one, but right now it is in limited use.

These issues are further complicated by federal regulations that prohibit the use of federal funds for the sterilization of "all minors and those considered mentally incompetent" (Blank, 1984). This lack of funding then limits access to such procedures and provides sterilization only to those who have private funds or insurance plans that cover such procedures. In the future, this inequity will need to be resolved.

INSTITUTIONALIZATION

Another crucial question concerning persons with handicaps is where they should live. Physicians significantly influence the choices parents make. One study in the 1960s revealed that 40% of general practitioners, 17% of pediatricians, and 11% of obstetricians believed that immediate institutionalization was appropriate for most children with retardation (Wolfensberger, 1967). Over 80% of the pediatricians and the obstetricians also stated that they believed it was up to them to decide whether or not to institutionalize the child; the decision was not the parents' to make.

More recently, professionals working with children with retardation have expressed the view that these children do best in the most normal situation possible (Allen & Allen, 1979). Realizing this, parents are sometimes faced with extremely difficult choices. A family may feel that they can no longer care for their child with severe retardation on a full-time basis. Yet, their community may not provide respite care, and the family may not have transportation to get their child to a good nonresidential program. Also, some families feel their child might receive better care if he or she were in a special setting on a 24-hour basis. Under much physical and emotional strain, the family may decide to place the child in a residential center. In making this decision, they may face criticism and judgment from professionals and relatives. Often a placement is not to be found. Either way, the family is in a bind. They feel drained if the child remains home, and they feel guilty if they send him or her away. The choice that is best for all concerned is not easy to make nor simple to implement.

A set of guidelines regarding placement may be helpful. Although years ago large institutions were the only alternatives available to families, this is no longer the case. Thus, the first guideline encourages families to explore and seek information on all the possibilities. Foster homes, group homes, or supervised apartments may be available in various communities. Second, the decision should be a joint one involving both parents and professionals caring for the child. This eases the burden on everyone. Third, if at all possible, the parents should continue to be involved with the child, visiting him or her and taking the child home on weekends. Finally, the need for continued placement should be reviewed by all concerned at regular intervals and a less restrictive environment chosen should this become appropriate.

EDUCATION FOR CHILDREN WITH HANDICAPS

At present, the majority of children with handicaps who live at home are in special education programs within their communities. In deciding on the establishment of these special programs, society must choose among various priorities. In 1975, Public Law 94-142 (the Education for All Handicapped Children Act) mandated states to set up "free and appropriate education" for every child with handicaps between the ages of 3 and 21 residing in the state (Jacobs & Walker, 1978). Most professionals in the field lauded this act as long overdue. Yet, some argue that while it sounded praiseworthy and beneficial, such blanket coverage did not really make sense. These individuals maintained that the amount of money available for human resources is limited. Therefore, they asked, should a large portion of this money be spent to set up individualized education programs for children who are incapable of learning academic skills (Fuchs, 1974)? Perhaps, they suggested, the money might be better spent providing nutrition to a disadvantaged child of normal intelligence. Others noted that the cost of training individuals with handicaps to reach their potential is much less than the cost of institutionalizing them. They also argued that there are many nonacademic, vocational, and "survival" skills that are very important and can be learned by these individuals. These skills then make them more adaptive as adults.

It is difficult to make funding decisions. Yet, they are being made on the federal, state, and local levels. Who gets served is becoming a major question. No longer are community leaders speaking about attempting to meet all human needs. Priorities are being established. The question is who decides what the priorities are.

SUMMARY

All of us must struggle with the ethical issues raised in this chapter. It is very difficult to make decisions on issues such as genetic screening and treatment, prenatal diagnosis, abortion, withholding treatment, sterilization, human experimentation, institutionalization, and educational programs for children with handicaps. Yet, these issues must be discussed openly and frankly. Society must make choices on what should get funded and what should not. Without a public discussion, ethical decisions are made by a select few. With discussion, more of us may have a chance to influence this decision-making process. Only in this way will we all be better served.

REFERENCES

Allen, D.F., & Allen, V.S. (1979). *Ethical issues in mental retardation: Tragic choices—living hope.* Nashville, TN: Abingdon.

Anderson, W.F., & Fletcher, J.C. (1980). Gene therapy in human beings: When is it ethical to begin? *New England Journal of Medicine, 303,* 1293–1296.

Annas, G.J. (1979). Denying the rights of the retarded: The Phillip Becker case. *Hastings Center Report, 9,* 18–20.

Annas, G.J. (1981). Sterilization of the mentally retarded: A decision for the courts. *Hastings Center Report, 11,* 18–19.

Annas, G.J. (1984). Ethics committees in neonatal care: Substantive protection or procedural diversion? *American Journal of Public Health, 74,* 843–845.

Annas, G.J. (1985). Baby Fae: The "anything goes" school of human experimentation. *Hasting Center Report, 15,* 15–17.

Atkinson, G.M. (1983). Deciding for others. *Linacre Quarterly, 50,* 75–92.

Bainbridge, J.S., Jr. (1983, May 29). More and more, courts grant fetuses legal rights. *Baltimore Sun,* pp. K1, K3.

Baines, R.A. (1979). Unequal protection for retarded? *Amicus, 4,* 128–132.

Bayles, M.D. (1981). Voluntary and involuntary sterilization: The legal precedents. In R. Macklin & W. Gaylin (Eds.), *Mental retardation and sterilization: A problem of competency and paternalism.* New York: Plenum Publishing Corp.

Beauchamp, T.L., & Walters, L. (Eds.). (1982). *Contemporary issues in bioethics* (2nd ed.). Belmont, CA: Wadsworth Publishing Co.

Blank, R.H. (1984). Human sterilization: Emerging technologies and reemerging social issues. *Science, Technology & Human Values, 9,* 8–20.

Bridge, P., & Bridge, M. (1981). The brief life and death of Christopher Bridge. *Hastings Center Report, 11,* 17–19.

Capron, A.M. (1985). When well-meaning science goes too far. *Hastings Center Report, 15,* 8–9.

Chamberlain, A., Rauh, J., Passer, A., et al. (1984). Issues in fertility control for mentally retarded female adolescents: I. Sexual activity, sexual abuse, and contraception. *Pediatrics, 73,* 445–450.

Churchill, L.R., & Siman, J.J. (1982). Abortion and the rhetoric of individual rights. *Hastings Center Report, 12,* 9–12.

Cook, J.W., Altman, K., & Haavik, S. (1978). Consent for aversive treatment: A model form. *Mental Retardation, 16,* 47–49.

Culliton, B.J. (1976). Genetic screening: States may be writing the wrong kinds of laws. *Science, 191,* 926–929.

Culliton, B.J. (1983). 'Baby Doe' regs thrown out by court. *Science, 220,* 479–480.

Davenport, K. (1985). The right to die: Sources of information. *Legal Reference Services Quarterly, 5,* 47–81.

Del Campo, C. (1984). Abortion denied—outcome of mothers and babies. *Canadian Medical Association Journal, 130,* 361–362, 366.

Denniston, L. (1985, June 18). Court to take on 'Baby Doe' issue. *Baltimore Sun,* p. 2A.

Derouin, J. (1982). *In Re: Guardianship of Eberhardy:* The sterilization of the mentally retarded. *Wisconsin Law Review, 6,* 1199–1227.

Diamond, E.F. (1982). Treatment versus nontreatment for the handicapped newborn. In D.J. Horan & M. Delahoyde (Eds.), *Infanticide and the handicapped newborn.* Provo, UT: Brigham Young University Press.

Drinan, R.J. (1970). Abortion and the law. In K. Vaux (Ed.), *Who shall live? Medicine, technology, ethics.* Philadelphia: Fortress Press.

Duff, R.S. (1981). Counseling families and deciding care of severely defective children: A way of coping with "medical Vietnam". *Pediatrics, 67,* 315–320.

Duff, R.S., & Campbell, A.G.M. (1973). Moral and ethical dilemmas in the special care nursery. *New England Journal of Medicine, 289,* 890–894.

Dunea, G. (1983). Squeal rules in the nursery. *British Medical Journal, 287,* 1203–1204.

Ellis, T.S. III. (1982). Letting defective babies die: Who decides? *American Journal of Law and Medicine, 7,* 393–423.

Ethics, of selective treatment of spina bifida: Report of a working-party. (1975). *Lancet, 1,* 85–88.

Evans, K.A. (1980). Sterilization of the mentally retarded—a review. *Canadian Medical Association Journal, 123,* 1066–1070.

Fletcher, J. (1975). Abortion, euthanasia, and care of defective newborns. *New England Journal of Medicine, 292,* 75–78.

Fletcher, J.C. (1981). Ethical issues in genetic screening and antenatal diagnosis. *Clinical Obstetrics and Gynecology, 24,* 1151–1168.

Fletcher, J.C., & Shulman, J.D. (1985). Fetal research: The state of the question. *Hastings Center Report, 15,* 6–12.

Fost, N. (1981). Counseling families who have a child with a severe congenital anomaly. *Pediatrics, 67,* 321–324.

Fost, N. (1982). Putting hospitals on notice. *Hastings Center Report, 12,* 5–8.

Freeman, J.M. (1973). To treat or not to treat: Ethical dilemmas of treating the infant with my-elomeningocele. *Clinical Neurosurgery, 20,* 134–146.

Fuchs, V.R. (1974). *Who shall live? Health, economics, and social choice.* New York: Basic Books.

Gallo, A. (1984). Spina bifida: The state of the art of medical management. *Hastings Center Report, 14,* 10–13.

Gaylin, W. (1982). The competence of children: No longer all or none. *Hastings Center Report, 12,* 33–38.

Goldstein, J., Freud, A., & Solnit, A.J. (1979). *Before the best interests of the child.* New York: Free Press.

Goldstein, J., Freud, A., & Solnit, A.J. (1979). *Beyond the best interests of the child.* New York: Free Press.

Gore, A., Jr. (1985). The need for a new partnership. *Hastings Center Report, 15,* 13.

Haavik, S.F., & Menninger, K.A. II. (1981). *Sexuality, law, and the developmentally disabled person:*

Legal and clinical aspects of marriage, parenthood, and sterilization. Baltimore: Paul H. Brookes Publishing Co.

Harrison, M.R., Golbus, M.S., & Filly, R.A. (1981). Management of the fetus with a correctable congenital defect. *Journal of the American Medical Association, 246*, 774–777.

Hefferman, B.T. (1984). The American Academy of Pediatrics and the Baby Doe rules. *New England Journal of Medicine, 310*, 51.

Holden, C. (1984). Federal court strikes down Baby Doe rules. *Science, 224*, 1078–1079.

Holder, A.R. (1983). Parents, courts, and refusal of treatment. *Journal of Pediatrics, 103*, 515–521.

Horan, D.J. (1975). Euthanasia, medical treatment and the mongoloid child: Death as a treatment of choice? *Baylor Law Review, 27*, 76–108.

Horan, D.J., & Delahoyde, M. (Eds.). (1982). *Infanticide and the handicapped newborn*. Provo, UT: Brigham Young University Press.

Iglehart, J.K. (1983). Transplantation: The problem of limited resources. *New England Journal of Medicine, 309*, 123–128.

Jacobs, F.H., & Walker, D. (1978). Pediatricians and the Education for All Handicapped Children Act of 1975 (Public Law 94-142). *Pediatrics, 61*, 135–137.

Janofsky J., & Starfield, B. (1981). Assessment of risk in research on children. *Journal of Pediatrics, 98*, 842–846.

Johnson, P.R. (1980). Selective nontreatment of defective newborns: An ethical analysis. *Linacre Quarterly, 47*, 39–53.

Jonsen, A.R. (1978). Research involving children: Recommendations of the National Commission for the Protection of Human Subjects of Biomedical and Behavioral Research. *Pediatrics, 62*, 131–136.

Joseph and Rose Kennedy Institute of Ethics. (1985). *Baby Fae: Ethical issues surrounding cross-species organ transplantation*. Washington, DC: Georgetown University.

Kolata, G.B. (1980). Mass screening for neural tube defects. *Hastings Center Report, 10*, 8–10.

Krauthammer, C. (1985). What to do about 'Baby Doe.' *New Republic, 193*, 16, 18–21.

Lorber, J. (1974). Selective treatment of myelomeningocele: To treat or not to treat? *Pediatrics, 53*, 307–308.

Low, M.B. (1978). The Education for All Handicapped Children Act of 1975: A pediatrician's viewpoint. *Pediatrics, 62*, 271–274.

McCormick, R.A. (1977). To save or let die: The dilemma of modern medicine. In R.F. Weir (Ed.), *Ethical issues in death and dying*. New York: Columbia University Press.

McCormick, R.A. (1985). Was there any real hope for Baby Fae? *Hastings Center Report, 15*, 12–13.

Macklin, R., & Gaylin, W. (Eds.). (1981). *Mental retardation and sterilization: A problem of competency and paternalism*. New York: Plenum Publishing Corp.

Mercola, K.E., & Cline, M.J. (1980). The potentials of inserting new genetic information. *New England Journal of Medicine, 303*, 1297–1300.

Milunsky, A., & Annas, G.J. (Eds.). (1976). *Genetics and the law*. New York: Plenum Publishing Corp.

Motulsky, A.G. (1983). Impact of genetic manipulation on society and medicine. *Science, 219*, 135–140.

Murray, T.H. (1985). The final, anticlimactic rule on Baby Doe. *Hastings Center Report, 15*, 5–9.

Neville, R. (1981). Sterilizing the mildly mentally retarded without their consent: The philosophical arguments. In R. Macklin & W. Gaylin (Eds.), *Mental retardation and sterilization: A problem of competency and paternalism*. New York: Plenum Publishing Corp.

Passer, A., Rauh, J., Chamberlain, A., et al. (1984). Issues in fertility control for mentally retarded female adolescents: II. Parental attitudes toward sterilization. *Pediatrics, 73*, 451–454.

Penrose, L.S., & Smith, G.F. (1966). *Down's anomaly*. London: J. & A. Churchill.

Perrin, J.C., Sands, C.R., Tinker, D.E., et al. (1976). A considered approach to sterilization of mentally retarded youth. *American Journal of Diseases in Children, 130*, 288–290.

Plamondon, A. (1979). An introduction to ethics. *Amicus, 4*, 118–119.

Powledge, T.M., & Fletcher, J. (1979). Guidelines for the ethical, social, and legal issues in prenatal diagnosis: A report from the Genetics Research Group of the Hastings Center, Institute of Society, Ethics and the Life Sciences. *New England Journal of Medicine, 300*, 168–172.

Ramsey, P. (1978). *Ethics at the edges of life: Medical and legal intersections*. New Haven, CT: Yale University Press.

Reemtsma, K. (1985). Clinical urgency and media scrutiny. *Hastings Center Report, 15*, 10–11.

Regan, T. (1983). *The case for animal rights*. Berkeley, CA: University of California Press.

Regan, T. (1985). The other victim. *Hastings Center Report, 15*, 9–10.

Reilly, P. (1977). *Genetics, law, and social policy*. Cambridge, MA: Harvard University Press.

Riga, P.J. (1984). The care of defective neonates, ethics committees, and federal intervention. *Linacre Quarterly, 51,* 255–276.

Robertson, J.A., & Fost, N. (1976). Passive euthanasia of defective newborn infants: Legal considerations. *Journal of Pediatrics, 88,* 883–889.

Robillard, D. (1979). For whose benefit are mentally retarded people being sterilized? *Canadian Medical Association Journal, 120,* 1433–1438, 1446.

Robinson, J., Tennes, K., & Robinson, A. (1975). Amniocentesis: Its impact on mothers and infants. A 1-year follow-up study. *Clinical Genetics, 8,* 97–106.

Rosenberg, N.S. (1980). Sterilization of mentally retarded adolescents. *Clearinghouse Review, 14,* 428–430.

Ruddick, W., & Wilcox, W. (1982). Operating on the fetus. *Hastings Center Report, 12,* 10–14.

Schmeck, H.M., Jr. (1985, June 18). Life, death, and the rights of handicapped babies. *New York Times,* pp. C1, C3.

Shaw, A. (1973). Dilemmas of "informed consent" in children. *New England Journal of Medicine, 289,* 885–890.

Shaw, A., Randolph, J.G., & Manard, B. (1977). Ethical issues in pediatric surgery: A nationwide survey of pediatricians and pediatric surgeons. *Pediatrics, 60,* 588–599.

Sheldon, R. (1985). The IRB's responsibility to itself. *Hastings Center Report, 15,* 11–12.

Sherlock, R. (1980). Selective non-treatment of defective newborns: A critique. *Ethics in Science & Medicine, 7,* 111–117.

Silverman, W.A. (1981). Mismatched attitudes about neonatal death. *Hastings Center Report, 11,* 12–16.

Sitomer, C.J. (1985, June 18). High court moves into uncharted church-state territory. *Christian Science Monitor,* p. 1.

Soskind, R.M., & Vitello, S.J. (1979). A right to treatment or a right to die? *Amicus, 4,* 120–127.

Steinbock, B. (1984). Baby Jane Doe in the courts. *Hastings Center Report, 14,* 13–19.

Sterilizing the mentally handicapped: Who can give consent? (1980). *Canadian Medical Association Journal, 122,* 234–240.

Strong, C. (1984). The neonatologist's duty to patient and parents. *Hastings Center Report, 14,* 10–16.

Sumner, L.W. (1981). *Abortion and moral theory.* Princeton, NJ: Princeton University Press.

U.S. Department of Health and Human Services, Office of Human Development Services. (1985). Child abuse and neglect prevention and treatment program: Final rule. *Federal Register, 50,* 14878–14901.

U.S. District Court, District of Columbia. (1983). American Academy of Pediatrics vs. Heckler. *Federal Supplement, 561,* 395–404.

Veatch, R.M. (1977). *Case studies in medical ethics.* Cambridge, MA: Harvard University Press.

Vining, E.P.G., & Freeman, J.M. (1978). Sterilization and the retarded female: Is advocacy depriving individuals of their rights? *Pediatrics, 62,* 850–852.

Weber, L.F. (1976). *Who shall live? The dilemma of severely handicapped children and its meaning for other moral questions.* New York: Paulist Press.

Wolfensberger, W. (1967). Counseling parents of the retarded. In A.A. Baumeister (Ed.), *Mental retardation: Appraisal, education, and retardation.* Chicago: Aldine Publishing Co.

Wright, E.E., & Shaw, M.W. (1981). Legal liability in genetic screening, genetic counseling, and prenatal diagnosis. *Clinical Obstetrics and Gynecology, 24,* 1133–1149.

Chapter 25

Public Benefits, Legal Services, and Estate Planning

John J. Capowski

Upon completion of this chapter, the reader will:
—Know many of the basic federally funded programs that provide assistance for children with handicaps and their families
—Be aware of the need for legal services and how to obtain them
—Understand the importance of and know a few basic points about estate planning for parents of children with handicaps

In addition to physical and emotional burdens, the presence in a family of a child with severe handicaps can create new financial problems and planning issues. For many families, knowing and availing themselves of federally funded public benefits is the only way for them to properly care for their child with handicaps and to maintain a reasonable standard of living for the rest of the family. The parents of a child with handicaps may also face difficult issues in establishing a plan for the care of the child following their death and in planning their will in such a way as to maximize the benefits of their estate for this child. This chapter focuses on the programs available for these families as well as the legal and financial issues involved in caring and planning for a child with handicaps. It also discusses both the need for and ways to obtain the legal expertise needed to resolve these issues.

PUBLIC BENEFITS

This section discusses some of the major programs available to families with children who have handicaps. Although this section is not all-inclusive, it does cover Special Education, Vocational Education, Vocational Rehabilitation, Social Security benefits, Supplemental Security Income (SSI), Medicaid, Medicare, and Crippled Children's Services.

John Capowski, J.D., is an Associate Professor at the University of Maryland School of Law.

Special Education

The Education for All Handicapped Children Act of 1975, P.L. 94-142 (20 U.S.C.A. §1401 et seq. (1985)), provides a process for assuring a free, appropriate public education for all children who require special education and related services to meet their unique needs. This education must not only be appropriate for the child but must take place in the least restrictive environment. For example, if the child could function within both a special education classroom and a regular classroom, the child should be placed in a regular class. Important things to remember about this program are: It is overseen by the U.S. Department of Education, administered by local school systems, and is free to all children, regardless of income or resources (20 U.S.C.A. §1412 (1978)). Although the program is generally available to children between the ages of 3 and 21 years of age (34 C.F.R. 300.122 (1985)), some states provide a special education for children under the age of 3 years.

Besides entitling students to an appropriate school placement, this program also offers a wide variety of related services, including physical therapy, occupational therapy, speech and language therapy, psychological counseling, and certain nursing services. These services and others that may be necessary to aid the child's educational progress become part of his or her individualized education program (IEP) (34 C.F.R. §300.340 (1985)).

To develop and implement an IEP, a number of steps are followed (34 C.F.R. §300.343 et seq. (1985)). Initially, a parent, teacher, or any other interested person can refer a child to a school or a school district for a special education plan to be developed for the child. Within 30 days of the application, the school district must obtain an evaluation of the child by appropriate professionals including psychologists, educators, physicians, and occupational or physical therapists. Parents must consent to the evaluation being done and should be involved in the evaluation process. They have the right to obtain their own evaluations from psychologists, speech therapists, and other professionals. A team meeting, including the parents, of those persons involved in the evaluation is held, at which time the school district decides if the child is handicapped and, if he or she is, develops an IEP based on the information presented during this meeting. If the parents agree with the plan, it is implemented. If the parents disagree, they have a right to appeal the school district's proposed plan and have a hearing. As at the team meeting, the parents can be represented at the hearing by an attorney or other advocate of their choice. Also, they have the right to present evidence and witnesses and to examine documents used in developing the plan as well as any witnesses called by the school district. The parents can accept or reject the decision made by the hearing officer after this proceeding. If they reject the decision, they can appeal the determination to the state education agency and the courts. Hearings on the implementation of individualized education programs are common, and parents should be diligent in ensuring that their children receive an appropriate public education in the least restrictive environment.

Vocational Education and Training

Like the Special Education Program, Vocational Education (20 U.S.C.A. §2301 et seq. (1976)) helps individuals with handicaps reach their potential. This program, which is federally funded and administered by the states, provides vocational and educational training to individuals with handicaps, regardless of their income. Although teenagers are most likely to use this program, individuals of any age are eligible.

Under this program, states can use federal funds for such things as vocational education programs and placement services for students who have completed such programs. States are also allowed to use the funds for work study programs and can pay private institutions to provide vocational training (34 C.F.R. §400.502 (1985)). Because of the variety of programs and the ways in which they are administered, one should contact local educational agencies to find out about application and appeals procedures.

Vocational Rehabilitation

The Rehabilitation Act of 1973, P.L. 93-112, established a federally funded program that is administered by the states and seeks to help persons with disabilities gain employment skills (29 U.S.C.A. §701 et seq. (1985)). With federal funds, the states provide a wide range of vocational rehabilitation services either directly or through nonprofit organizations. To be eligible for the program, individuals must have a reasonable chance of employment after rehabilitation, despite having a physical or mental disability (34 C.F.R. §361.1 (1985)). In addition, only individuals with limited income and resources are eligible for the program, and these financial eligibility requirements vary from state to state. However, Supplemental Security Income recipients (see section on "Supplemental Security Income") are automatically financially eligible but need to meet some additional requirements. Their disability must be so severe that they could be expected to qualify for SSI for most of the rest of their lives, but the disability must not be so progressive that they would be incapacitated before the vocational rehabilitation is completed (34 C.F.R. §361.124 (1985)). As mentioned earlier, great variety exists in the vocational rehabilitation assistance available under this program. Besides vocational training, diagnosis and evaluation of the individual's rehabilitation potential is provided by the program as well as counseling, guidance, and referral and placement services. The program also provides treatment such as corrective surgery, prosthetic devices, and psychological counseling. Transportation to and from rehabilitation services and technological aids such as teletype machines for deaf persons are also available. For deaf and/or blind individuals, the vocational rehabilitation program may provide support services such as interpreters, readers, and orientation and mobility services. The program can also assist with the general cost of living during the period of rehabilitation, regardless of the specific handicapping condition (29 U.S.C.A. §723 (1985)).

Social Security Benefits

One thinks of Social Security benefits as being given to individuals who have worked for many years and have since become disabled or retired, but children may also be eligible for benefits, and special treatment is given to children with handicaps and their parents. Eligibility for a worker or a family member can occur when a person who has worked for a number of years and contributed to the Social Security fund

384 / CHILDREN WITH HANDICAPS

dies, retires, or becomes disabled. The number of years one needs to have worked to become eligible or to make one's family eligible for benefits under the disability program varies with the individual's age. However, retirement benefits can begin at age 62; higher benefits are received when one waits until age 65 to retire. To be eligible because of disability, claimants must be unable to perform their past work as well as all other jobs that they could perform given their age, education, and work experience. The standard for judging disability is a strict one.

As mentioned, when a wage earner becomes eligible for benefits or dies, members of his or her family may also be eligible. Children under 18 years of age and those who are over 18 but under 19 and are full-time students can receive benefits (20 C.F.R. §404.352 (1985)). Also, and this provision is especially important for the handicapped offspring of wage earners, children who are over 18 years of age and who become disabled before the age of 22 are eligible for benefits (20 C.F.R. §404.350 (1985)). The test for disability for the children of wage earners is the same as that for the wage earner. As with adults, the child's impairment(s) must have existed or be expected to exist for a continuous period of 12 months and must make the individual unable to "engage in substantial gainful activity" (20 C.F.R. §404.1505 (1985)). To meet this standard, the individual can show that his or her impairment meets or equals a list of impairments found in Volume 20 of the Code of Federal Regulations (20 C.F.R. Pt. 404, Subpt. P, App.1 (1985)) or that the individual's age, education, and work experience would result in a finding of disability. In the case of an individual who has not worked, skills developed in school and through hobbies are considered.

The presence of a child in the family who is eligible for benefits can also make the spouse of a deceased wage earner entitled to what are called mother's and father's benefits. When the surviving spouse or surviving divorced spouse is caring for an insured child who is under age 16 or who is disabled, the spouse may be entitled to mother's or father's benefits (20 C.F.R. §404.339 and §404.340 (1985)). A few other eligibility requirements apply. For example, the widow or widower must not remarry, and the marriage must have lasted a certain length of time, depending on the nature of the spouse's death. Even so, this public benefit can be a significant resource for widows and widowers caring for young or disabled children.

The first step one needs to take to obtain Social Security benefits is to apply at a Social Security District Office. Besides having Social Security numbers and such documents as marriage and birth records, when a claim of disability is involved, the claimant should also bring to the application interview the names and addresses of hospitals and doctors who are treating the child with disabilities. Some claimants may find it helpful to have their doctors review the listing of disabling impairments found in Volume 20 of the Code of Federal Rules to see if the individual's impairment meets the requirements of the listing. If it does, a letter setting out the specifics of the condition and the way in which it meets the code's listing of impairments should be of great help.

Disability claims are frequently denied at this initial stage, and claimants should seriously consider appealing the case to the stages beyond the application. After an initial determination denying the claim, one can ask for an appeal, called a recon-sideration. After the reconsideration stage, one has the right to a hearing before an administrative law judge. This hearing is the first time the claimant actually appears before the individual making the decision, and approximately 50% of denied claims are granted by these judges (Mashaw, Goetz, Goodman, et al., 1978). If the decision of the administrative law judge is unfavorable, claimants can ask the Appeals Council of the Social Security Administration to review the hearing officer's decision and, if the claim is again denied, they can appeal to a federal court. A lawyer can be of assistance at any stage in the process; such assistance is especially helpful at the hearing and Appeals Council stages and almost mandatory for the federal court appeal.

Supplemental Security Income

The Supplemental Security Income, or SSI program, has many characteristics in common with the Social Security system. It is a federal program that is partly state administered, and it provides monthly cash assistance to eligible individuals. Like the Social Security program, it assists those who are over 65, blind, or disabled (20 C.F.R. §416.202 (1985)). However, unlike the Social Security program, only persons with limited income and resources are eligible for SSI. In addition, SSI does not require that claimants or their relatives have contributed to a fund like Social Security's.

To be found disabled, children under the age of 18 must meet a number of eligibility requirements (20 C.F.R. §416.924 (1985)). The child must have a medically determinable physical or mental impairment or impairments that compare in severity to those that would make an adult disabled. To meet this test, the impairment(s) must have lasted or be expected to last 12 months and either be included in the listing of impairments found in the Code of Federal Regulations or be medically equal to a listed impairment. The listing of impairments (20 C.F.R. Pt. 404, Subpt. P, App. 1 (1985)) includes a wide range of handicapping conditions such as epilepsy, asthma, cerebral palsy, mental retardation, and autism. When a child is found eligible for SSI, the amount of the benefit is determined by the income, resources, and SSI eligibility of the persons with whom the child is living. In the case of a child living in a household with parents who are ineligible for SSI, a portion of the parent's income is considered or "deemed" available for the use of the child. In deciding how much income of an ineligible parent is deemed available, the needs of ineligible children are also considered (20 C.F.R. §416.1160 (1985)). Parents' income and resources, unless actually available to the disabled individual, are not an eligibility factor after he or she reaches age 21 (20 C.F.R. §416.1165 (1985)). A number of steps are followed to determine the level of financial assistance for eligible children. Consulting either the regulations or an advocate should be of help to parents in determining whether or not the SSI award is correct.

Both the application and appeals process for Supplemental Security Income are nearly identical to those for Social Security. In addition, some individuals may be provisionally certified as eligible for benefits and receive payments pending a final determination. As with Social Security, there are many initial denials of claims, and individuals should not be discouraged from appealing early denials of eligibility.

Medicaid

The Medicaid program (42 U.S.C.A. §1396 et seq. (1983)) is a federally established and partially federally funded program that pays the cost of medical assistance for persons receiving federal cash assistance such as SSI, and for others of low income who cannot meet the costs of medical expenses. Eligible individuals receive a Medicaid card that can be used much like a credit card to obtain a wide range of medical services. The card is presented to health care providers who seek reimbursement from the state, which both administers and supplements the cost of the program.

Changes made in the program during the early years of the Reagan administration give the states wide latitude in both determining eligibility and in deciding what medical services should be provided. Because of this, benefits vary greatly from state to state. The discussion here simply provides general information on the types of persons who may be eligible for Medicaid and the types of services available through the program.

There are two major classifications of persons who are eligible for Medicaid benefits: the "categorically" eligible and those termed the "medically needy." The categorically eligible are those individuals who meet or are very close to meeting the federal requirements for cash benefits under the Supplemental Security Income program or the Aid to Families with Dependent Children (AFDC) program, the latter being the federal program most persons think of as welfare. The medically needy are those individuals who are ineligible for a federal cash program but who have high medical expenses.

Although all those who receive AFDC must be covered under state Medicaid programs, the states can choose one of two options for covering persons eligible for SSI. Under one option, states may provide Medicaid to SSI recipients. In addition, states may also provide Medicaid to persons who receive only an optional cash supplement and not the basic SSI grant. Under a second option, states may limit Medicaid eligibility to the aged, blind, or disabled who meet eligibility requirements more restrictive than those under the SSI program. However, states that elect this option must deduct medical expenses, SSI, and optional state supplements from the individual's income in determining eligibility for Medicaid. For this reason, there is no fixed ceiling on income under the second option (42 C.F.R. §435.1(d)(3)(1984)).

Besides the states having options in dealing with persons who are eligible for SSI, states have an extraordinary flexibility in deciding who will receive benefits among the medically needy—those who are not eligible for federal cash programs such as SSI or AFDC but who have high medical expenses (42 C.F.R. §435.300 et seq. (1984)). The states may provide Medicaid only to certain groups such as the aged, blind, disabled, and families with dependent children who do not receive federal cash assistance and whose income and resources are insufficient to pay the cost of health care. However, if a state decides to assist any group of medically needy persons, it must provide medical assistance to young persons and pregnant women who would be included among those considered categorically needy except that they have more income and resources. So, any state that provides assistance for those considered medically needy must offer it to medically needy disabled children, regardless of their eligibility for SSI.

Services as well as eligibility requirements vary according to whether one is categorically needy or medically needy. For those who are categorically needy, the benefits include physician's services, inpatient hospital services, outpatient hospital services, laboratory and X ray services, home health services, and skilled nursing facility services for individuals 21 years of age and older. Although states must supply these services, they also can elect to supply a wide range of additional medical care. This care may include clinic services, dental services, prescribed drugs, dentures, prosthetic devices, and eyeglasses. Of special importance to children with handicaps are physical and occupational therapy; services for individuals with speech, hearing, or language disorders; inpatient psychiatric services; and diagnostic, screening, preventive, and rehabilitative services (42 C.F.R. §440.10 et seq. (1984)).

States have even greater discretion in deciding what services, if any, they supply to the medically needy. If the state plan covers the medically needy, it must provide, at a minimum, ambulatory services for individuals under age 18 and individuals entitled to institutional services, obstetric care for pregnant women, and home health services to any individual entitled to skilled nursing facility care.

To receive Medicaid, one needs to apply at the state agency that administers the program. In most states, this is the department of social services or state health agency. Persons applying for SSI at Social Security offices should inquire about their state's procedures and eligibility standards for Medicaid. Because of the complexity of the Medicaid program, disputes over eligibility as well as the adequacy of payment often occur. To challenge the state agency's decision, individuals are entitled to a hearing and may be able to have adverse hearing determinations reviewed in court (42 C.F.R. §431.220 et seq. (1984)). Again, because of the complexity of the program, the assistance of a trained advocate or lawyer familiar with the Medicaid program is often very helpful.

Medicare

Although one usually thinks of Medicare (42 U.S.C.A. §1395 et seq. (1983)) as a program that helps pay the hospital and other medical expenses of the elderly, this federally funded and state administered program also assists with the health care costs of disabled children and others under the age of 65. For persons under 65 years of age to be eligible for Medicare, they need to be entitled or "deemed entitled" for 25 consecutive months to Social Security disability benefits as an insured individual, child, widow, or widower who is "under a disability" (see discussion of Social Security benefits). "Deeming" is complicated and the regulations should be checked on this (42 C.F.R. §408.12(c) (1984)). Other individuals under the age of 65 also qualify for benefits if they qualify as beneficiaries with disabilities under the Railroad Retirement Act (42 C.F.R.(a)(2) §408.12 (1984)).

Medicare insurance is composed of two major types: hospital insurance, which is often called Part A, and medical insurance, which is referred to as Part B. Although there is no cost for most persons covered by Medicare hospital insurance, medical insurance, or Part B, is a supplementary program, and all individuals must pay a premium to be covered and receive its benefits.

Hospital insurance, Part A, helps pay for medically necessary inpatient hospital care. In addition, the program subsidizes the cost of inpatient care in a skilled nursing facility and home care by a home health agency when either of these two types of services is needed following hospitalization. Although Medicare hospital insurance helps pay for these expenses, the number of days covered or, in the case of home health care, the number of visits, is limited for each hospital admission the individual has. After the limit has been reached, an individual can again become entitled for hospital insurance by remaining out of the hospital or skilled nursing facility for a specific amount of time, currently approximately 2 months.

Medical insurance, Part B, covers a wide range of health services, and although the insurance covers the full cost of many services and medical devices, individuals often need to pay a percentage of the costs. To cover the cost of this remainder as well as the deductible in the Medicare program, other insurance from a private insurance company is often available. The services covered include physicians' services, medical supplies furnished in a doctor's office, outpatient hospital services and supplies, diagnostic X-ray and laboratory tests, and rental and purchase of medical equipment including wheelchairs, prosthetic devices, and artificial limbs. Medical insurance also helps pay for the costs of outpatient physical therapy and speech pathology services.

To receive Medicare benefits, individuals may apply to their local Social Security District Office. Some individuals are automatically eligible for benefits and should receive information about the program in the mail shortly before they become eligible for coverage. Persons of low income can receive both Medicaid and Medicare. Medicaid will pay the costs of covered medical care not paid for by the Medicare program. A full review process, comparable to that available to individuals denied Social Security benefits, is available to persons who are found ineligible for either Part A or Part B of Medicare (42 C.F.R. §405.701 (1984)). This review process is also available for individuals who are dissatisfied with a hospital insurance, or Part A, determination where the amount of the claim equals $100 or more. Claims that involve $1,000 or more are entitled to court review (42 C.F.R. §405.730 (1984)).

In a dispute over medical insurance coverage, individuals have a right to have the Medicare carrier, which is a private insurance company, review the initial determination (42 C.F.R. §405.807 (1984)). Following that review, individuals have a right to a hearing where the amount in controversy is $100 or more. The hearing takes place before a hearing officer designated by the carrier; no judicial review is available to challenge the amount of a Part B claim.

Crippled Children's Services

The Crippled Children's Services (CCS) program was initiated as part of the Social Security Act of 1935 to locate children who have severe handicaps or who have conditions that lead to "crippling" and to provide them with diagnostic, medical, and corrective services as well as hospitalization and aftercare (Davis & Schoen, 1978). The program has established Crippled Children's agencies in states and many U.S. territories. These state administered programs receive funding under the Maternal and Child Health services block grant but also receive significant funds from state and local governments, as well as various foundations.

Because the CCS programs are state administered, receive funding from many sources, and are given great freedom because of block grant funding, there is tremendous variation among state programs as to the medical problems covered, financial eligibility requirements, and services provided (Ireys, Hauck, & Perrin, 1985). Despite these differences, programs generally attempt to alleviate undue hardship on families with children with special needs. In addition, the states share the view that the CCS program should be the payor of last resort. That is, other available public and private benefits or entitlements must be used before the CCS program pays the cost of care.

As mentioned, there is wide variation in the services provided by the states. Some states provide only diagnostic and minimal treatment services, while others provide a full range of medical services, support services, supplies, and other assistance necessary for proper treatment and care. Examples of assistance provided under the programs include physician's services, hospital care, dental care, medication, medical supplies and equipment, speech pathology, occupational and physical therapy, transportation, meals, and lodging.

Even in states that provide a wide range of services, whether or not this full range is available to individual children may depend on the condition the child has as well as its severity. Most programs provide services for financially eligible children who have major chronic illnesses or mental disabilities. Conditions such as cerebral palsy, cystic fibrosis, sickle cell anemia, hemophilia, diabetes mellitus, and disabilities requiring orthopedic treatment or surgical intervention are examples of the disorders that are often covered. Acute illness, prematurity, and emotional and psychological conditions are generally excluded from coverage. Age is also a factor, and most CCS programs limit their coverage to persons under a specific age, for example 18 or 21 years, but particular illnesses may be covered regardless of the individual's age.

Crippled Children's Services focus their services on the medically needy, and most states have specific financial eligibility guidelines. Although some of these eligibility limits are generous in comparison to those established for other public benefit programs—for example, California will provide services to four-member families with an adjusted gross income of $40,000 (West's California Health and Safety Code, §255 (1985))—three-fourths of the children served are from families at or below 150% of the poverty level.

Many different systems are used by the states for determining financial eligibility, and a variety of factors are included in them. For example, some states provide a wider range of services for individuals at lower income levels. Others have established sliding fee scales that allow families with higher incomes to receive services while paying a reduced fee for them. Some programs have higher income eligibility cutoffs for highly complex conditions and multiple impairments (Force, 1985).

To receive assistance from CCS, one usually needs to apply to the local office of the state health agency, since the great majority of CCS programs are housed within these agencies. A small number are under social service departments and education agencies, and one CCS program is under the auspices of a state university. Application and appeals procedures are similar to those that apply for other state benefit programs. After an initial denial, one can usually obtain a review or reconsideration of that decision and, if still dissatisfied, request a hearing. One can generally appeal an adverse hearing decision to the state court.

ADVOCACY AND LEGAL ASSISTANCE

Problems of public benefit eligibility and quality of care affect many children with handicaps and their families. Although these issues can often be resolved informally, there are many situations in which the assistance of a lawyer or legal advocate is of great benefit.

To assist with the legal issues facing children with handicaps, a number of resources exist, many of which are available at little or no cost to eligible individuals. Most lawyers regularly representing individuals in public benefit claims work for local offices of the Legal Services Corporation. The corporation, with federal funding, oversees the operation of legal aid and legal services offices throughout the United States. These offices are located in every major city, and many also exist to service rural areas. Because these offices specialize in representing persons who cannot afford legal counsel, attorneys working in them are usually very knowledgeable about public benefits eligibility and the procedures for obtaining these benefits. Unfortunately, the services of these programs are available only to persons of limited income and resources. As a general rule, individuals are eligible for assistance from these programs if their incomes do not exceed 125% of the federal poverty income guidelines. However, other factors such as medical expenses, existing debts, employment expenses, and the expenses associated with the physical infirmity of family members are normally considered.

In addition to legal services programs, there is a federally funded protection and advocacy agency in each state (see Appendix C). The purpose of these agencies is to provide information and assistance to persons with developmental disabilities, and the types of cases and assistance available varies from agency to agency. Many agencies have no financial eligibility requirements and serve persons with developmental disabilities with a broad range of information and legal help.

Individual advocacy or legal assistance may also be obtained from local chapters of organizations that deal with specific handicapping conditions. For example, local chapters of groups such as the Association for Retarded Citizens of the United States, United Cerebral Palsy, and the Epilepsy Foundation of America are all places to turn for information about benefits available to persons with these specific disabilities. If no trained advocates or lawyers are on the staff, information on what legal resources are available in the community is usually provided. The national offices of these and other similar groups provide legislative assistance and may be helpful places to turn for general information and assistance (see Appendix C).

Another resource is a local law school, which is likely to have a clinical program in which law students, under the supervision of attorneys, represent individuals in a wide variety of civil and criminal problems. Many of these programs handle public benefit cases, and some specialize in particular areas such as Social Security disability, special education, and rights of persons who are institutionalized. Eligibility criteria as well as the cases handled vary dramatically from program to program, but law school clinical programs are certainly another resource to which individuals with handicaps and their families can turn for effective legal assistance.

In many areas, private attorneys have formed groups of lawyers who provide free legal assistance to persons who cannot afford counsel. These groups of attorneys may be connected with legal services programs, may have formed groups of their own as volunteer lawyer services, or may operate under the auspices of a city, county, or state bar association.

In addition to obtaining legal services through any one of these groups, individuals can always seek out the assistance of a private attorney to handle a case. In most instances, the private attorney will charge a fee for his or her services but, in some cases, the fee is a percentage of the client's recovery or may be obtained from the government agency one is suing. For example, in Social Security claims, attorneys can request that a portion of the client's retroactive or back benefits be paid to the attorney as a fee if the case is won. Acts such as the Equal Access to Justice Act (5 U.S.C.A. §594 (1983)) and the Rehabilitation Act of 1973 allow attorneys to recover their fees against the government (29 U.S.C.A. §794a (1985)).

An attorney who is experienced in a particular field can often provide both more efficient and more effective legal services. For this reason, specialized agencies are often good places to turn for assistance with public benefit and disability issues. Private attorneys who have worked for legal services programs are often more experienced in these areas than other practitioners. However, many practitioners specialize in public benefit areas such as Social Security and can effectively represent any individual's case.

Deciding whether or not to obtain counsel and at what stage may be difficult. The assistance of an advocate early on in the applications process can often smooth the process and make sure that helpful and complete information is given to an agency from the start. However, many claims are granted without an attorney's intervention and, at early stages in the process, the time and expense needed to obtain counsel may not be justified. Yet, it is clear that the assistance of an attorney is extraordinarily helpful at all hearings and is virtually a necessity for any court proceeding. Although administrative hearings are informal in comparison to court proceedings, persons not familiar with them will benefit greatly from the presence of either a trained advocate or an attorney.

While the parents of children with handicaps are sometimes faced with problems where the assistance of counsel is necessary, they undoubtedly confront many situations where they need to serve as advocates for themselves and their children. Disputes over such issues as the quality of care in an institution or a particular portion of an individualized education plan may not be significant enough for one to obtain a lawyer but may require the efforts of parents as advocates for their children.

To be effective advocates, individuals should first clearly establish what the need or problem is that they wish to address and what facts have given rise to it. In addition, they should collect information on what assistance they would like to obtain and what agency might provide this help. Before approaching the agency, individuals should obtain as much information as they can about the type of assistance they seek and develop a list of questions that can be used in this process. Different approaches work for different persons, and it is difficult to describe a particular procedure that all advocates should follow. However, it is important to keep notes about one's contacts with the agency and, when an agreement is reached, it is helpful to embody that agreement in a letter to the agency. As a final step in the advocacy process, it is important to keep in touch with the agency to make sure that the terms of the agreement one has reached have been followed. Parents' groups can be extremely helpful to individuals working as their children's advocates. For example, a group of parents whose children have similar handicaps or whose children are at a particular residential facility usually has some members whose experience at advocacy is helpful to others in the group. In addition, a parents' group is able to monitor a particular program or institution in a way that individual parents simply cannot. Besides the advocacy, monitoring, and emotional support such parents' groups can provide, many groups have become active in lobbying, testifying at public hearings, and in pursuing litigation around major developmental disability law issues.

ESTATE PLANNING

The purposes of this section are to alert the parents of children with handicaps to the importance of estate planning and to raise some of the issues that should be discussed with an attorney during the planning and preparation of a will and any other estate plan. Although some persons with limited assets and diligent research may be able to prepare a will for themselves, estate planning is a complex area. In addition to the law varying from state to state as to such things as the formalities needed to create a valid will and the ways in which property is distributed to relatives when an individual dies without a will, the area is made far more complex by the tax issues, at least for larger estates, that permeate estate planning. The presence in the family of a child with handicaps adds an additional level of complexity. Although the parents of children with handicaps can in many cases represent those children's interest in public benefit claims, the area of estate planning is not a place for the do-it-yourselfer.

One goal for parents in estate planning is to make sure that an individual, couple, or group will make decisions for a minor or a person with handicaps that would be in the best interest of this person and similar to the decisions that would have been made by the parents. One vehicle for achieving this goal is a guardianship of the person. For an individual with handicaps, the guardian of the person would see that appropriate services are provided to that individual, would coordinate these services, and would make certain that all necessary and available assistance is provided. The guardian might also make decisions about whether or not the individual is to live with another family, reside in a public or private institution, or live in some other residential placement. In some states, parents with children with handicaps have formed groups for the express purpose of employing social workers and other trained professionals to serve as guardians for handicapped individuals. One such group is the Maryland Trust for Retarded Citizens. Parents who reside in an area where no such group exists or where the groups do not cover the child's handicap might consider joining with others to set up this type of program.

In addition to appointing a guardian of the person to oversee the care of the person with handicaps, parents may decide to establish a guardianship of the property of the child. The same individual might serve as both the guardian of the child and his or her property, but it is often advantageous to have separate persons or institutions serve these functions; one may have more knowledge about the individual needs of the particular person while the other might be highly sophisticated in financial matters. However, the amount of funds available may not justify the expense of having two guardians. Guardianships can be requested from a court during the lives of the parents, or provisions can be set out in a will requesting that guardianships be established and that certain persons be named guardians. An advantage to a guardianship is that decisions made by the guardian are subject to supervision by the court.

Although a guardianship of the property is an appropriate method for administering the funds available to an individual with handicaps, another vehicle, the trust, has significant advantages over the guardianship. Simply put, a trust is a relationship in which one person holds the title to real or personal property and has an obligation to keep or use that property for the benefit of another. Like a guardianship of the property, one of the major purposes of a trust is to provide for the financial needs of the person who has a handicap, the beneficiary. However, the trust may also serve to insulate assets from being taken by the state to pay for the cost of care in a public institution. In addition, a trust may keep assets and income from being considered when the state or federal government determines a beneficiary's eligibility for public benefits. In many cases, assets left directly to a child with handicaps and the income from them can make the child ineligible for public benefits.

When the cost of administering a trust would be great in relationship to the assets in it, parents may decide to establish an "informal trust." For example, parents can arrange to have assets in their will pass to a sibling of the individual with handicaps and have an understanding with that sibling that the funds are to be used for the person with handicaps. Although this arrangement can insulate the funds from state attachment and public benefit eligibility determinations, the funds can be diverted from their intended purpose by the death, divorce, or bankruptcy of the sibling. Because of the risks involved in an "informal trust," the use of a formal trust document should be thoroughly considered. A trust may be established either while the parents are alive, termed inter-vivos trusts, or by a will, called testamentary trusts. Although most trusts established for persons with handicaps are testamentary trusts, parents with significant assets may wish to discuss with their attorneys the possibility of establishing an inter-vivos trust. Inter-vivos trusts can be either revocable or irrevocable, and the benefits of each might also be reviewed.

The considerations in choosing a trustee are similar to those that are important in selecting a guardian of property. An individual trustee may have more time to devote to administering the trust than would a corporate trustee. In addition, an individual trustee, because of a more personal relationship with the person with handicaps and his or her family, may be willing to serve with no compensation. This might be a determinative factor where the value of the trust is small.

On the other hand, a corporate trustee, such as a bank or trust company, is likely to be more knowledgeable about administering trusts, more sophisticated on investment information and, by pooling the resources of many trusts, able to minimize risks by diversifying investments. However, corporate trustees are reluctant to oversee smaller trusts, and their minimum annual fees could significantly deplete the income of such trusts.

To insulate the trust from cost of care claims and to ensure that the person with handicaps will not be made ineligible for various public benefits because of the bequests, the attorney needs to be up-to-date on the state law dealing with the invasion of trusts as well as knowledgeable about the income and resource eligibility requirements of the various public benefits from which the person with handicaps might benefit. Based on this information, the attorney, in drafting the trust instrument, must be careful to use language that will have the greatest chance of maintaining public benefit eligibility and insulating the trust assets. In most cases, phrasing that allows the trustee discretion in distributing and using the income of the trust, rather than language that directs the income to be distributed to the beneficiary is more likely to achieve this goal. In addition, the trust language might specifically state that the parent desires that the income of the trust not be used to diminish public benefits eligibility.

While the attorney needs to use care in choosing the language for setting up the trust, he or she should also consider with the parents the circumstances under which the trust might be terminated and draft language to achieve this purpose. Reasons for termination of the trust might include changes in public benefits law, the needs of the siblings of the person with handicaps, improvement in the condition of the person with handicaps, and depletion of the assets of the trust.

In obtaining representation, the parents of a child with handicaps need to make attorneys aware of any special needs their family has. In representing children with handicaps, the lawyer needs to be a counselor as well as an attorney-at-law.

SUMMARY

To help with the cost of caring for a child with handicaps, parents should be aware of state and federal public benefits programs. These programs can provide financial support, medical assistance, education, and training for the child with handicaps. Although parents are often able to obtain these benefits without the assistance of a trained advocate, the aid of an attorney or paralegal may be necessary. The area of estate planning is a complex one and is made more so by the need to provide for a child with handicaps. This is an area where the parents of children with handicaps should seek the help of trained counsel.

REFERENCES

Anderson, W., Chitwood, S., & Hayden, D. (1982). *Negotiating the special education maze: A guide for parents and teachers*. Englewood Cliffs, NJ: Prentice-Hall.

Apolloni, T. (1985). Effective advocacy: How to be a winner. *Exceptional Parent, 15*, 14–19.

Apolloni, T., & Cooke, T.P. (Eds.). (1984). *A new look at guardianship: Protective services that support personalized living*. Baltimore: Paul H. Brookes Publishing Co.

ASTHO Foundation. (1984). Selected services of state crippled children's agencies. Services for mothers and children. In *Public health agencies, 1982* (Vol. 3). Kensington, MD: ASTHO Foundation.

Ballard, J. (1982). *Special education in America: Its legal and governmental foundations*. Reston, VA: Council for Exceptional Children.

Bersani, H. (1985). Advocacy: The role of parents' groups. *Exceptional Parent, 15*, 28–30.

Buchanan, R.J., & Minor, J.D. (1985). *Legal aspects of health care reimbursement*. Rockville, MD: Aspen Systems Corp.

Capowski, J.J. (1983). Accuracy and consistency in categorical decisionmaking: A study of Social Security's medical-vocational guidelines—two birds with one stone or pigeon holing claimants? *Maryland Law Review, 42*, 329–386.

Commerce Clearing House. (1984). *1985 Social Security benefits, including Medicare*. Chicago: Commerce Clearing House.

Cremins, J.J. (1983). *Legal and political issues in special education*. Springfield, IL: Charles C Thomas.

Cutler, B.C. (1981). *Unraveling the special education maze. An action guide for parents*. Champaign, IL: Research Press.

Dane, E. (1985). Professional lay advocacy in the education of handicapped children. *Social Work, 30*, 505–510.

Davis, K., & Schoen, C. (1978). *Health and the war on poverty*. Washington, DC: Brookings Institution.

Force, J. (1985). *Survey of states' financial eligibility policies—Crippled Children's Services*. Unpublished manuscript.

Ireys, H.T., Hauck, R. J-P., & Perrin, J.M. (1985). Variability among state Crippled Children's Service programs: Pluralism thrives. *American Journal of Public Health, 75*, 375–381.

Leviton, S. (1983). *Special education resources manual*. Baltimore: University of Maryland School of Law.

Lybarger, B.E., & Onerheim, N. (1985). *An advocate's guide to surviving the SSI System*. Boston: Massachusetts Poverty Law Center.

Maged, G., & Stage, M.E. (Eds.). (1984). *Little max: Creating maximum benefits for children, elderly, poor, and disabled people*. Boston: Massachusetts Poverty Law Center.

Mashaw, J., Goetz, C., Goodman, F., et. al. (1978). *Social Security hearings and appeals: A study of the Social Security Administration Hearing System*. Lexington, MA: Lexington.

Meers, G.D. (Ed.). (1980). *Handbook of special vocational needs education*. Rockville, MD: Aspen Systems Corp.

National Institute on Legal Problems of Educating the Handicapped. (1984). *The fifth national institute on legal problems of educating the handicapped* (5th ed.). Chicago: National Institute on Legal Problems of Educating the Handicapped.

Phillips, J.N., Moore, R.J., Jr., Morton, K.A., et al. (1983). *Estate planning for families with handicapped dependents*. Baltimore: Maryland Institute for Continuing Professional Education of Lawyers.

Pullin, D. (1982). *Special education, a manual for advocates*. Cambridge, MA: Center for Law and Education, Guttman Library.

Silva, N. Jorge da. (1981). *A new approach to understanding PL 94-142: Procedural safeguards*. Novata, CA: Academic Therapy Publications.

Summers, J.A. (Ed.). (1986). *The right to grow up: An introduction to adults with developmental disabilities*. Baltimore: Paul H. Brookes Publishing Co.

Sweeney, D., & Lyko, J. (1980). *Practice manual for Social Security claims*. New York: Practicing Law Institute.

Abruptio placenta   Premature detachment of a normally situated placenta.

Acetabulum   The cup-shaped cavity of the hip bone that holds the head of the femur.

Acetaminophen   A medication used to control fever and pain; it has a different chemical structure than aspirin and fewer side effects.

Achondroplasia   *See* Syndromes, Appendix B.

Acid-base balance   In metabolism, the balance of acid to base necessary to keep the pH of the blood neutral.

Acoustic impedance audiometry   A test used to evaluate middle ear functioning.

Actin   Protein involved in muscle contraction.

Adrenalin   A potent stimulant of the autonomic nervous system; it increases blood pressure, heart rate, and other physiological changes needed for a "fight or flight" response.

Afferent   In the nervous system, *afferent* refers to the signals sent from the periphery to the brain.

Akinetic   A form of seizure associated with a sudden loss of muscle tone.

Alleles   Alternate forms of a gene that may exist at the same site on the chromosome.

Alveoli   Small air sacs in the lungs. Carbon dioxide and oxygen are exchanged through their walls.

Amblyopia   Dimness of vision with no detectable organic cause.

Ambulatory   Able to walk.

Amnioscopy   A prenatal diagnostic procedure in which the fetus is seen by use of a fibro-optic light source.

Amniotic fluid   Fluid that surrounds and protects the developing fetus; this fluid is sampled through amniocentesis.

Amphetamine   A drug that stimulates the central nervous system. Examples include Dexedrine and Ritalin.

Anemia   Disorder in which the blood has either too few red blood cells or too little hemoglobin; adjective: anemic.

Anencephaly   Birth defect in which either the whole brain or all the brain except the most primitive regions is missing.

Aneurysm   A localized swelling of an artery or vein.

Anorexia   A severe loss of appetite.

Anoxia   Lack of oxygen in body tissues.

Anterior fontanel   The membrane-covered space on the top of the head; also called the *soft spot*. It generally closes over by 18 months of age.

Anterior horn cells   Cells in the spinal column that transmit impulses from the pyramidal tract to the peripheral nervous system.

Antibody   A protein formed in the bloodstream to fight infection.

Anticonvulsant   Any medication used to control seizures.

Antihistamine   A drug that counteracts the effects of histamines, substances involved in allergic reactions.

Aorta   The major artery of the body. It originates in the left ventricle of the heart and carries oxygenated blood to the rest of the body.

Aphasia   Decreased expressive or receptive language often due to traumatic injury or stroke; adjective: aphasic.

Apnea Episodic arrest of breathing.

Aqueous humor The fluid in the eyeball that fills the space between the lens and the cornea.

Arcuate fasciculus A nerve tract that connects Wernicke's and Broca's areas of the brain. It is involved in the control of language.

Arthrogryposis *See* Syndromes, Appendix B.

Asphyxia Interference with circulation and oxygenation of the blood that leads to loss of consciousness and possible brain damage.

Aspirated Inhaled.

Aspiration pneumonia A lung inflammation caused by inhaling a foreign body, such as food, into the lungs.

Ataxia An unbalanced gait caused by loss of cerebellar control; adjective: ataxic.

Athetoid Pertaining to repeated, involuntary, writhing movements most prominent in the hands.

Atonic Loss of normal muscle tone.

Atresia Congenital absence of a body part.

Atrium A small cavity—for example, an upper chamber in the heart; plural: atria.

Atrophy A wasting away.

Audiometry The testing of hearing.

Auditory sequential memory Ability to repeat a sequence of words or numbers one hears.

Autoimmune Reaction in which one's immune system attacks other parts of the body.

Autonomic nervous system The part of the nervous system that regulates certain automatic functions of the body—for example, heart rate, sweating, and bowel movement.

Autosomal dominant trait A genetic trait carried on the autosomes. The disorder appears when one of a pair of chromosomes contains the abnormal gene; statistically, it is passed on from the affected parent to half of the children.

Autosomal recessive trait A genetic trait carried on the autosomes. Both asymptomatic parents must carry the trait to produce an affected child. This child has two abnormal genes. The risk of recurrence is 25%.

Autosome Any of the first 22 pairs of chromosomes; all chromosomes are autosomes except for the two sex chromosomes.

Banding pattern A series of dark and light bars that appear on chromosomes after they are stained. Each chromosome has a distinct banding pattern.

Beri-beri Disease caused by thiamine deficiency.

Bicornuate uterus Two-chambered uterus.

Bilirubin A yellow pigment produced by the breakdown of red blood cells in the liver; elevated levels of it lead to jaundice.

Blastocyst The embryonic group of cells that exists at the time of implantation.

Bolus A round mass of chewed food or medication that is ready for swallowing.

Brachial artery The principal artery of the forearm.

Bradycardia Slowing of the heart rate, usually below 60 beats a minute.

Brain stem The primitive portion of the brain that lies between the cerebrum and the spinal cord.

Brain stem auditory evoked response (BAER) A test to evaluate the processing of sound by the brain stem.

Braxton-Hicks Usually painless, irregular contractions that occur intermittently throughout pregnancy.

Bruxism Repetitive grinding of the teeth.

Butyrophenones Drugs that affect neurochemicals in the brain and are used to control behavior.

Caffeine A central nervous system stimulant found in coffee, tea, and cola.

Calcified Hardened through the laying down of calcium salts.

Callus A disorganized network of bone tissue formed around the edges of a fracture.

Carcinogen A cancer-producing substance.

Carotid artery The principal artery of the neck. It carries blood to the front part of the brain.

Cataract A clouding of the lens of the eye.

Celiac disease *See* Syndromes, Appendix B.

Central nervous system The portion of the nervous system that consists of the brain and spinal cord. It is primarily involved in voluntary movement and thought processes.

Centrioles Tiny organelles that migrate to the opposite poles of a cell during cell division and align the spindles.

Cephalocaudal From head to tail; refers to neurological development that proceeds from the head downward.

Cephalohematoma A swelling of the scalp containing blood; often found in newborn infants. It is usually not harmful.

Cerebral palsy A disorder of movement and posture due to a nonprogressive defect of the immature brain.

Cervical Pertaining to the neck.

CHARGE association *See* Syndromes, Appendix B.

Chemotherapy Treatment or control of a disease, usually cancer, by the use of chemical agents.

Choreoathetosis A form of cerebral palsy marked by variable muscle tone and involuntary movements of the arms and legs; adjective: choreoathetoid.

Chorionic Relating to the outermost covering of the fetus.

Chorionic gonadotrophin The hormone secreted by the embryo that prevents its expulsion from the uterus. A pregnancy test measures the presence of this hormone in the urine.

Chorioretinitis An inflammation of the retina and choroid that produces severe visual loss.

Choroid The middle layer of the eyeball between the sclera and the retina.

Choroid plexus Cells that line the ventricles of the brain and produce cerebrospinal fluid.

Chromatid Term given to chromosomes during cell division.

Cilia Hairlike projections attached to the surface of a cell.

Clonus Alternate muscle contraction and relaxation in rapid succession.

Cobalt Chemical element whose radioactive isotope is used in the treatment of cancer.

Cochlea The snail-shaped structure in the inner ear containing the organ of hearing.

Concave Having a curved, indented surface.

Congenital Present at or before birth.

Conjunctiva The membrane lining the eyelids and covering the eyeball.

Contracture Irreversible shortening of muscle fibers that causes decreased joint mobility.

Convex Having a curved, elevated surface such as a dome.

Convulsion A seizure; it most commonly involves a series of involuntary contractions of voluntary muscles.

Cornea The transparent, domelike covering of the iris.

Corpus callosum The bridge of white matter connecting the two cerebral hemispheres.

Cortex The gray matter that lies at the outer portion of the cerebrum; adjective: cortical.

Craniofacial Relating to the skull and the bones of the face.

Creatine phosphokinase (C-PK) An enzyme released by damaged muscle cells. Its level is elevated in muscular dystrophy.

Cretinism *See* Syndromes, Appendix B.

Cri-du-chat syndrome *See* Syndromes, Appendix B.

Crossing over The exchange of genetic material between two closely aligned chromosomes during the first meiotic division; abnormal cause of genetic diversity.

Cystic fibrosis Autosomal recessive disorder involving recurrent lung infections and malabsorption of food. *See* Syndromes, Appendix B.

Cytomegalovirus A viral disease with symptoms that may mimic mononucleosis, or it may be asymptomatic. It can also lead to severe fetal malformations similar to congenital rubella.

Deciduous Describes baby teeth which are shed.

Deletion Loss of genetic material from a chromosome.

Dentin The principal substance of the tooth surrounding the tooth pulp and covered by the enamel.

Deoxyribonucleic acid (DNA) A fundamental component of living tissue; it contains the genetic code.

Depolarization Changing the electrical charge of a cell.

Detoxification The conversion of a toxic compound to a nontoxic material.

Digit Finger or toe.

Diopter The unit of refractive power of a lens.

Duodenum Upper part of the small intestine.

Dysarthria Improper articulation of speech from problems in muscle control that result from damage to the central or peripheral nervous system.

Dyspraxia Inability to perform coordinated movements, with no apparent problem in the muscles or nerves.

Dystocia Structural abnormalities of the uterus that may cause premature or prolonged labor.

E. coli Bacteria normally found in the digestive tract. Certain kinds can cause infections ranging from diarrhea to sepsis.

Edema An abnormal accumulation of fluid in the tissues of the body.

Edetate calcium disodium (EDTA)   A drug used to bind ingested heavy metals, especially lead. EDTA must be given by injection.

Efferent   Nerve impulse that goes to a nerve or muscle from the central nervous system.

Electrolyte   Mineral contained in the blood.

Electromyogram   An electrical test of muscle contraction.

Ellis–van Creveld syndrome   *See* Syndromes, Appendix B.

Encephalitis   Inflammation or infection of the brain, usually viral in origin.

Encephalopathy   An acute or chronic disorder of the brain often caused by intoxication.

Endocarditis   Inflammation of the lining of the heart.

Endorphins   The body's natural opiates, probably involved in the perception of pain and pleasure.

Epidemiology   The study of factors determining the frequency and distribution of diseases—for example, an outbreak of food poisoning; adjective: epidemiological.

Epiglottis   A lidlike structure that hangs over the entrance to the windpipe and prevents aspiration into the lungs during swallowing.

Epithelial   Pertaining to the skin.

Equinus   Involuntary extension of the foot. This position is often found in spastic cerebral palsy.

Esophagus   Tube extending from the pharynx to the stomach.

Estimated date of confinement (EDC)   Expected date of delivery.

Eustachian tube   The canal that leads from the middle ear to the pharynx.

Extract   A concentrated preparation.

Fibro-optic   A flexible light source that can be used to examine internal body organs.

Flagellum   Whiplike projection of a cell that gives it mobility. The sperm is one example of a cell having a flagellum; plural: flagella.

Flexor   A muscle whose primary function is flexion at a joint.

Flora   Bacteria normally residing within the intestine, such as *E. coli*.

Folic acid   A vitamin needed for certain enzyme reactions. Its use may help prevent the development of spina bifida in high risk women.

Forebrain   The front portion of the brain during fetal development.

Fovea centralis   The small pit in the center of the macula; the area of clearest vision.

Frejka pillow   A cushion used to spread an infant's legs in the treatment of congenital hip dislocation.

Fundal plication   An operation in which the opening from the esophagus to the stomach is tightened.

Fundus uteri   The upper portion of the uterus where the fallopian tubes attach.

Galactosemia   *See* Syndromes, Appendix B.

Gastroenteritis   Stomach flu.

Gastroesophageal reflux   The backward flow of food from the stomach into the esophagus.

Gastrostomy   An operation in which an artificial opening is made into the stomach through the wall of the abdomen.

Genotype   The genetic composition of an individual (e.g., blood type).

Germ cell   The cells involved in reproduction, that is, the sperm and the egg.

Glaucoma   A disease caused by increased intraocular pressure.

Glucose   A sugar, also called sucrose, contained in fruits and other carbohydrates.

Gluten   The protein of wheat and other grains. People with celiac disease are unable to digest this protein.

Glycogen   The chief carbohydrate stored in the body, primarily in the liver and muscle.

Goiter   Enlargement of the thyroid gland leading to hypothyroidism.

Goniotomy   An operation to treat glaucoma that decreases pressure by providing an opening for the release of fluid from the anterior chamber of the eye.

Grand mal   A form of seizure in which there is a sudden loss of consciousness immediately followed by a generalized convulsion.

Gyri   Convolutions of the surface of the brain; singular: gyrus.

Habilitation   The training of children with developmental disabilities in new skills.

Hallermann-Streiff syndrome   *See* Syndromes, Appendix B.

Helix   The coiled structure of DNA.

Hematocrit   Percentage of red blood cells in whole blood, normally about 35%–40%.

Herpesvirus   A virus leading to symptoms that range from cold sores to vaginal infections to encephalitis; also a cause of fetal malformations and sepsis in early infancy.

Heterozygote   A carrier of a recessive genetic disorder.

Homeostasis   Equilibrium of fluid, chemical, and temperature regulation in the body.

Homocystinuria   *See* Syndromes, Appendix B.

Huntington's disease *See* Syndromes, Appendix B.
Hybrid Offspring of parents of dissimilar species.
Hydrocephalus A condition characterized by the abnormal accumulation of cerebrospinal fluid within the ventricles of the brain. This leads to an enlargement of the head.
Hyperbilirubinemia Excess of bilirubin in the blood.
Hypertelorism Widely spaced eyes.
Hypocalcemia Abnormally low levels of calcium in the blood.
Hypoglycemia Low blood sugar; often found in premature infants and infants of diabetic mothers.
Hypothermia Low body temperature; especially a risk in the newborn infant.
Hypothyroidism Deficiency of thyroid hormone. *See* Syndromes, Appendix B.
Hypotonia Decreased muscle tone; adjective: hypotonic.
Hypoxia Reduction of oxygen content in body tissues.
Ileum Lower portion of the small intestine.
Immunoglobulin An antibody.
Implantation The attachment and imbedding of the fertilized egg into the mucous lining of the uterus.
Incontinence Absence of bowel or bladder control.
Indomethacin Drug used to treat arthritis. It is also used to close a patent ductus arteriosus in premature infants.
Intracerebral Within the brain.
Intracranial Within the skull.
Intravenous The administration of medication directly into a vein.
Intraventricular Within the ventricle of the brain.
Intubation The insertion of a tube through the nose or mouth into the trachea to provide artificial ventilation.
In utero Occurring during fetal development.
Iris The circular, colored membrane behind the cornea, perforated by the pupil.
Islet cells Cells in the pancreas that produce insulin and control blood sugar levels. These cells do not function in individuals who have diabetes.
Jaundice Yellowing of the skin and whites of the eyes caused by an accumulation of bilirubin in the blood. This is often found in liver disease and Rh incompatibility; also called *icterus*.
Karyotype Photograph of the chromosomal makeup of a cell; in a human, there are 23 pairs of chromosomes in a normal karyotype.
Kernicterus *See* Syndromes, Appendix B.
Ketosis The buildup of acid in the body due to starvation or diabetes.
Kinesthetic Relating to the ability to perceive movement; noun: kinesthesia.
Labyrinth The inner ear, made up of the vestibular apparatus and the cochlea.
Lacrimal Pertaining to tears.
Lactose Milk sugar composed of glucose and galactose.
Laser therapy A new form of operation using a light source.
Lateral ventricle Cavity in the interior of the cerebral hemisphere.
Lecithin Fat compound found in surfactant.
Lens The biconvex, translucent body that rests in front of the vitreous humor and refracts light.
Lesion Injury or loss of function.
Lissencephaly An abnormality of the brain in which few gyri are formed. This is associated with some forms of mental retardation.
Locus ceruleus An area of the brain involved in attention.
Lumbar Pertaining to the lower back.
Lumbar puncture The tapping of the subarachnoid space to obtain cerebrospinal fluid from the lower back region. This procedure is used to diagnose meningitis.
Lymphocyte A type of white blood cell.
Macula The area of the eye that contains the greatest concentration of cones and the fovea centralis.
Mandible Lower jaw bone.
Mastoid Bone resting behind the ear.
Maxilla Upper jaw bone.
Megavitamin therapy See Orthomolecular therapy.
Meiosis Reductive cell division occurring only in eggs and sperm in which the daughter cells receive half (23) the number of chromosomes of the parent cells (46).
Meninges The three membranes covering the brain and spinal cord.

Meningitis Infection of the meninges.

Meningomyelocele *See under* Spina bifida, Syndromes, Appendix B.

Menses The menstrual flow.

Mental retardation Intellectual functioning at least two standard deviations below the mean.

Methotrexate Drug that interferes with folic acid metabolism; folic acid is essential for cell division. This drug is used in chemotherapy but may cause fetal malformations.

Methylmalonic aciduria *See* Syndromes, Appendix B.

Microcephaly A small head; more than two standard deviations below the average size; adjective: microcephalic.

Milligram One thousandth of a gram.

Milliliter One thousandth of a liter; equal to about 15 drops.

Millisievert A unit of measuring radiation exposure.

Mitosis Cell division in which two daughter cells of identical composition to the parent cell are formed; each contains 46 chromosomes.

Modem Device that allows individuals to connect their computers through phone lines.

Mononucleosis A viral illness whose symptoms include fever, malaise, sore throat, swollen lymph nodes, and an enlarged spleen.

Morpheme The smallest linguistic unit of meaning.

Morula The group of cells formed by the division of a fertilized egg.

Mosaicism The presence of two genetically distinct types of cells in one individual—for example, a child with Down syndrome who has some cells containing 46 chromosomes and some cells containing 47 chromosomes.

Mucopolysaccharide Product of metabolism that may accumulate in certain disorders and cause mental retardation.

Mucosa The mucous-membrane that lines organs such as the mouth, stomach, and vagina; adjective: mucosal.

Multiple sclerosis A degenerative nervous system disease leading to loss of myelin, progressive spasticity, and paralysis; it occurs in adults.

Mutation A change in the genetic material that occurs by chance.

Myelination The production of a coating called *myelin* around an axon. This quickens neurotransmission.

Myoclonic Repetitive contractions of muscles. This occurs in infantile spasms.

Myosin Protein necessary for muscle contraction.

Myringotomy The surgical incision of the eardrum.

Nasogastric tube A plastic feeding tube placed in the nose and extended into the stomach.

Neural tube The precursor of the spinal column.

Neuroectoderm Fetal skin cells that differentiate to form the retina and central nervous system.

Neurotoxin A chemical that damages the central nervous system.

Neurotransmitter A chemical released at the synapse that permits transmission of an impulse from one nerve to another.

Nondisjunction Failure of a pair of chromosomes to separate during mitosis or meiosis, resulting in an unequal number of chromosomes in the daughter cells.

Nucleotide One of the compounds that form DNA, for example, adenine, guanine, cytosine, and thymine.

Ocular Pertaining to the eye.

Ophthalmologist Physician specializing in treatment and diseases of the eye.

Ophthalmoscope An instrument containing a mirror and a series of magnifying lenses used to examine the interior of the eye.

Opsin The protein in rods and cones necessary for vision.

Opticokinetic Pertaining to movement of the eyes.

Optometrist A professional who examines eyes and prescribes glasses.

Organ of Corti A series of hair cells in the cochlea that form the beginning of the auditory nerve.

Orthodontist Dentist who specializes in the correction of irregularities of the teeth or the improper alignment of the jaw.

Orthomolecular therapy The use of at least 10 times the required amount of vitamins; also called *megavitamin therapy*.

Orthopedic Relating to bones or joints.

Orthosis An orthopedic appliance used to support, align, prevent, or correct deformities or to improve the functioning of movable parts of the body.

Ossicles The three small bones in the middle ear: the stapes, incus, and malleus.

Osteoarthritis Degenerative joint disease.

Osteoblast Cell type that produces bony tissue.

Osteoclast Cell type that absorbs and removes bone.

Osteogenesis imperfecta *See* Syndromes, Appendix B.

Oxygenation The provision of sufficient oxygen for bodily needs.

Palatal Relating to the palate, the back portion of the roof of the mouth.

Parkinson's disease A progressive, neurological disease usually affecting older people that is associated with tremor, slowed movements, and muscular rigidity.

Pavlik harness A device used to correct congenital hip dislocation.

Penicillamine A drug used to bind ingested heavy metals, particularly lead and copper. This drug may be given orally.

Periodontal Pertaining to the gums and bony structures that surround the teeth.

Periosteum Fibrous tissue covering and protecting all bones.

Peripheral nervous system The parts of the nervous system that are outside the brain and spinal cord.

Phagocyte A cell that ingests microorganisms or other foreign particles.

Phalanges Bones of the fingers or toes.

Pharyngeal *See* **pharynx.**

Pharynx The back of the throat; adjective: pharyngeal.

Phenothiazines Drugs that affect neurochemicals in the brain and are used to control behavior.

Phenylketonuria *See* Syndromes, Appendix B.

Phocomelia Defective development of the limbs so that the hands and/or feet are attached close to the body and resemble flippers.

Phoneme The smallest unit of sound in speech.

Phonetic Pertaining to articulated sounds.

Phonics The sounding out of words.

Pica The hunger for nonfood items.

Placenta The organ of nutritional interchange between the mother and the embryo. It has both maternal and embryonic portions and is disc-shaped and about 7 inches in diameter. The umbilical cord attaches in the center of the placenta. The placenta is also called the *afterbirth;* adjective: placental.

Placenta previa Condition in which the placenta is implanted in the lower segment of the uterus extending over the cervical opening. This often leads to bleeding during labor.

Polyneuropathy A disorder that involves damage to many peripheral nerves (e.g., Guillain-Barré syndrome).

Postural Relating to the positioning of the body.

Presbyopia A decrease in the accommodation of the lens of the eye that occurs with aging.

Prone Lying on one's stomach.

Prophylactic Preventive agent.

Propionic acidemia *See* Syndromes, Appendix B.

Psychosis A psychiatric disorder characterized by hallucinations, delusions, loss of contact with reality, and unclear thinking; adjective: psychotic.

Pulmonary Pertaining to the lungs.

Pupil The aperture in the center of the iris.

Purine A type of organic molecule found in RNA and DNA.

Quickening The first signs of life felt by the mother as a result of fetal movements in the fourth or fifth month of pregnancy.

Rachitic rosary Beadlike processes along the ribs that are associated with rickets.

Rad A measure of radioactivity.

Radiotherapy Treatment of disease, usually cancer, by using X rays.

Receptive aphasia Impairment of receptive language due to a disorder of the central nervous system.

Refracted Deflected.

Reticular activating system The area of the brain stem that is involved in the control of awareness and attention.

Retina The photosensitive nerve layer of the eye.

Retinitis pigmentosa *See* Syndromes, Appendix B.

Retinoblastoma A tumor of the retina.
Retinoscope An instrument used to detect errors of refraction in the eye.
Retraction The drawing back of a part of the body.
Retrovirus A virus involved in the transfer of DNA in gene therapy.
Ribonucleic acid (RNA) A molecule essential for protein synthesis within the cell.
Ribosome Intracellular structure concerned with protein synthesis.
Rooting A reflex in newborns that makes them turn their mouths toward the breast or bottle to feed.
Rubella German measles.
Rumination After swallowing, the regurgitation of food followed by chewing another time.
Salicylate A chemical found in many food substances and in aspirin.
Schizophrenia A form of psychosis.
Sclera The white, outer coating of the eyeball.
Scoliosis Curvature of the spine.
Sepsis Bacterial infection spread throughout the bloodstream; also called *blood poisoning*.
Sex chromosomes Those chromosomes that determine gender, the X and Y chromosomes.
Shunt A surgical passage between two blood vessels, two spaces, or two organs. An example is the ventriculo-peritoneal shunt used to drain cerebrospinal fluid in hydrocephalus.
Siblings Brothers and sisters.
Spastic Increased muscle tone so that muscles are stiff and movements are difficult; noun: spasticity.
Spasticity *See* Spastic.
Sphincter Circular muscle surrounding an opening in the body.
Sphingomyelin A fatty component of surfactant.
Spina bifida A developmental defect of the spine. *See* Syndromes, Appendix B.
Sporadic In the context of this book, sporadic refers to a disease that occurs by chance and carries little risk of recurrence.
Stereoscopic The blending together of two images of the same object from two slightly different viewpoints.
Sternum The breast plate.
Steroids Medications used to treat severe inflammatory diseases and infantile spasms; also refers to certain natural hormones in the body.
Strabismus Squint; deviation of the eye inward or outward.
Subarachnoid Beneath the arachnoid membrane, or middle layer, of the meninges.
Subcutaneous Under the skin.
Subdural Resting between the outer (dural) and middle (arachnoid) layers of the meninges.
Subluxation Partial dislocation.
Sulci Furrow of the brain; singular: sulcus.
Surfactant Material that coats the alveoli in the lungs, keeping them open. A deficiency of it leads to respiratory distress syndrome in premature infants.
Suture A stitch made to close a wound—also, for example, used to treat an incompetent cervix.
Synapse The minute space separating one neuron from another. Neurochemicals breach this gap.
Syntax The way in which words are put together to form meaning.
Syphilis A venereal disease.
Systemic Pertaining to the whole body.
Teratogen An agent that causes malformations in a developing embryo; adjective: teratogenic.
Thalamotomy *See* **ventrolateral thalamotomy.**
Thalamus The part of the brain involved in refining muscle movement.
Tonic Continuous increased muscle tone.
Tonic-clonic Spasmodic alternation of muscle contraction and relaxation; characteristic of grand mal seizures.
Tonometer An instrument for measuring intraocular pressure and determining the presence of glaucoma.
Torsion dystonia *See* Syndromes, Appendix B.
Toxemia Also called preeclampsia; the combination of high blood pressure, protein in the urine, and edema that may occur in the third trimester of pregnancy, especially in teenagers and women over 35.
Toxoplasmosis An infectious disease caused by a microorganism; it may be asymptomatic in adults but can lead to severe fetal malformations.
Trachea Windpipe.

Trachoma   Parasitic infection of the eye that causes blindness in children. This is seen only in developing countries.

Translocation   The transfer of a fragment of one chromosome to another chromosome.

Trauma   A wound or injury.

Treacher-Collins syndrome   *See* Syndromes, Appendix B.

Triglycerides   One of the types of fats found in food. A diet high in these is thought to be linked to heart disease.

Turner's syndrome   *See* Syndromes, Appendix B.

Twinning   The production of twins.

Umbilicus   The navel.

Urea   End product of protein metabolism.

Uterine fibroid tumors   Benign fibrous growths within the uterus. They may take up space within the uterus and lead to fetal deformities.

Varicella   The virus that causes chickenpox and herpes.

Varus osteotomy   The surgical cutting of the femur.

Vascular   Pertaining to blood vessels.

Ventricle   A small cavity, especially in the heart or the brain.

Ventriculo-peritoneal shunt   Plastic tube connecting a cerebral ventricle with the abdominal cavity; this is used to treat hydrocephalus.

Ventrolateral thalamotomy   A neurosurgical procedure in which a small area of the thalamus is destroyed. This is used to treat torsion dystonia and certain forms of cerebral palsy.

Vestibular apparatus   Three ring-shaped bodies located in the labyrinth of the ear that are involved in maintenance of balance.

Villus   Tiny vascular projection coming from the embryo that becomes part of the placenta; plural: villi.

Visual sequential memory   Ability to retain a sequence of pictures one sees.

Vitreous humor   The gelatinous portion of the eye located between the lens and the retina.

Werdnig-Hoffmann syndrome   *See* Syndromes, Appendix B.

X-linked recessive trait   A trait transmitted by a gene located on the X chromosome; also called *sex-linked*. It is passed on by a carrier mother to an affected son.

Zonular fibers   The fibers that keep the lens of the eye in place; contraction and relaxation of these fibers permit accommodation of the lens.

REFERENCES

Chapman medical dictionary for the non-professional. (1984). Woodbury, NY: Barron's Educational Series.

Dorland's pocket medical dictionary (23rd ed.). (1982). Philadelphia: W.B. Saunders Co.

Franks, R., & Swartz, H. (1977). *Simplified medical dictionary.* Oradell, NJ: Medical Economics Co. Book Division.

Stedman, T.L. (1982). *Illustrated Stedman's medical dictionary* (24th ed.). Baltimore: Williams & Wilkins Co.

Taber's cyclopedic medical dictionary (14th ed.). (1984). Philadelphia: F.A. Davis Co.

Appendix B

Syndromes

Children with certain rare disorders look alike. For example, children with Down syndrome share common features and look like brothers and sisters. When a combination of physical traits or malformations is inherited in the same way and carries a similar prognosis, the condition is called a *syndrome*.

This appendix lists a number of syndromes often associated with developmental disabilities. Their principal characteristics, pattern of inheritance, frequency of occurrence, risk of recurrence, and availability of prenatal diagnosis are noted. Inheritance is described as being autosomal recessive (AR), autosomal dominant (AD), X-linked (XL), or **sporadic** (SP), that is, not inherited. In most cases, no specific treatment is available to correct these defects. In those cases where treatment is available, it, too, is included in the description.

Achondroplasia Stature less than 50 inches, relatively large head, disproportionately short limbs, normal intelligence. *Inheritance:* AD. *Incidence:* 1/10,000; recurrence risk, 50%. *Prenatal diagnosis:* Available. (*See* Chapter 2, p. 16, and Chapter 13, Figure 13.3, p. 170.)
  Reference: Elejalde, B.R., De Elejalde, M.M., Hamilton, P.R., et al. (1983). Prenatal diagnosis in two pregnancies of an achondroplastic woman. *American Journal of Medical Genetics, 15,* 437–439.

Anencephaly Malformation of the brain in which the area above the brain stem is not formed; incompatible with prolonged survival. *Inheritance:* SP. *Incidence:* 6/10,000; recurrence risk, 3%–5%. *Prenatal diagnosis:* Ultrasound; measurement of alpha fetoprotein in amniotic fluid. (*See* Chapter 4, pp. 44, and Chapter 5, p. 60.)
  References: Ferguson-Smith, M.A. (1983). The reduction of anencephalic and spina bifida births by maternal serum alphafetoprotein screening. *British Medical Bulletin, 39,* 365–372.
  Pietrzyk, J.J. (1980). Neural tube malformations: Complex segregation analysis and recurrence risk. *American Journal of Medical Genetics, 7,* 293–300.

Apert syndrome Microcephaly, bony sutures closed so head appears flat, syndactyly (webbed hands and feet), frequent mental retardation. *Inheritance:* AD. *Incidence:* 1/160,000; recurrence risk, 50%. *Prenatal diagnosis:* Fetoscopy.
  Reference: Leonard, C.O., Daikoku, N.H., & Winn, K. (1982). Prenatal fetoscopic diagnosis of the Apert syndrome. *American Journal of Medical Genetics, 11,* 5–9.

Arthrogryposis multiplex congenita Multiple joint contractures. Muscles are wasted. *Cause:* Neuromuscular disorder or insufficient amniotic fluid. *Inheritance:* SP or AR, depending on cause. *Incidence:* Unknown. *Treatment:* Casting of joints. *Prenatal diagnosis:* Unavailable. (*See* Chapter 13, p. 170.)
  Reference: Symposium: Arthrogryposis multiplex congenita. (1985). *Clinical Orthopedics, 194,* 1–123.

Batten disease (Ceroid lipofuscinosis) Gray matter progressive nervous system disease. Child develops normally until 6 months to 2 years of age and then starts to lose skills. Eventually seizures, mental retardation, and blindness occur. Fatal outcome. *Inheritance:* AR. *Incidence:* 1/100,000; recurrence risk, 25%. *Prenatal diagnosis:* Available.
  References: Kristensen, K., & Lou, H.C. (1983). Central nervous system dysfunction as early

sign of neuronal ceroid lipofuscinosis (Batten's disease). *Developmental Medicine and Child Neurology, 25,* 588–590.

Wolfe, L.S., & Ng-Ying-Kin, N.M. (1982). Batten disease: New research findings on the biochemical defect. *Birth Defects, 18,* 233–239.

Cat cry syndrome *See* Cri-du-chat syndrome.

Celiac disease (Sprue) Malabsorption syndrome that leads to a failure to gain weight; passage of loose, foul-smelling stools. *Cause:* Intolerance of cereal products (gluten). *Inheritance:* ?AR. *Incidence:* 1/3,300. *Treatment:* Restriction of intake of foods containing gluten. *Prenatal diagnosis:* Unavailable. (*See* Chapter 10, p. 133.)
    Reference: Lebenthal, E., & Branski, D. (1981). Childhood celiac disease—A reappraisal. *Journal of Pediatrics, 98,* 681–690.

CHARGE association Coloboma (absence of part of iris or retina), Heart disease, Atresia chonae (blockage of nasal passage), Retarded growth and development, Genital anomalies, and Ear anomalies and/or deafness. *Inheritance:* AR. *Treatment:* Supportive. *Prenatal diagnosis:* Unavailable. (*See* Chapter 15, p. 200.)
    Reference: Pagon, R.A., Graham, J.M., Zonana, J., et al. (1981). CHARGE association. *Journal of Pediatrics, 99,* 223–227.

Cornelia de Lange syndrome Small-for-dates, microcephaly, mental retardation, excessive facial and body hair, congenital heart defects. *Cause:* Looks like a chromosomal disorder, but no chromosomal abnormality has been found. *Inheritance:* SP. *Incidence:* Less than 1/10,000; recurrence risk, 4%. *Prenatal diagnosis:* Unavailable.
    Reference: Preus, M., & Rex, A.P. (1983). Definition and diagnosis of the Brachmann-de Lange syndrome. *American Journal of Medical Genetics, 16,* 301–312.

Cretinism *See* (Congenital) Hypothyroidism.

Cri-du-chat syndrome Small-for-dates, growth retardation, catlike cry in infancy, mental retardation, congenital heart defects, microcephaly. *Cause:* Partial deletion of short arm of chromosome #5. *Incidence:* 1/20,000. *Prenatal diagnosis:* Chromosome analysis of fetal cells. (*See* Chapter 1, pp. 7–8.)
    Reference: Niebuhr, E. (1978). The cri-du-chat syndrome: Epidemiology, cytogenetics, and clinical features. *Human Genetics, 44,* 227–275.

Cystic fibrosis Malabsorption, failure to thrive, recurrent lung infections, normal intelligence. *Inheritance:* AR. *Incidence:* 1/2,000; recurrence risk, 25%. *Prenatal diagnosis:* Restriction enzyme analysis of fetal cells. (*See* Chapter 9, p. 117, and Chapter 10, p. 133.)
    Reference: DiSant' Agnese, P.A., & Davis, P.B. (1976). Research in cystic fibrosis. *New England Journal of Medicine, 295,* 481–485, 534–541.

(Fetal) Dilantin syndrome Small-for-dates, microcephaly, mild mental retardation, abnormalities of face and limbs. *Cause:* Maternal intake of Dilantin in first trimester. *Incidence:* 10% of women receiving Dilantin in first trimester. *Prenatal diagnosis:* Unavailable. (*See* Chapter 4, p. 46.)
    Reference: Hanson, J.W., & Smith, D.W. (1975). The fetal hydantoin syndrome. *Journal of Pediatrics, 87,* 285–290.

Down syndrome Hypotonia, short stature, mental retardation, small nose and low nasal bridge, upward slant to the eyes, short stubby fingers, simian crease, ventricular septal defects. *Cause:* Trisomy 21 (94%), mosaicism (2.4%), and translocation (3.6%). *Incidence: See* Chapter 3, Figure 3.1, p. 26. *Prenatal diagnosis:* Chromosome analysis of fetal cells. (Also, *see* Chapter 1, Figure 1.3, p. 5, Chapter 2, p. 18, and Chapter 16, p. 228.)
    Reference: Smith, D.W., & Wilson, A.A. (1973). *The child with Down's syndrome (mongolism).* Philadelphia: W.B. Saunders Co.

Duchenne muscular dystrophy Progressive muscle weakness and wasting, enlargement of thigh muscles, respiratory difficulty, heart failure, often mild mental retardation. Survival beyond 20 years is unusual. *Inheritance:* XL. *Incidence:* 1/100,000; recurrence risk, 50% in males only. *Prenatal diagnosis:* Can determine sex of the child by amniocentesis. (*See* Chapter 2, p. 17, and Chapter 13, pp. 178–179.)
    Reference: Dubowitz, V. (1978). *Muscle disorders in childhood.* Philadelphia: W.B. Saunders Co.

Edwards syndrome *See* Trisomy 18.

Ellis-van Creveld syndrome Short stature, short limbs, extra fingers, neonatal teeth, undeveloped nails, missing teeth with delayed eruption, heart defect, occasional mental retardation. *Inheritance:* AR. (*See* Chapter 11, p. 139.)
    Reference: Smith, D.W., with assistance of Jones, K.L. (1982). *Recognizable patterns of*

human malformation: Genetic, embryologic, and clinical aspects (3rd ed.). Philadelphia: W.B. Saunders Co.

Fetal alcohol syndrome   Small-for-dates, mild-moderate mental retardation, congenital heart defects, droopy eyelids, microcephaly, joint abnormalities. *Cause:* Excessive alcohol intake during pregnancy. *Incidence:* One-third of chronic alcoholics have children with this syndrome. *Prenatal diagnosis:* Unavailable. (*See* Chapter 4, pp. 47–48.)
   Reference: Smith, D.W. (1979). The fetal alcohol syndrome. *Hospital Practice, 14,* 121–128.

Galactosemia   Enlarged liver and jaundice in newborn period, mental retardation, cataracts, increased risk of infection. *Cause:* Inability to metabolize the sugar galactose. *Inheritance:* AR. *Incidence:* 1/40,000; recurrence risk, 25%. *Treatment:* Galactose-free diet. *Prenatal diagnosis:* Enzyme analysis of fetal cells and newborn screening available. (*See* Chapter 8, p. 100.)
   Reference: Cornblath, M., & Schwartz, R. (1976). *Disorders of carbohydrate metabolism in infancy* (2nd ed.). Philadelphia: W.B. Saunders Co.

Hallermann-Streiff syndrome   Short stature, unusual facial appearance, small eyes with cataracts, undeveloped or missing teeth, thin hair, feeding and respiratory problems, occasional mental retardation. *Inheritance:* AR. *Prenatal diagnosis:* Unavailable. (*See* Chapter 11, p. 139.)
   Reference: Judge, C., & Chalcanovskis, J.F. (1971). The Hallermann-Streiff Syndrome. *Journal of Mental Deficiency Research, 15,* 115–120.

Homocystinuria   Inborn error of metabolism associated with mental retardation, dislocated lenses, and increased risk of blood clots in the arteries. *Inheritance:* AR. *Incidence:* Less than 1/100,000. *Treatment:* Pyridoxine (Vitamin B_6) and betaine. *Prenatal diagnosis:* Enzyme analysis of fetal cells. (*See* Chapter 8, p. 100.)
   Reference: Mudd, S.H., & Levy, H.L. (1983). Disorders of transsulfuration. In J.B. Stanbury, J.B. Wyngaarden, D.S. Fredrickson, et al. (Eds.), *The metabolic basis of inherited disease* (5th ed.). New York: McGraw-Hill Book Co.

Huntington's disease   Choreic movement disorder and progressive neurological disease. Generally manifests itself in adulthood as dementia. *Inheritance:* AD. *Incidence:* 1/20,000; recurrence risk, 50%. *Prenatal diagnosis:* Unavailable.
   Reference: Goebel, H.H., Herpert, Z.R., Scholz, W., et al. (1978). Juvenile Huntington's chorea: Clinical, ultrastructural and biochemical studies. *Neurology, 28,* 23–31.

Hurler's syndrome   Short stature, progressive mental retardation, coarse facial appearance, clouding of the cornea, deafness, liver and spleen enlargement, bony abnormalities of spine and limbs. *Cause:* Enzyme deficiency of alpha iduronidase. *Inheritance:* AR. *Incidence:* 1/100,000; recurrence risk, 25%. *Prenatal diagnosis:* Enzyme analysis of fetal cells. (*See* Chapter 8, p. 105.)
   Reference: Kleijer, W.J., Thompson, E.J., & Niermeijer, M.F. (1983). Prenatal diagnosis of the Hurler syndrome: Report on 40 pregnancies at risk. *Prenatal Diagnosis, 3,* 179–186.

(Congenital) Hyperammonemia   Vomiting, lethargy, and coma in newborn period or early childhood. If untreated, infants die or suffer mental retardation. *Cause:* Defect in one of the five urea cycle enzymes leading to buildup of ammonia. *Inheritance:* AR (except ornithine transcarbamylase enzyme deficiency [OTC], which is XL). *Incidence:* 1/30,000; recurrence risk, 25%, except OTC, which is 50% in males. *Treatment:* Protein restriction and sodium benzoate/sodium phenylacetate. *Prenatal diagnosis:* Enzyme analysis of amniotic fluid plus DNA studies. (*See* Chapter 8, pp. 100, 102–103.)
   Reference: Batshaw, M.L. (1984). Hyperammonemia. *Current Problems in Pediatrics, 14,* 1–69.

(Congenital) Hypothyroidism (Cretinism)   Hoarse cry, large-for-dates, umbilical hernia, floppy tone, mental retardation. *Cause:* Deficiency in production of thyroid hormone. *Inheritance:* AR. *Incidence:* 1/6,000; recurrence risk, less than 5%. *Treatment:* Thyroid hormone. *Prenatal diagnosis:* Unavailable, but newborn screening is available. (*See* Chapter 8, pp. 100, 103, and Chapter 9, p. 113.)
   References: Hulse, J.A. (1984). Outcome for congenital hypothyroidism. *Archives of Disease in Childhood, 59,* 23–29.
   New England Congenital Hypothyroidism Collaborative. (1984). Characteristics of infantile hypothyroidism discovered on neonatal screening. *Journal of Pediatrics, 104,* 539–544.

Kernicterus   Mental retardation, choreoathetoid cerebral palsy, staining of secondary teeth, upward gaze paralysis, high-frequency hearing loss. *Cause:* Rh incompatibility. *Prevention:* The drug RhoGAM is given to the mother after delivery of the first affected child. *Prenatal diagnosis:* Measurement of level of bilirubin in amniotic fluid. (*See* Chapter 6, p. 79, Chapter 7, p. 92, Chapter 16, p. 229, and Chapter 21, p. 309.)

Reference: Ahdab-Barmada, M., & Moossy, J. (1984). The neuropathology of kernicterus in the premature neonate: Diagnostic problems. *Journal of Neuropathology and Experimental Neurology, 43,* 45–56.

Ketotic hyperglycinemia *See* Methylmalonic aciduria.

Klinefelter's syndrome (XXY syndrome) Low-normal intelligence, long limbs, thin appearance. Small penis and testes, sterility. *Cause:* Nondisjunction of X chromosome. *Incidence:* 1/5,000. *Prenatal diagnosis:* Chromosome analysis of fetal cells. (*See* Chapter 2, p. 20.)
References: Caldwell, P.D., & Smith, D.W. (1972). The XXY syndrome in childhood: Detection and treatment. *Journal of Pediatrics, 80,* 250–258.
Theilgaard, A. (1984). A psychological study of the personalities of XYY− and XXY− men. *Acta Psychiatrica Scandinavica (Suppl.), 315,* 1–133.

Lesch-Nyhan syndrome Progressive nervous system disorder, self-injurious behavior, profound mental retardation, progressive choreoathetoid cerebral palsy. *Cause:* Enzyme deficiency in **purine** metabolism. *Inheritance:* XL. *Incidence:* Unknown; recurrence risk, 50% in males only. *Prenatal diagnosis:* Enzyme analysis of fetal cells.
References: Christie, R., Bay, C., Kaufman, I.A., et al. (1982). Lesch-Nyhan disease: Clinical experience with 19 patients. *Developmental Medicine and Child Neurology, 24,* 293–306.
Wilson, J.M., & Kelley, W.N. (1984). Molecular genetics of the HPRT-deficiency syndromes. *Hospital Practice, 19,* 81–100.

Maple syrup urine disease Vomiting, lethargy, and coma in the first week of life. Urine smells like maple syrup. If untreated, leads to mental retardation or death. *Cause:* Enzyme deficiency affecting branch chain amino acids. *Inheritance:* AR. *Incidence:* 1/125,000; recurrence risk, 25%. *Treatment:* Special low protein diet. *Prenatal diagnosis:* Amniocentesis and enzyme analysis. (*See* Chapter 8, pp. 100, 102.)
References: Clow, C.L., Reade, T.M., Scriver, C.R., et al. (1981). Outcome of early and long-term management of classical maple syrup urine disease. *Pediatrics, 68,* 856–862.
Moser, H.W. (1977). Maple syrup urine disease. In P.J. Vinken & G.W. Bruyn (Eds.), *Handbook of clinical neurology, Vol. 29: Metabolic and deficiency diseases of the nervous system.* Amsterdam: North Holland Publishing Co.

Marfan syndrome Tall, thin stature, spiderlike limbs, dislocation of lens, aortic **aneurysms,** intelligence usually normal. *Inheritance:* AD. *Incidence:* 1/66,000; recurrence risk, 50%. *Prenatal diagnosis:* Unavailable.
Reference: Pyeritz, R.E., & McKusick, V.A. (1979). The Marfan syndrome: Diagnosis and management. *New England Journal of Medicine, 300,* 772–777.

Meningomyelocele *See* Spina bifida.

Menkes (Kinky hair) syndrome Small for gestational age, progressive neurological disorder, sparse, steely hair, profound mental retardation. *Inheritance:* XL. *Incidence:* 1/40,000. *Cause:* Defect in copper metabolism. *Prenatal diagnosis:* Evaluation of copper metabolism in fetal cells.
Reference: Horn, N. (1983). Menkes X-linked disease: Prenatal diagnosis and carrier detection. *Journal of Inherited Metabolic Disease, 6 (Suppl. 1),* 59–62.

Metachromatic leukodystrophy Progressive nervous system disease, profound mental retardation, loss of reflexes. Fatal. *Cause:* Enzyme deficiency of arylsulfatase A. *Inheritance:* AR. *Incidence:* 1/40,000; recurrence risk, 25%. *Prenatal diagnosis:* Enzyme analysis of fetal cells.
Reference: Dulaney, J.T., & Moser, H.W. (1983). Sulfatide lipidosis: Metachromatic leukodystrophy. In J.B. Stanbury, J.B. Wyngaarden, D.S. Fredrickson, et al. (Eds.), *The metabolic basis of inherited disease* (5th ed.). New York: McGraw-Hill Book Co.

(Fetal) Methotrexate (aminopterin) syndrome Small-for-dates, cleft palate, anencephaly, mental retardation, skeletal malformations. *Cause:* Maternal intake of this anticancer agent during pregnancy. *Incidence:* About 50% in women taking this drug during pregnancy. *Prenatal diagnosis:* Increased alpha fetoprotein levels in amniotic fluid. (*See* Chapter 4, p. 47.)
Reference: Shaw, E.B., & Steinback, H.L. (1968). Aminopterin-induced fetal malformations. *American Journal of Diseases of Children, 115,* 477–482.

Methylmalonic aciduria Inborn error of metabolism leading to an abnormal accumulation of methylmalonic acid. If untreated, results in mental retardation and repeated episodes of vomiting, lethargy, and coma associated with acidosis and hypoglycemia. *Inheritance:* AR. *Incidence:* 1/100,000; recurrence risk, 25%. *Treatment:* Protein-restricted diet. About 50% of the cases respond to vitamin B_{12}. Prenatal treatment of mother has also been useful. *Prenatal diagnosis:* Enzyme analysis of fetal cells and methylmalonic acid in amniotic fluid. (*See* Chapter 8, pp. 100, 106.)

Reference: Rosenberg, L.E. (1983). Disorders of propionate and methylmalonate metabolism. In J.B. Stanbury, J.B. Wyngaarden, D.S. Fredrickson, et al. (Eds.), *The metabolic basis of inherited disease* (5th ed.). New York: McGraw-Hill Book Co.

Muscular dystrophy *See* Duchenne muscular dystrophy.

Neurofibromatosis Intelligence usually normal but increased incidence of school problems, café-au-lait spots over body; nerve tumors develop on body and in eyes and ears. *Inheritance:* AD. *Incidence:* 3/10,000; recurrence risk, 50%. *Prenatal diagnosis:* Unavailable.

Reference: Riccari, V.M. (1981). Von Recklinghausen neurofibromatosis. *New England Journal of Medicine, 305,* 1617–1627.

Noonan syndrome Short stature, mental retardation, congenital heart defects, webbed neck, sometimes mistaken for Turner's syndrome. *Inheritance:* AD. *Incidence:* Possibly 1/1,000; recurrence risk, 50%. *Prenatal diagnosis:* Unavailable.

Reference: Theintz, G., & Savage, M.O. (1982). Growth and pubertal development in five boys with Noonan's syndrome. *Archives of Disease in Childhood, 57,* 13–17.

Osteogenesis imperfecta Increased susceptibility to fractures that results in bony deformities, blue-colored sclera, and translucent skin; normal intelligence, but often children are deaf. X rays show thin bones. *Inheritance:* AD. *Incidence:* 1/50,000; recurrence risk, 50%. *Prenatal diagnosis:* In the congenital type, X rays of the fetus show multiple fractures; type that has later onset (tarda) is undiagnosable prenatally. (*See* Chapter 13, p. 171.)

Reference: Binder, H., Hawks, L., Graybill, G., et al. (1984). Osteogenesis imperfecta: Rehabilitation approach with infants and young children. *Archives of Physical Medicine and Rehabilitation, 65,* 537–541.

Phenylketonuria (PKU) Blond hair, blue eyes, profound mental retardation, hyperactivity. *Cause:* Enzyme deficiency of phenylalanine hydroxylase. *Inheritance:* AR. *Incidence:* 1/14,000; recurrence risk, 25%. *Treatment:* Dietary restriction of phenylalanine leads to normal intellectual functioning. *Diagnosis:* Prenatal diagnosis unavailable, but newborn screening available. (*See* Chapter 4, p. 42, and Chapter 8, pp. 99, 100, 101–102.)

Reference: Tourian, A., & Sidbury, J.B. (1983). Phenylketonuria and hyperphenylalaninemia. In J.B. Stanbury, J.B. Wyngaarden, & D.S. Fredrickson, et al. (Eds.), *The metabolic basis of inherited disease* (5th ed.). New York: McGraw-Hill Book Co.

Prader-Willi syndrome Severe obesity, small testes and penis, mental retardation, floppiness in infancy. *Cause:* Partial deletion of chromosome #15, found in half of cases. *Inheritance:* AD. *Incidence:* Unknown. *Prenatal diagnosis:* Chromosome analysis of fetal cells in families with #15 deletion. (*See* Chapter 9, p. 112.)

Reference: Clarren, S.K., & Smith, D.W. (1977). Prader-Willi syndrome: Variable severity and recurrence risk. *American Journal of Diseases of Children, 131,* 798–800.

Propionic acidemia Inborn error of metabolism associated with the accumulation of organic acids; leads to recurrent episodes of vomiting, lethargy, and coma. Intelligence is often impaired. *Inheritance:* AR. *Treatment:* Special amino acid diet and biotin. *Prenatal diagnosis:* Enzyme analysis of fetal cells.

Reference: Wolf, B., Hsia, Y.E., Sweetman, L., et al. (1981). Propionic acidemia: A clinical update. *Journal of Pediatrics, 99,* 835–846.

Retinitis pigmentosa A group of diseases associated with retinal degeneration and progressive blindness; starts with night blindness in adolescence or adult life. *Cause:* Unknown. *Inheritance:* AR in most cases. *Incidence:* 1/200. *Prenatal diagnosis:* Unavailable. (*See* Chapter 15, p. 206.)

Reference: Carr, R.E. (1982). Retinitis pigmentosa: Recent advances. *Progress in Clinical and Biological Research, 82,* 135–146.

Reye's syndrome Acute **encephalopathy** following viral illness. Mortality rate: 20%. Reversible liver abnormalities and blood clotting disturbance, brain swelling. *Cause:* Virus and toxin; aspirin implicated. *Incidence:* Less than 1/100,000; recurrence risk, less than 1%.

Reference: Glasgow, J.F. (1984). Clinical features and prognosis of Reye's syndrome. *Archives of Disease in Childhood, 59,* 230–235.

(Congenital) Rubella syndrome Small-for-dates, mental retardation, microcephaly, cataracts, high-frequency hearing loss, chorioretinitis, congenital heart disease. *Cause:* Maternal exposure to rubella in the first trimester of pregnancy. *Incidence:* Less than 1/10,000. *Prenatal diagnosis:* Can establish fetal exposure to rubella. (*See* Chapter 4, pp. 48–49.)

Reference: Hardy, J.B. (1973). Clinical and developmental aspects of congenital rubella. *Archives of Otolaryngology, 98,* 230–236.

Rubinstein-Taybi syndrome Short stature, large beaked nose, very broad thumbs and large toes, mental retardation, microcephaly. *Cause:* Unknown. *Inheritance:* AR. *Prenatal diagnosis:* Unavailable.
Reference: Simpson, N.E., & Brissenden, J.E. (1975). The Rubinstein-Taybi syndrome. *American Journal of Human Genetics, 25,* 225–229.

Sotos syndrome (Cerebral gigantism) Large head, prominent forehead, jutting narrow jaw, coarse-looking facial appearance, prenatal onset of excessive growth, advanced bone age, usually moderate-severe mental retardation. *Inheritance:* AD. *Prenatal diagnosis:* Unavailable.
Reference: Sotos, J.F., Dodge, P.R., Muirhead, D., et al. (1964). Cerebral gigantism in childhood: A syndrome of excessively rapid growth with acromegalic features and a nonprogressive neurologic disorder. *New England Journal of Medicine, 271,* 109–116.

Spina bifida (Meningomyelocele) Malformation of the spinal column with cystic swelling around the spine. Paralysis occurs below lesion. Hydrocephalus common. Intelligence may be normal. *Cause:* Unknown. *Incidence:* 0.6/1,000; recurrence risk, 3%–5%. *Prenatal diagnosis:* Ultrasound; amniocentesis and measurement of alpha fetoprotein in the amniotic fluid. (*See* Chapter 4, Figure 4.3, p. 43.)
References: Charney, E.B., Weller, S.C., Sutton, L.N., et al. (1985). Management of the newborn with myelomeningocele: Time for a decision-making process. *Pediatrics, 75,* 58–64.
Freeman, J.M. (Ed.). (1974). *Practical management of meningomyelocele.* Baltimore: University Park Press.

Sturge-Weber syndrome Benign tumor made up of blood vessels over half of face and in brain; seizures and mental retardation. *Inheritance:* AD. Recurrence risk: 50%. *Prenatal diagnosis:* Unavailable.
Reference: Enjolras, O., Riche, M.C., & Merland, J.J. (1985). Facial port-wine stains and Sturge-Weber syndrome. *Pediatrics, 76,* 48–51.

Tay-Sachs disease Progressive nervous system disorder, profound mental retardation, deafness, blindness, seizures. Rapidly fatal. *Cause:* Enzyme deficiency of hexosaminidase A. *Inheritance:* AR. *Incidence:* 1/3,000 in Ashkenazic Jews; 1/360,000 in non-Jews; recurrence risk, 25%. *Prenatal diagnosis:* Carrier detection (blood test) and measurement of enzyme in fetal cells. (*See* Chapter 2, pp. 11, 13–15, and Chapter 18, p. 255.)
Reference: Kaback, M.M., Rimoin, D.L., & O'Brien, J.S. (Eds.). (1977). *Tay-Sachs disease: Screening and prevention.* New York: A.R. Liss.

Thalidomide embryopathy Phocomelia (shortened limbs), usually normal intelligence. *Cause:* Ingestion of thalidomide during first trimester of pregnancy. *Prenatal diagnosis:* Not required as thalidomide is no longer used. (*See* Chapter 4, Figure 4.5, p. 46.)
Reference: McBride, W.G. (1961). Thalidomide and congenital abnormalities. *Lancet, 2,* 1358.

Torsion dystonia (Dystonia musculorum deformans) Progressive movement disorder, normal intelligence. *Inheritance:* AD and AR forms exist. *Incidence:* 1/20,000 in Ashkenazic Jews; recurrence risk, 50% or 25% depending on inheritance pattern. *Prenatal diagnosis:* Unavailable. (*See* Chapter 12, p. 157, and Chapter 13, p. 179.)
Reference: Wachtel, R.C., Batshaw, M.L., Eldridge, R., et al. (1982). Torsion dystonia. *Johns Hopkins Medical Journal, 151,* 355–361.

Treacher-Collins syndrome Unusual facial appearance with malformed ears and conductive hearing loss, absence of lower eyelashes, cleft palate. Intelligence is usually normal. *Inheritance:* AD. *Treatment:* Surgical repair of most of the malformations is possible. *Prenatal diagnosis:* Unavailable. (*See* Chapter 16, p. 228.)
References: Johnston, C., Taussig, L.M., Koopmann, C., et al. (1981). Obstructive sleep apnea in Treacher-Collins syndrome. *Cleft Palate Journal, 18,* 39–44.
Shprintzen, R.J., & Berkman, M.D. (1979). Pharyngeal hypoplasia in Treacher-Collins syndrome. *Archives of Otolaryngology, 105,* 127–131.

Trisomy 18 Small-for-dates, mental retardation, low-set ears, clenched hands with overriding fingers, congenital heart defects. Limited survival: 90% die by 1 year of age. *Incidence:* 3/10,000; recurrence risk, 2%. *Prenatal diagnosis:* Chromosome analysis of fetal cells.
Reference: Hodes, M.E., Cole, J., Palmer, C.G., et al. (1978). Clinical experience with trisomies 18 and 13. *Journal of Medical Genetics, 15,* 48–60.

Trisomy 21 *See* Down syndrome.

Tuberous sclerosis Café-au-lait spots, acnelike lesions in small children, mental retardation, infantile spasms, calcium deposits in the brain. *Inheritance:* AD. *Incidence:* 1/100,000; recurrence risk, 50%. *Prenatal diagnosis:* Unavailable.

Reference: Pampiglione, G., & Moynahan, E.J. (1976). The tuberous sclerosis syndrome: Clinical and EEG studies in 100 children. *Journal of Neurology, Neurosurgery, and Psychiatry, 39,* 663–673.

Turner's syndrome (XO syndrome) Short stature (less than 5 feet), female, broad chest with widely spaced nipples, atrophied ovaries (sterile), webbed neck, congenital heart disease, usually normal intelligence. *Cause:* Nondisjunction. *Incidence:* 1/10,000. *Prenatal diagnosis:* Amniocentesis and chromosome analysis. *(See* Chapter 1, p. 7, Chapter 2, p. 20, and Chapter 20, p. 285.)
Reference: Palmer, C.G., & Reichmann, A. (1976). Chromosomal and clinical findings in 110 females with Turner syndrome. *Human Genetics, 35,* 35–49.

VATER syndrome Vertebral defects, Anal atresia, Tracheoesophageal connection, Esophageal stricture, and Renal (kidney) malformation. *Cause:* SP. *Incidence:* Unknown; recurrence risk, less than 5%. *Prenatal diagnosis:* Unavailable.
References: Aleksic, S., Budzilovich, G., Greco, M.A., et al. (1984). Neural defects in Say-Gerald (VATER) syndrome. *Child's Brain, 11,* 255–260.
Temtamy, S.A., & Miller, J.D. (1974). Extending the scope of the VATER association: Definition of the VATER syndrome. *Journal of Pediatrics, 85,* 345–349.

Von Recklinghausen's disease *See* Neurofibromatosis.

Werdnig-Hoffmann syndrome A form of spinal-muscular atrophy that leads to respiratory difficulties and severe muscle weakness in infancy. Survival is unusual past childhood. Intelligence: normal. *Inheritance:* AR. *Treatment:* Supportive. *Prenatal diagnosis:* Unavailable. (*See* Chapter 13, p. 177.)
Reference: Dubowitz, V.D. (1978). *Muscle disorders in childhood.* Philadelphia: W.B. Saunders, Co.

XYY syndrome Subtle abnormalities including tall stature, mild mental retardation, and aggressive behavior. *Cause:* Nondisjunction of sex chromosome. *Prenatal diagnosis:* Chromosome analysis of fetal cells. (*See* Chapter 2, p. 20.)
Reference: Hakola, H.P., & Iivanainen, M. (1978). Pneumoencephalographic and clinical findings of the XYY syndrome. *Acta Psychiatrica Scandinavica, 58,* 360–370.

GENERAL REFERENCES

Bergsma, D. (Ed.). (1979). *Birth defects compendium.* New York: A.R. Liss.

Holmes, L.B., Moser, H.W., Halldorsson, S., et al. (1972). *Mental retardation: An atlas of diseases with associated physical abnormalities.* New York: Macmillan Co.

McKusick, V.A. (1983). *Mendelian inheritance in man* (6th ed.). Baltimore: Johns Hopkins University Press.

Smith, D.W., with assistance of Jones, K.L. (1982). *Recognizable patterns of human malformation: Genetic, embryologic, and clinical aspects* (3rd ed.). Philadelphia: W.B. Saunders Co.

Appendix C

Resources for Children with Handicaps

NATIONAL ORGANIZATIONS

Listed below are a number of national organizations that provide services in the area of developmental disabilities. A brief description of the purpose of the organization follows each listing. This section is a representative sample and is not intended to be all-inclusive. We have tried to make addresses and phone numbers as current as possible. We apologize if readers find any of these have changed.

ACCESSIBILITY

Barrier-Free Design Centre, 357 Bay St., Tenth Floor, Toronto, Ontario, M5H 2T7, Canada (416-364-9079)

Nonprofit organization that operates a referral service for individuals, organizations, and professionals seeking expert advice on how to make homes or buildings accessible to persons with disabilities.

In Door Sports Club, Inc., 1145 Highland St., Napoleon, OH 43545 (419-592-5756)

Educates the public to promote and support opportunities that provide accessibility for persons with disabilities everywhere; interested in opportunities for rehabilitation and employment.

AUTISM

Autism Services Center, 101 Richmond St., Huntington, WV 25702 (304-525-8014)

Provides information, advocacy, training, consultation, seminars, and a summer camp for individuals with autism.

Institute for Child Behavior Research, 4182 Adams Ave., San Diego, CA 92116 (619-281-7165)

Information and referral for parents, teachers, physicians, and students working with children with autism and similar developmental disabilities.

National Society for Children and Adults with Autism, 1234 Massachusetts Ave., NW, Suite 1017, Washington, DC 20005 (202-783-0125)

Provides comprehensive services to individuals with autism and their families, including information, support, promotion of education and diagnostic services and facilities, and research.

CEREBRAL PALSY

American Academy for Cerebral Palsy and Developmental Medicine, 2315 Westwood Ave., P.O. Box 11083, Richmond, VA 23230 (804-355-0147)

Multidisciplinary scientific society that fosters professional education, research, and interest in the problems associated with cerebral palsy. Provides information to the public.

United Cerebral Palsy Associations, Inc., 66 E. 34th St., New York, NY 10016 (212-481-6300)

Direct services to children and adults with cerebral palsy that include medical diagnosis, evaluation and treatment, special education, career development, counseling, social and recreational programs, and adapted housing for persons with disabilities.

CLEFT LIP AND PALATE

American Cleft Palate Association and Educational Foundation, 331 Salk Hall, University of Pittsburgh, Pittsburgh, PA 15261 (412-681-9620)

Multidisciplinary professional organization that provides educational materials for parents, teachers, teenagers, and others. Also publishes a newsletter for parents.

COMPUTERS

ComputAbility Corporation, 101 Route 46 E., Pine Brook, NJ 07058 (201-882-0171)

Provides hardware adaptations and specialized software programs to aid persons with special needs in their use of computers. Will send free catalog.

Disabled Children's Computer Group (DCCG), Fairmont School, 724 Kearney St., El Cerrito, CA 94530 (415-528-DCCG)

Offers workshops for parents, teachers, and children that provide hands-on experience with computers; has a library of catalogs, articles, and books that relate to computers, disability, and special education. Interested in talking to parents or others who want to set up a similar organization in their community.

LINC Resources, Inc., 3857 N. High St., Columbus, OH 43214 (614-263-5462)

Offers marketing services for special education instructional materials; operates database of software programs for special education.

Trace Research and Development Center, 1500 Highland Ave., S-151, Madison, WI 53705-2280 (608-262-6966; TDD: 608-263-5408)

Conducts research and development in the areas of communication and computer access for individuals with disabilities. Disseminates information and has a reprint service on a variety of topics.

CYSTIC FIBROSIS

Cystic Fibrosis Foundation, 6000 Executive Blvd., Suite 510, Rockville, MD 20852 (301-881-9130)

Provides referral for diagnostic services and medical care; offers professional and public information and supports research and professional training.

DENTAL CARE

National Foundation of Dentistry for the Handicapped, 1250 14th St., Suite 610, Denver, CO 80202 (303-573-0264)

Maintains preventive dental health programs for persons with developmental disabilities in nine states; operates some dental house-call programs that serve homebound individuals; publishes guidelines for care and provides information.

EDUCATION

Center for Innovation in Teaching the Handicapped, 2805 E. 10th St., Room 150, Bloomington, IN 47405 (812-335-5847; 812-335-5849)

Conducts research for developing instructional materials for special education teachers.

Council for Exceptional Children, 1920 Association Dr., Reston, VA 22091 (703-620-3660)

Provides information to teachers, administrators, and others concerned with the education of gifted children and children with handicaps. Maintains a library and database on literature in special education; provides information and assistance on legislation.

National Association of Private Schools for Exceptional Children, 2021 K. St., NW, Suite 315, Washington, DC 20006 (202-296-1800)

National organization of private schools that promotes communication among these schools and informs the public about schools across the country; publishes a directory of schools that includes the services they offer and for whom.

National Information Center for Educational Media (NICEM), P.O. Box 40130, Albuquerque, NM 87196, (Toll free: 800-421-8711)

Provides database of educational audiovisual materials including motion pictures, filmstrips, audiotapes, slides, etc.

Task Force on Education for the Handicapped, 812 East Jefferson Blvd., South Bend, IN 46617 (219-234-7101; Indiana toll free: 800-332-4433)

Coalition of concerned parents, professionals, and persons with handicaps who are dedicated to the right to a free, appropriate public education for all children with handicaps.

TASH: The Association for Persons with Severe Handicaps, 7010 Roosevelt Way, NE, Seattle, WA 98115 (206-523-8446)

Advocates high-quality education for persons with handicaps; disseminates research findings and practical applications for education habilitation; encourages sharing of experience and expertise.

EPILEPSY

Epilepsy Foundation of America, 4351 Garden City Dr., Suite 406, Landover, MD 20785 (301-459-3700)

Provides programs of information and education, advocacy, support of research, and the delivery of needed services to person with epilepsy and their families.

EQUIPMENT

Independent Living Aids, Inc., 11 Commercial Ct., Plainview, NY 11803 (516-681-8288)

Provides, at a cost, aids that make daily tasks easier for those with physical disabilities. Will send free catalog.

PAM Assistance Centre, 601 W. Maple St., Lansing, MI 48906 (517-371-5897)

Provides free information from up-to-date ABLEDATA database on aids and equipment available for individuals with handicaps.

FEDERAL

Clearinghouse on the Handicapped, Office of Special Education and Rehabilitative Services, U.S. Dept. of Education, Room 3119, Switzer Bldg., Washington, DC 20202 (202-732-1245; 202-732-1248)

National information and referral center for questions relating to different handicaps.

National Information Center for Handicapped Children and Youth, P.O. Box 1492, Washington, DC 20013 (703-522-3332)

Federal center established as part of PL 94-142. Provides information on many handicaps through fact sheets and newsletters; offers advice to people working in groups and connects people with similar problems across the country. Services are available to children with handicaps, families, and professionals.

President's Committee on Employment of the Handicapped, 1111 20th St., NW, Washington, DC 20036 (202-653-5029)

One of oldest presidential committees in the United States. Promotes acceptance of persons with physical and mental handicaps in the world of work. Involves the public and the private sector. Promotes the elimination of barriers, both physical and attitudinal, to the employment of persons with handicaps.

GENERAL

ACCENT on Living, P.O. Box 700, Bloomington, IL 61701 (309-378-2961)

Computerized retrieval system that has information on a variety of topics including employment, aids for independent living, laws and legislation, special education, home management, housing and architectural barriers, special facilities, etc.

American Academy of Pediatrics, 141 Northwest Point Rd., P.O. Box 927, Elk Grove Village, IL 60007 (312-228-5005)

Professional membership association for board-certified pediatricians that offers professional continuing education, health education materials, and other programs.

American Association for the Advancement of Science, Project on Science, Technology, and Disability, 1333 H St., NW, Washington, DC 20005 (202-326-6667 [Voice or TDD])

Seeks to increase the number of minorities, women, and individuals with handicaps in the natural, social, and applied sciences and engineering, and the opportunities available to these groups; also seeks to further the participation of these groups in policy making, advisory, and managerial positions.

American Association of University Affiliated Programs for Persons with Developmental Disabilities, 8605 Cameron St., #406, Silver Spring, MD 20910 (301-588-8252)

Represents the professional interests of the national network of 51 University Affiliated Facilities (UAFs) that serve persons with developmental disabilities in 37 states.

Avenues, P.O. Box 5192, Sonora, CA 95370 (209-533-1468)
Publishes a semiannual newsletter that provides lists of parents, interested doctors, and experienced medical centers that are concerned with persons with disabilities.

Center on Human Policy, Syracuse University, 406 Huntington Hall, Syracuse, NY 13210 (315-423-3851)
Advocacy and research organization committed to the rights of persons with disabilities; holds local, regional, and national workshops on rights; offers advice and backup assistance to individuals and advocacy groups.

Council for Disability Rights, 343 S. Dearborn, #318, Chicago, IL 60604 (312-922-1093 [Voice/TTY])
Provides information and workshops on rights of persons with disabilities; information and referral services; evening hotline for persons with disabilities and/or family members; monthly newsletter.

Federation of the Handicapped, Inc., 211 W. 14th St., New York, NY 10011 (212-242-9050)
Services include vocational training and job placement for adults with severe disabilities.

Gesell Institute of Human Development, 310 Prospect St., New Haven, CT 06511 (203-789-1911)
Multidisciplinary team that provides primary health care and preventive medicine; also offers consultation on ways to influence the course of chronic disease; has departments on vision, psychological evaluations, and developmental assessments.

Information Center for Individuals with Disabilities, 20 Park Plaza, Suite 330, Boston, MA 02116 (617-727-5540; TTY: 727-5236; MA toll free: 800-462-5015)
Information, referral, and problem-solving assistance for persons with disabilities, families, friends, and professionals.

Mainstream, Inc., 1200 15th St., NW, Washington, DC 20005 (202-833-1136 [Voice/TDD])
Provides information and technical assistance to employers and organizations for persons with handicaps on mainstreaming such persons into the workplace. Provides placement services to job-ready handicapped persons in Washington, DC, and Dallas, TX, metro areas.

March of Dimes Birth Defects Foundation, 1275 Mamaroneck Ave., White Plains, NY 10605 (914-428-7100)
Awards grants to institutions and organizations to develop genetic services, perinatal care in high-risk pregnancies, prevention of premature delivery, parent support groups, and other community programs.

Mobility International, 62 Union St., London SEI Ltd., England (01-403-5688); In USA: P.O. Box 3551, 1870 Onyx #E, Eugene, OR 97403 (503-343-1284)
International exchange programs for individuals with disabilities and other young people.

National Association of Developmental Disabilities Councils, 1234 Massachusetts Ave., NW, Suite 103, Washington, DC 20005 (202-347-1234)
Organization of councils that exist in each state; these councils provide information on resources and services for persons with developmental disabilities and their families.

National Clearinghouse in Maternal and Child Health, 3520 Prospect St., NW, Ground Floor, Washington, DC 20057 (202-625-8410)
Dissemination of publications and fact sheets to the public and professionals in the field; develops and maintains database of topics, agencies, and organizations related to maternal and child health.

National Easter Seal Society, 2023 W. Ogden Ave., Chicago, IL 60612 (312-243-8400; toll free: 800-221-6827)
Oldest nonprofit health care agency that provides direct services to people with disabilities, advocacy, public health education, organization and funding, and support of research.

National Organization for Rare Disorders, Inc., P.O. Box 8923, New Fairfield, CT 06812 (203-746-6518)
Clearinghouse for information about rare disorders; encourages and promotes research; represents people with rare diseases who are not otherwise represented; educates the public and the medical profession about these diseases.

National Organization on Disability, 2100 Pennsylvania Ave., NW, #234, Washington, DC 20037 (202-293-5960; TDD: 293-5968)
Promotes the acceptance and understanding of the needs of citizens with disabilities through a national network of communities and organizations; facilitates exchange of information regarding resources available to persons with disabilities.

National Rehabilitation Clearinghouse, 115 Old USDA Bldg., Oklahoma State University, Stillwater, OK 74078 (405-624-7650)

Provides training materials for professionals in rehabilitation and related professions.

National Rehabilitation Information Center (NARIC), The Catholic University of America, 4407 Eighth St., NE, Washington, DC 20017 (202-635-5826; TDD: 202-635-5884)

Rehabilitation information service and research library; also has database of information on commercially available products that aid rehabilitation and independent living.

P.R.I.D.E. Foundation, 1159 Poquonnock Rd., Groton, CT 06340 (203-445-1448; CT toll free: 800-962-0707)

Primary objective is to provide dressing, grooming, and home management assistance to persons with disabilities and the elderly.

GENETICS

National Down Syndrome Society, 70 W. 40th St., New York, NY 10018 (212-764-3070; outside NY: 800-221-4602)

Conducts research, promotes public awareness and education, and provides services to families about Down syndrome.

National Down Syndrome Congress, 1800 Dempster St., Park Ridge, IL 60068-1146 (1-800-232-NDSC [outside IL]; 312-823-7550 [IL])

Provides a wide referral/resource system in the United States and 40 foreign countries; publishes two journals and literature available to the public; serves as a clearinghouse on all aspects of Down syndrome; monitors research; provides legislative awareness and pursues public awareness.

National Genetics Foundation, 555 West 57th St., New York, NY 10019 (212-586-5800)

Provides information on genetic diseases, genetic counseling, and genetic services to families and individuals. Offers a computerized analysis of an individual's health history, known as a Family Health Profile (small fee for this service).

National Society of Genetic Counselors, Dept. of Pediatrics, University of California, Irvine Medical Center, 101 City Dr., S., Orange, CA 92668 (714-634-5791)

Professional organization of genetic counselors. Can provide referral to nearest source for genetic counseling and services.

The National Tay-Sachs & Allied Diseases Association, 385 Elliot St., Newton, MA 02164 (617-964-5508)

Promotes genetic screening programs nationally; has updated listing of Tay-Sachs prevention centers in a number of countries; provides educational literature to general public and professionals; peer group support for parents.

HEARING, SPEECH, AND LANGUAGE

Academy of Rehabilitative Audiology, c/o M.A. Henoch, Ph.D., Division of Communication Disorders, NTSU, Denton, TX 76203 (817-565-2262)

Provides rehabilitative services to persons with hearing impairment.

Alexander Graham Bell Association for the Deaf, 3417 Volta Pl., NW, Washington, DC 20007 (202-337-5220)

Umbrella organization for International Organization for the Education of the Hearing Impaired (IOEHI), International Parents' Organization (IPO), and Oral Deaf Adults Section (ODAS). Provides general information and information on resources.

American Society for Deaf Children, 814 Thayer Ave., Silver Spring, MD 20910 (301-585-5400 [Voice/TDD])

Provides information and support to parents and families with children who are deaf or who have hearing impairment.

American Speech-Language-Hearing Association, 10801 Rockville Pike, Rockville, MD 20852 (301-897-5700 [Voice/TTY])

Professional and scientific organization; certifying body for professionals providing speech, language, and hearing therapy; conducts research in communication disorders; publishes several journals.

The Deafness Research Foundation, 55 East 34th St., New York, NY 10016 (212-684-6556)

Solicits funds for the support of research into the causes, treatment, and prevention of deafness and other hearing disorders.

Hearing Aid Helpline, 20361 Middlebelt Rd., Livonia, MI 48152 (313-478-2610; outside MI: 800-521-5247)

Information on how to proceed when hearing loss is suspected; free consumer kit, facts about hearing aids, and a variety of literature on hearing-related subjects is available.

International Parents' Organization, 3417 Volta Pl., NW, Washington, DC 20007 (202-337-5220)

Provides materials and correspondence to parents of children with hearing impairment; gives support to parents wanting "oral options" for their children.

National Center for Stuttering, Inc., 200 E. 33rd St., New York, NY 10016 (212-532-1460; toll free: 800-221-2483)

Provides free information for parents of young children just starting to show symptoms of stuttering; runs training programs for speech professionals in current therapeutic approaches; provides treatment for people over 7 years of age who stutter.

National Information Center on Deafness, Gallaudet College, 800 Florida Ave., NE, Washington, DC 20002 (202-651-5109; TDD: 651-5976)

Provides information related to deafness; has a multitude of resources and experts available for individuals with hearing impairment, their families, and professionals. Collects information about resources around the country.

LEARNING DISABILITIES

Association for Children and Adults with Learning Disabilities, 4156 Library Rd., Pittsburgh, PA 15234 (412-341-1515)

Encourages research and the development of early detection programs, disseminates information, serves as an advocate, and works to improve education for individuals with learning disabilities.

Association of Learning Disabled Adults, P.O. Box 9722, Friendship Station, Washington, DC 20016 (301-593-1035 [home phone; please use sparingly])

Self-help group of adults with learning disabilities; provides technical assistance to anyone wishing to organize a group of adults with learning disabilities.

Foundation for Children with Learning Disabilities, 99 Park Ave., New York, NY 10016 (212-687-7211)

Committed to increasing public awareness of learning disabilities; provides free information to interested parents, friends, and professionals on learning disabilities.

The Orton Dyslexia Society, 724 York Rd., Baltimore, MD 21204 (301-296-0232; toll free: 800-222-3123)

Devoted to the study, treatment, and prevention of dyslexia; disseminates information on dyslexia and has two regular publications.

LEGAL

ACLU Children's Rights Project, 132 W. 43rd St., New York, NY 10036 (212-944-9800)

Nationwide test-case litigation program designed to protect and expand the statutory and constitutional rights of children, in particular those in foster care.

Children's Defense Fund, 122 C St., NW, Washington, DC 20001 (202-628-8787; toll free: 800-424-9602)

Provides information about legislation in health care, child welfare, and special education.

Mental Health Law Project, 2021 L St., NW, Suite 800, Washington, DC 20036 (202-467-5730)

Legal advocacy program that works to define, establish, and protect the rights of children and adults with mental disabilities, using test-case litigation, federal policy advocacy, and training and technical assistance for legal services lawyers and other advocates nationwide.

National Center for Law and the Deaf, Gallaudet College, 800 Florida Ave., NE, Washington, DC 20002 (202-651-5454 [Voice/TDD])

Provides a variety of legal services to persons with hearing impairment, including representation, counseling, information, and education.

MENTAL RETARDATION

American Association on Mental Deficiency, 1719 Kalorama Rd., NW, Washington, DC 20009 (202-387-1968)

Professional organization that promotes cooperation among those involved in services, training, and research in mental retardation. Encourages research, dissemination of information, development of appropriate community-based services, and the promotion of preventive measures designed to further reduce the incidence of mental retardation.

Association for Retarded Citizens of the United States, 2501 Avenue J, Arlington, TX 76011 (817-640-0204)

National advocacy organization working on behalf of individuals with mental retardation and their families; has 1,600 local units across the United States.

The Joseph P. Kennedy, Jr., Foundation, 1350 New York Ave., NW, Suite 500, Washington, DC 20005 (202-393-1250)

Promotes public awareness, develops innovative models of treatment, and provides seed money for programs in mental retardation. Also sponsors Let's Play to Grow (LPTG) clubs, which provide training to parents in play skills, community support, and an opportunity for children to learn and develop through play and recreation.

King County Advocates for Retarded Citizens, 2230 8th Ave., Seattle, WA 98121 (206-622-9292; 206-622-9324 [Parent-to-Parent Support])

Conducts support groups for parents and grandparents of children with disabilities. Publishes national newsletter for and about grandparents of children with special needs.

National Association of Private Residential Facilities for the Mentally Retarded, 6269 Leesburg Pike, Suite B5, Falls Church, VA 22044 (703-536-3311)

Publishes directory of members each year; also publishes monthly newsletter and has alert system that is used to inform members about important legislation.

National Association of State Mental Retardation Program Directors, 113 Oronoco St., Alexandria, VA 22314 (703-683-4202)

Organization consisting of one representative from each state. Publishes two newsletters; provides information on state and national trends, statistics, and programs in the field of developmental disabilities.

MUSCULAR DYSTROPHY

Muscular Dystrophy Association, 810 Seventh Ave., New York, NY 10019 (212-586-0808)

Voluntary health care agency that fosters research and direct care for individuals with muscular dystrophy; concerned with conquering muscular dystrophy and other neuromuscular diseases.

NUTRITION

National Nutrition Consortium, Inc., 24 Third St., NE, Suite 200, Washington, DC 20002 (202-547-4819)

Nonprofit scientific and educational organization; facilitates communication among the food and nutrition professional community, training of food and nutrition students in public policy and government activities, and involvement in public affairs around issues of interest to the food and nutrition professional.

OCCUPATIONAL THERAPY

The American Occupational Therapy Association, Inc., 1383 Piccard Dr., Rockville, MD 20850 (301-948-9626)

Professional organization of occupational therapists; provides services including accreditation of educational programs, certification of practitioners, and public education.

PARENTS

American Council of the Blind Parents, 1211 Connecticut Ave., NW, Suite 506, Washington, DC 20036 (202-833-1251)

Provides services to parents of children with visual impairment as well as professionals. Purposes are to provide exchange of information among parents, to educate the public, and to monitor developments in technology, education, legislation, etc. Helps sighted parents and parents with visual impairment with childrearing problems.

Closer Look, Parents' Campaign for Handicapped Children and Youth, 1201 16th St., NW, Washington, DC 20036 (202-822-7900; Learning Disabled Teen Hotline, toll free: 800-522-3458)

National information center that serves parents of children with handicaps; primary purpose is to help families help themselves as they face the challenges of raising a child who has a disability.

Compassionate Friends, P.O. Box 3696, Oak Brook, IL 60521 (312-990-0010)

National and worldwide organization that supports and aids parents in the positive resolution of the grief experienced upon the death of their child; fosters the physical and emotional health of bereaved parents and siblings.

The Exceptional Parent, 605 Commonwealth Ave., Boston, MA 02215 (617-536-8961)

This magazine provides straightforward, practical information for families and professionals involved in the care of children and young adults with disabilities; many articles are written by parents.

National Association of Mothers of Special Children (MSC), 9079 Arrowhead Ct., Cincinnati, OH 45231 (513-521-0670)

Offers emotional support, information, and socialization to mothers of special children; helps to start new chapters across the country.

PACER Center, Inc. (Parent Advocacy Coalition for Educational Rights), 4826 Chicago Ave., S., Minneapolis, MN 55417 (612-827-2966 [Voice/TDD])

Parent information and training center on public school issues that relate to PL 94-142. Also has a handicap awareness program that uses puppets in a presentation for nonhandicapped students to increase awareness and facilitate mainstreaming.

Parent Educational Advocacy Training Center, 228 S. Pitt St., Alexandria, VA 22301 (703-836-2953)

Professionally staffed organization that helps parents to become effective advocates for their children with school personnel and the educational system.

PARENTELE, 5538 North Pennsylvania St., Indianapolis, IN 46220 (317-259-1654)

Communication network among parents of persons with handicaps and the professionals who serve them. Publishes quarterly newsletter. Also, the Parent Information Resource Council, Inc., houses a library and handles inquiries from parents and professionals.

Project COPE, 9160 Monte Vista Ave., Montclair, CA 91763 (714-985-3116; 714-621-3884)

Serves as a link between parents who are raising children with handicapping conditions and new parents seeking understanding and hope. Professionally trained and supervised parent volunteers contact new parents at their request. No fees are charged.

Team of Advocates for Special Kids (TASK), 1800 E. La Veta, Orange, CA 92666 (714-771-6542)

Central resource center that offers parent information, legal rights information, and assistance; has bilingual materials. Conducts an advocacy training course; publishes a bimonthly newsletter. Has a peer support group and a speakers' bureau.

PHYSICAL THERAPY

American Physical Therapy Association, 1111 N. Fairfax St., Alexandria, VA 22314 (703-684-2782)

Professional membership association of physical therapists. Operates clearinghouse for questions on physical therapy and disabilities. Publishes bibliographies on a wide range of topics.

RECREATION

American Alliance for Health, Physical Education, Recreation and Dance, 1900 Association Dr., Reston, VA 22091 (703-476-3400)

Association of professionals in physical education, sports and athletics, health and safety education, recreation and leisure, and dance. Supports and disseminates research, promotes better public understanding of these professions, and supports and provides opportunities for professional growth to members.

American Athletic Association of the Deaf, 3916 Lantern Dr., Silver Spring, MD 20902 (202-224-8637)

Promotes sports competition on a local, national, and international level for deaf persons and those with hearing impairment.

Boy Scouts of America, Scouting for the Handicapped Division, 1325 Walnut Hill La., Irving, TX 75038-3096 (214-580-2127)

Provides educational, recreational, and therapeutic resource programs through the Boy Scouts of America.

Girl Scouts of the U.S.A., 830 Third Ave., New York, NY 10022 (212-940-7500)

Open to all girls ages 5 through 17 (or kindergarten through grade 12). Runs camping programs, sports and recreational activities, and service programs. Mainstreams children with disabilities into regular Girl Scout troop activities.

National Handicapped Sports & Recreation Association, 1145 19th St., NW, Suite 717, Washington, DC 20036 (301-652-7505)

Provides year-round sports and recreational opportunities to persons with orthopedic, spinal cord, neuromuscular, and visual impairments through a national network of local chapters.

National Wheelchair Athletic Association, 3617 Betty Drive, Suite S, Colorado Springs, CO 80907 (303-597-8330)

Governing body of various sports of wheelchair athletics including swimming, archery, fencing, weightlifting, track & field, slalom, and table tennis. Publishes a newsletter; no membership fee for individuals under 16 years old.

Special Olympics, 1350 New York Ave., NW, Suite 500, Washington, DC 20005-4709 (202-393-1250)

Largest year-round sports organization for children and adults with mental retardation; sanctioned by the United States Olympic Committee. Local, area, and regional games are held throughout the United States and in 70 other countries.

Special Recreation, Inc., 362 Koser Ave., Iowa City, IA 52240 (319-337-7578; 319-353-6808)

National organization dedicated to serving the recreational rights and recreational needs of persons with disabilities.

U.S. Government Printing Office, Washington, DC 20402

Publishes guide entitled *Access National Parks,* available for a nominal fee, that lists all national parks and describes the services each park offers visitors with disabilities—for example, sign language interpreters at Yosemite Park.

SCOLIOSIS

Scoliosis Research Society, 444 N. Michigan Ave., Chicago, IL 60611 (312-822-0970; 312-665-3165—Office of the Secretary)

Conducts research on the etiology and treatment of scoliosis and spinal disorders.

SELF-ADVOCACY

American Coalition of Citizens with Disabilities, Inc. (ACCD), 1012 14th St., NW, Suite 901, Washington, DC 20005 (202-628-3470 [Voice/TDD])

Organization of persons with disabilities and other interested individuals that works to promote better situations for persons with disabilities in the areas of housing, employment, education, transportation, recreation, etc.

Coalition on Sexuality and Disability, Inc., 853 Broadway, Room 611, New York, NY 10003 (212-242-3900 [answering service; staff person will return call])

Organization committed to assisting persons with disabilities to achieve full integration into society with confidence in their sexuality. Offers seminars and workshops on sexuality and disability; advocates for persons with disabilities.

Little People of America, Inc., P.O. Box 633, San Bruno, CA 94066 (415-589-0695)

Nationwide, voluntary organization dedicated to helping people of short stature. Provides fellowship, moral support, and information to "little persons."

United Together, 348 Haworth, University of Kansas, Lawrence, KS 66045 (913-864-4950)

National self-advocacy network for persons with disabilities. Works to promote the full participation in life of persons with all kinds of disabilities. Publishes a quarterly newsletter.

SIBLINGS

The Sibling Information Network, Dept. of Educational Psychology, Box U-64, The University of Connecticut, Storrs, CT 06268 (203-486-4032/4034)

Assists individuals and professionals interested in serving the needs of families of individuals with disabilities; disseminates bibliographic material and directories; places people in touch with each other; publishes a newsletter written for and by siblings or parents.

SICKLE CELL DISEASE

Howard University Center for Sickle Cell Disease, 2121 Georgia Ave., NW, Washington, DC 20772 (202-636-7916)

Screening and counseling for sickle cell disease; provides services to both adults and children, including medical treatment and psychosocial intervention.

National Association for Sickle Cell Disease, Inc., 4221 Wilshire Blvd., Suite 360, Los Angeles, CA 90010-3503 (213-936-7205; toll free: 800-421-8453)

Provides education, screening, genetic counseling, technical assistance, tutorial services, vocational rehabilitation, and research support in the United States and Canada.

SPINA BIFIDA

Spina Bifida Association of America, 1700 Rockville Pike, Suite 540, Rockville, MD 20852 (301-770-SBAA)

Provides information and referral for new parents and literature on spina bifida; supports a public awareness program; advocates for individuals with spina bifida and their families; supports research; conducts conferences for parents and professionals.

SYNDROMES

American Tuberous Sclerosis Association (ATSA), P.O. Box 44, Rockland, MA 02370 (617-878-5528; toll free: 800-446-1211)

Provides information and referral services, counseling, public and professional education; supports research in tuberous sclerosis.

Cornelia de Lange Syndrome Foundation, Inc., 60 Dyer Ave., Collinsville, CT 06022 (203-693-0159)

Supports parents and children affected by Cornelia de Lange syndrome, encourages research, and disseminates information to increase public awareness through a newsletter and informational pamphlet.

Gaucher's Disease Registry, 4418 E. Chapman Ave., #139, Orange, CA 92669 (714-532-2212)

Publishes bimonthly newsletter, operates support groups, and provides referrals to organizations for appropriate services.

Guillain-Barré Syndrome Support Group, P.O. Box 262, Wynnewood, PA 19096 (215-896-6372; 215-649-7837)

Provides emotional support to patients and their families; fosters research, educates the public about the disorder, develops nationwide support groups, and directs persons with this syndrome to resources.

International Rett's Syndrome Association, Inc., 8511 Rose Marie Dr., Ft. Washington, MD 20744, (301-248-7031)

Provides information and referral, support to families, and acts as a liaison with professionals. Also facilitates research on Rett's syndrome.

The National Neurofibromatosis Foundation, Inc., 141 5th Ave., 7th Fl., New York, NY 10010 (212-460-8980)

Supplies information to laypersons and professionals; offers genetic counseling and support groups throughout the United States.

Osteogenesis Imperfecta Foundation, Inc., P.O. Box 245, Eastport, NY 11941 (516-325-8992)

Supports research on osteogenesis imperfecta and provides information to those with this disorder, their families, and other interested persons.

Prader-Willi Syndrome Association, 5515 Malibu Dr., Edina MN 55436, (612-933-0113)

National organization that serves as a clearinghouse for any information on Prader-Willi syndrome; shares information with parents, professionals, and other interested persons.

Tourette Syndrome Association, 42-40 Bell Blvd., Bayside, NY 11361 (212-224-2999)

Offers information, referral, advocacy, education, research, and self-help groups to those affected by this syndrome.

VISION

American Foundation for the Blind, Inc., 15 W. 16th St., New York, NY 10011, (212-620-2020)

Works in cooperation with other agencies, organizations, and schools to offer services to blind persons and those with visual impairments; provides consultation, public education, referrals, information, talking books, and adaptation of equipment for persons with visual impairment.

American Printing House for the Blind, 1839 Frankfort Ave., Louisville, KY 40206 (502-895-2405)

Publishing house for persons with visual handicaps; books in braille, large type, and recordings are available. Nonprofit.

Associated Services for the Blind, 919 Walnut St., Philadelphia, PA 19107, (215-627-3501)

Provides custom transcription of print materials in large print, audiotape, or braille; operates retail store for aids and materials for blind persons; provides social services counseling and support groups for blind persons and their families.

Association for Education and Rehabilitation of the Blind and Visually Impaired, 206 N. Washington St., Alexandria, VA 22314, (703-548-1884; 703-836-6060)

Inservice training primarily through conferences and publications for educators and those involved in rehabilitation of blind and low-vision persons.

International Institute for Visually Impaired, 0-7, Inc., 1975 Rutgers, East Lansing, MI 48823 (517-332-2666)

Information clearinghouse for parents and teachers of infants and young children who are blind or visually impaired.

National Association for Visually Handicapped, 22 W. 21st St., 6th Fl., New York, NY 10010 (212-889-3141)

Provides informational literature, guidance and counseling, and referral services for parents of partially sighted children and those who work with them. Publishes free large-print newsletter.

National Braille Association, Inc., 1290 University Ave., Rochester, NY 14607 (716-473-0900)

Produces and distributes braille reading materials for visually impaired persons. Collection consists of college-level textbooks, technical materials, and some materials of general interest.

National Federation of the Blind, 1800 Johnson St., Baltimore, MD 21230 (301-659-9314)

Offers advocacy services for the blind in such areas as discrimination in housing and insurance. Operates a job referral and listing system to help blind individuals find competitive employment. Runs an aids and appliances department to assist blind persons in independent living. Has a scholarship program for blind college students and a loan program for blind persons who are going into business for themselves.

National Library Service for the Blind and Physically Handicapped, Library of Congress, 1291 Taylor St., NW, Washington, DC 20542 (202-287-5100)

Administers a free library program of braille and recorded books for eligible readers with visual impairment and physical handicaps throughout the United States and for American citizens living abroad.

National Society to Prevent Blindness, 79 Madison Ave., New York, NY 10016-7896 (212-684-3505)

Voluntary health agency committed to the reduction of cases of blindness.

PROTECTION AND ADVOCACY AGENCIES

Listed below are the protection and advocacy agencies mandated by law to serve and protect the rights of persons with disabilities.

Alabama

Alabama Developmental Disabilities Advocacy Program, 918 Fourth Ave., Tuscaloosa, AL 35401 (205-348-4998)

Alaska

Protection and Advocacy for the Developmentally Disabled, Inc., Rm. 204, Alaska Sportsman Mall, 1514 Cushman St., Fairbanks, AL 99701 (907-456-1070; 907-456-1079; ZENITH 6600 [statewide toll free])

Arizona

Arizona Center for Law in the Public Interest, 112 N. Fifth Ave., Phoenix, AZ 85002 (602-252-4904; toll free: 800-352-5335)

Arkansas

Advocacy Services, Inc., Suite 504, Medical Arts Bldg., 12th and Marshall, Little Rock, AR 72202 (501-371-2171)

California

Protection and Advocacy, Inc., 1400 K. St., Suite 307, Sacramento, CA 95814 (916-447-3324; toll free: 800-952-5746)

Colorado

Legal Center for Handicapped Citizens, 1060 Bannock St., Suite 316, Denver, CO 80204 (303-573-0542)

Connecticut

Office of Protection and Advocacy for Handicapped and Developmentally Disabled Persons, 401 Trumbull St., Hartford, CT 06103 (203-566-7616; 203-566-2101 [teletype]; statewide toll free: 800-842-7303)

Delaware

Community Legal Aid Society, Inc., Developmental Disabilities Protection and Advocacy System, 913 Washington St., Wilmington, DE 19801 (302-575-0660; statewide toll free: 800-292-7980)

District of Columbia

Information Center for Handicapped Individuals, 605 G St., NW, #202, Washington, DC 20001 (202-347-4986)

Florida

Governor's Commission on Advocacy for Persons with DD, Office of the Governor, Tallahassee, FL 32301 (904-488-9070; statewide toll free: 800-342-0823)

Georgia

Georgia Advocacy Office, Inc., 1447 Peachtree St., NE, Suite 811, Atlanta, GA 30309 (404-885-1447; toll free: 800-282-4538)

Guam

The Advocacy Coordinating Office for the Developmentally Disabled, P.O. Box 8319, Tamuning, Guam 96911 (809-477-7280)

Hawaii

Protection & Advocacy Agency of Hawaii, 1580 Makaloa St., Suite 860, Honolulu, HI 96814 (808-949-2922; toll free: EPO 7777)

Idaho

Idaho's Coalition of Advocates for the Disabled, Inc., 1510 W. Washington, Boise, ID 83702 (208-336-5353; toll free: 800-632-5125)

Illinois

Illinois DD Advocacy Authority, 206 S. Sixth St., Springfield, IL 62701 (217-544-5750)

Indiana

Indiana Protection & Advocacy Service Commission for the Developmentally Disabled, 964 N. Pennsylvania St., Suite 1-A, Indianapolis, IN 46204 (317-232-1150; toll free: 800-622-4845)

Iowa

Protection and Advocacy Division, Iowa Civil Rights Commission, 507 10th St., 8th Floor, The Colony Bldg., Des Moines, IA 50319 (515-281-8081; statewide toll free: 800-532-1465)

Kansas

Kansas Advocacy & Protection Services for the DD, Inc., The Denholm Bldg., 513 Leavenworth, Suite 2, Manhattan, KS 66502 (913-776-1541; toll free: 800-432-8276)

Kentucky

Office of Public Advocacy, Division for Protection & Advocacy, 2nd Floor, State Office Bldg. Annex, Frankfort, KY 40601 (502-564-2967; toll free: 800-372-2988)

Louisiana

Advocate for the Developmentally Disabled, 333 St. Charles Ave., Rm. 1221, New Orleans, LA 70130 (504-522-2337; toll free: 800-662-7705)

Maine

Advocates for the DD, Cleveland Hall, Winthrop St., P.O. Box 88, Hallowell, ME 04347 (207-289-2395; toll free: 800-452-1948; 207-289-2394 [Augusta area])

Maryland

Maryland Disability Law Center, 2510 St. Paul St., Baltimore, MD 21218 (301-383-3400; 301-234-4227 TTY)

Massachusetts

DD Law Center of Massachusetts, 294 Washington St., Suite 840, Boston, MA 02108 (617-426-7020)

Michigan

Michigan Protection and Advocacy Service for Developmentally Disabled Citizens, 230 N. Washington Sq., Suite 200, Lansing, MI 48933 (517-487-1755)

Minnesota

Minnesota Developmental Disabilities Protection & Advocacy Network, 222 Grain Exchange Bldg., 323 Fourth Ave., S., Minneapolis, MN 55415 (612-338-0968)

Mississippi

Advocacy Office, Inc., Suite 100, Watkins Bldg., 510 George St., Jackson, MS 39201 (601-944-0485)

Missouri

Missouri Developmental Disabilities Protection and Advocacy Services, Inc., 211 B Metro Dr., Jefferson City, MO 65101 (314-893-3333)

Montana

Developmental Disabilities/Montana Advocacy Program, Inc., 1219 8th Ave., Helena, MT 59601 (406-449-3889; statewide toll free: 800-332-6149)

Nebraska

Nebraska Advocacy Services for Developmentally Disabled Citizens, Inc., Lincoln Ctr. Bldg., 215 Centennial Mall S., Room 422, Lincoln, NE 68508 (402-474-3183)

Nevada

Developmental Disabilities Advocates Office, 495 Apple St., Reno NV 89502 (702-784-6375; statewide toll free: 800-992-5715; FTS 4705911)

New Hampshire

DD Advocacy Center, Inc., 2½ Beacon St., P.O. Box 19, Concord, NH 03301 (603-228-0432; toll free: 800-852-3336)

New Jersey

Office of Advocacy for the Developmentally Disabled; CN 850, Trenton, NJ 08625 (609-292-9742; toll free: 800-792-8600)

New Mexico

P & A System for New Mexicans with DD, Suite 300, 510 Second St., NW, Albuquerque, NM 87102 (505-243-8831)

New York

Protection & Advocacy Bureau, New York State Commission on Quality of Care for the Mentally Disabled, 99 Washington Ave., Suite 730, Albany, NY 12210 (518-473-7378)

North Carolina

Governor's Advocacy Council for Persons with Disabilities, North Carolina Dept. of Administration, 107 Howard Bldg., 116 W. Jones St., Raleigh, NC 27611 (919-733-3111)

North Dakota

Protection & Advocacy Project for the Developmentally Disabled, Governor's Council on Human Resources, State Capital, 13th Floor, Bismarck, ND 58505 (701-224-2972; toll free: 800-472-2670)

Ohio

Ohio Legal Rights, 8 E. Long St., Suite 320, Columbus, OH 43215 (614-461-1318; toll free: 800-282-9181)

Oklahoma

Protection & Advocacy Agency for DD, 9726 E. 42nd St., Osage Bldg., Suite 133, Tulsa, OK 74145 (918-664-5883)

Oregon

Oregon Developmental Disabilities Advocacy Center, 621 S.W. Morrison, Room 713, Portland, OR 97205 (503-243-2081; statewide toll free: 800-452-1694)

Pennsylvania

Developmental Disabilities Advocacy Network (DDAN), Inc., 3540 N. Progress Ave., Harrisburg, PA 17110 (717-657-3320; toll free: 800-692-7443)

Puerto Rico

Protection & Advocacy, Puerto Rico Dept. of Consumer Affairs, Minillas Governmental Center, North Bldg., P.O. Box 41059 Minillas Sta., Santurce, PR 00904 (809-727-8536)

Rhode Island

Rhode Island Protection & Advocacy System (RIPAS), Inc., 70 S. Main St., Providence, RI 02903 (401-831-3150)

South Carolina

South Carolina P & A System for the Handicapped, Inc., 2360-A Two Notch Rd., Columbia, SC 29204 (803-254-1600)

South Dakota

South Dakota Advocacy Project, Inc., 111 W. Capitol Ave., Pierre, SD 57501 (605-224-8294; statewide toll free: 800-742-8108)

Tennessee

Tennessee State Planning Office, James K. Polk State Office Bldg., 505 Deaderick St., Suite 1800, Nashville, TN 37219 (615-741-1676)

Texas

Advocacy, Inc., 1006 E. 50th St., Austin, TX 78751 (512-475-5543; statewide toll free: 800-252-9108 [Voice/TTY])

Utah

Legal Center for the Handicapped, 455 E. 400 S., Suite 300, Salt Lake City, UT 84111 (801-363-1347; toll free: 800-662-9080)

Vermont

Vermont DD Law Project, 180 Church St., Old Courthouse, Burlington, VT 05401 (802-863-2881)

Virgin Islands

Committee on Advocacy for the Developmentally Disabled, Inc., P.O. Box 734, Fredericksted, St. Croix, U.S. Virgin Islands 00840 (809-772-1200)

Virginia

State Protection and Advocacy Office, Suite 100, 9th St. Office Bldg., Richmond, VA 23219 (804-786-4185; toll free: 800-552-3961)

Washington

Troubleshooters for the Disabled, 1600 W. Armory Way, Seattle, WA 98119 (206-284-1037)

West Virginia

West Virginia Advocates for the Developmentally Disabled, Inc., 1021 Quarrier St., Suite 411, Charleston, WV 25301 (304-346-0847; statewide toll free: 800-642-9205)

Wisconsin

Wisconsin Coalition for Advocacy, 2 W. Mifflin, Suite 200, Madison, WI 53703 (608-251-9600; statewide toll free: 800-363-9053)

Wyoming

Developmental Disabilities Protection and Advocacy System, Inc., 508 Hynds Bldg., Cheyenne, WY 82001 (307-632-3496; toll free: 800-442-2744)

UNIVERSITY AFFILIATED PROGRAMS

Listed below are the university affiliated programs that provide diagnostic and treatment services to children with handicaps and their families.

Alabama

Center for Developmental & Learning Disorders (CDLD), University of Alabama-Birmingham, 1720 Seventh Ave., S., Birmingham, AL 35233 (205-934-5471)

California

Division of Clinical Genetics & Developmental Disabilities, Dept. of Pediatrics, College of Medicine, University of California-Irvine, Irvine, CA 92717 (714-634-5791)

University Affiliated Facility, Mental Retardation Program, University of California-Los Angeles, 760 Westwood Plaza, Los Angeles, CA 90024 (213-825-0395)

University Affiliated Training Program, Center for Child Development and Developmental Disorders, Children's Hospital of Los Angeles, 4650 Sunset Blvd., Los Angeles, CA 90027 (213-669-2151)

Colorado

Rocky Mountain Child Development Center, University of Colorado Health Sciences Center, Box C234, 4200 E. Ninth Ave., Denver, CO 80262 (303-394-7224)

District of Columbia

Georgetown University Child Development Center, CG-52 Bles Bldg., 3800 Reservoir Rd., NW, Washington, DC 20007 (202-625-7675)

Florida

Mailman Center for Child Development, University of Miami School of Medicine, P.O. Box 016820, Miami, FL 33101 (305-547-6635)

Georgia

University Affiliated Facility, University of Georgia, 850 College Station Rd., Athens, GA 30610 (404-542-8970)

Illinois

Illinois Institute for Developmental Disabilities, 1640 W. Roosevelt Rd., Chicago, IL 60608 (312-996-1590)

Indiana

Developmental Training Center, Indiana University, 2853 E. Tenth St., Bloomington, IN 47405 (812-335-6508)

Riley Child Development Program, Riley Hospital, Rm. A578, 702 Barnhill Dr., Indianapolis, IN 46223 (317-264-2051)

Iowa

University Hospital School, The University of Iowa, Iowa City, IA 52242 (319-353-5972)

Kansas

Kansas University Affiliated Facility-Central Office, Bureau of Child Research, 223 Haworth Hall, University of Kansas, Lawrence, KS 66045 (913-864-4295)

Kansas University Affiliated Facility-Kansas City, Children's Rehabilitation Unit, Kansas University Medical Center, 39th & Rainbow Blvd., Kansas City, KS 66103, (913-588-5900)

Kansas University Affiliated Facility-Lawrence, 348 Haworth Hall, University of Kansas, Lawrence, KS 66045 (913-864-4950)

Kansas University Affiliated Facility-Parsons, 2601 Gabriel, Parsons, KS 67357 (316-421-6550)

Kentucky

University of Kentucky Human Development Program, 114 Porter Bldg., 730 S. Limestone, Lexington, KY 40506-0205 (606-257-1715)

Louisiana

Human Development Center, Louisiana State University Medical Center, 1100 Florida Ave., New Orleans, LA 70119 (504-949-7541)

Maine

University Affiliated Handicapped Children's Program, Eastern Main Medical Center, 489 State St., Bangor, ME 04401 (207-947-3711, ext. 2573)

Maryland

Kennedy Institute for Handicapped Children, 707 N. Broadway, Baltimore, MD 21205 (301-522-2100)

Massachusetts

Developmental Evaluation Clinic, Children's Hospital Medical Center, 300 Longwood Ave., Boston, MA 02115 (617-735-6501)

Eunice Kennedy Shriver Center for Mental Retardation, Walter E. Fernald State School, 200 Trapelo Rd., Waltham, MA 02254 (617-893-3500)

Minnesota

Gillette Development Disabilities Program, Gillette Children's Hospital, 200 E. University Ave., St. Paul, MN 55101 (612-291-2848)

Mississippi

University Affiliated Program of Mississippi, 1102 Robert E. Lee Bldg., Jackson, MS 39201 (601-359-1290)

Missouri

University Affiliated Facility for Developmental Disabilities, University of Missouri-Kansas City, 2220 Holmes St., Kansas City, MO 64108 (816-474-7770)

Montana

Montana University Affiliated Program, 401 Social Science Bldg., University of Montana, Missoula, MT 59812 (406-243-5467)

Nebraska

Meyer Children's Rehabilitation Institute, University of Nebraska Medical Center, 444 S. 44th St., Omaha, NE 68131 (402-559-6430)

New Jersey

University Affiliated Facility, University of Medicine & Dentistry of New Jersey, Rutgers Medical School, Box 101, Trailer 3, Piscataway, NJ 08854 (201-931-7888)

New York

Rose F. Kennedy Center, Albert Einstein College of Medicine, Yeshiva University, 1410 Pelham Pkwy. S., Bronx, NY 10461 (212-430-2440)

Developmental Disabilities Center, St. Lukes-Roosevelt Hospital, 428 W. 59th St., New York, NY 10019 (212-870-6844)

University Affiliated Diagnostic Clinic for Developmental Disorders, University of Rochester Medical Center, Box 671, 601 Elmwood Ave., Rochester, NY 14642 (716-275-2986)

Mental Retardation Institute, Westchester County Medical Center, Valhalla, NY 10595 (914-347-4514)

North Carolina

Division for Disorders of Development and Learning, Biological Sciences Research Center 220H, University of North Carolina-Chapel Hill, Chapel Hill, NC 27514 (919-966-5171)

Ohio

University Affiliated Cincinnati Center for Developmental Disorders, Pavilion Bldg., Elland & Bethesda Aves., Cincinnati, OH 45229 (513-559-4623)

The Nisonger Center, The Ohio State University, McCampbell Hall, 1580 Cannon Dr., Columbus, OH 43210 (614-422-8365)

Oregon

Center on Human Development, University of Oregon, 901 E. 18th St., Eugene, OR 97403 (503-686-3591)

Child Development & Rehabilitation Center, Crippled Children's Division, Oregon Health Sciences University, P.O. Box 574, Portland, OR 97207 (503-225-8362)

Pennsylvania

Developmental Disabilities Program, Temple University, Ritter Annex, 13th St. & Columbia Ave., Philadelphia, PA 19122 (215-787-1356)

Rhode Island

Child Development Center, Rhode Island Hospital, 593 Eddy St., Providence, RI 02902 (401-277-5681)

South Carolina

UAF Program of South Carolina-USC, Center for Developmental Disabilities, Benson Bldg., Pickens St., University of South Carolina, Columbia, SC 29208 (803-777-4839)

UAF Program of South Carolina, Human Development Center, Winthrop College, Rock Hill, SC 29733 (803-323-2244)

South Dakota

Center for the Developmentally Disabled, Julian Hall, University of South Dakota, Vermillion, SD 57069 (605-677-5311)

Tennessee

Child Development Center, University of Tennessee, 711 Jefferson Ave., Memphis, TN 38105 (901-528-6511)

Texas

University Affiliated Center, University of Texas Health Sciences Center, Suite 748, 6011 Harry Hines Blvd., Dallas, TX 75235 (214-688-2883)

Utah

Exceptional Child Center, UMC 68, Utah State University, Logan, UT 84322 (801-750-1982)

Washington

Child Development and Mental Retardation Center, University of Washington, Seattle, WA 98195 (206-543-3224)

West Virginia

University Affiliated Center, 807 Allen Hall, P.O. Box 6122, West Virginia University, Morgantown, WV 26506-6122 (304-293-4692)

Wisconsin

Clinical Services Unit, Waisman Center, University of Wisconsin, 1500 Highland Ave., Madison, WI 53706 (608-263-5776)

Appendix D

Lifesaving Techniques

The two most common lifesaving techniques are cardiopulmonary resuscitation, or CPR, and the manual thrust, also called the Heimlich maneuver. The methods of each of these techniques are explained in this appendix.

PRINCIPLES OF CARDIOPULMONARY RESUSCITATION

The most common causes of loss of consciousness are fainting and seizures. In neither of these instances is CPR needed, and, in fact, the inappropriate use of CPR can actually be dangerous. Therefore, the rescuer should always try to arouse the person before beginning CPR. If the victim responds, CPR is not necessary. To determine whether the victim can be aroused, the rescuer should shake and/or shout at the person. While the rescuer is doing this, he or she can also call for assistance and place the person in a supine position, best suited for the performance of CPR.

Open the Airway

Once the rescuer has determined the need for CPR, the next step is to make sure nothing is obstructing the victim's airway. The tongue is the most common obstacle in an unconscious person. To remove this obstruction, one needs to pull the mandible, or jaw bone, forward. Since the tongue is attached to this bone, pulling the jaw also pulls the tongue forward and opens the airway. Either of two methods, the head tilt or the chin pull, can be used to accomplish this. In the head tilt, one hand is placed on the forehead and the other under the neck; the head is gently extended (Figure D.1). In most instances, the tongue will then swing free, and the airway will open. If, however, the victim is quite floppy, this method may not work. In that case, the chin pull is performed by placing the tips of the fingers under the jaw bone and jutting the chin forward (see Figure D.1). Again, the tongue is pulled away from the back of the throat, and the airway is opened (Morikawa, Safer, & De Carlo, 1961).

Check for Breathing and a Pulse

After the airway is opened, the rescuer should establish whether or not the victim is breathing and has a pulse. To check for breathing, the rescuer places his or her ear near the victim's mouth and watches the victim's chest to see if it rises and falls while he or she also listens for air escaping from the mouth and nose. The rescuer may feel the victim's moist breath on his or her cheek. If the person is not breathing, artificial ventilation must be started at once.

At the same time that the rescuer is determining whether or not the person is breathing, he or she should also check to see if the victim has a pulse. To do this, the rescuer slides his or her fingers down beside the thyroid cartilage (part of the windpipe) and feels for the pulse over the **carotid artery** (Figure D.2). This is the easiest place in which to feel the pulse, and its central location gives some indication of the blood flow to the brain. In an infant, feeling for the pulse in the **brachial artery**, located in the middle of the forearm, is simpler than feeling for a pulse in a baby's chubby neck (see Figure D.2). If no pulse is evident, closed-chest compression as well as artificial ventilation must begin immediately. While artificial ventilation can be done by itself, chest compression must always be accompanied by artificial ventilation.

Artificial Ventilation

Artificial ventilation involves a number of steps. First, an airtight seal is formed over the victim's mouth and nose. To accomplish this, the rescuer places his or her open mouth over the victim's mouth and, at the

433

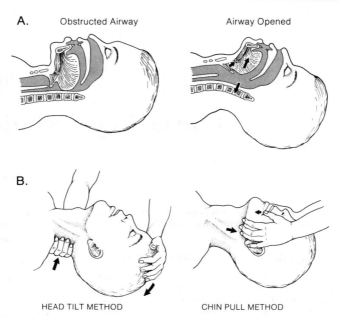

Figure D.1.   The airway. A) Obstructed airway must be opened by pulling the tongue away from the back of the throat. B) Either the head tilt or the chin pull will accomplish this.

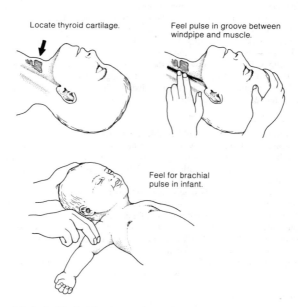

Figure D.2.   Pulse. Method of feeling for the carotid pulse in the adult and the brachial pulse in the child.

same time, pinches the victim's nose closed. While doing this, the rescuer must remember to continue holding the head in a tilted position to ensure an open airway (Figure D.3).

For an infant or small child, the rescuer's mouth usually can cover both the child's mouth and nose. If both of these openings are not covered, the air blown into the mouth will simply come out the nose instead of going into the victim's lungs (see Figure D.3). The infant's back should be supported (lying down) with the flat of the rescuer's hand.

Once an airtight seal is formed, four quick breaths are given to expand and oxygenate the lungs. To make sure this is successful, two indications should be checked: 1) the victim's chest rises and falls with each breath; and 2) the rescuer can hear and feel air escaping when he or she removes his or her mouth. If these signs are not present, the airway is probably obstructed. When the airway seems blocked, the rescuer must first make sure the chin is jutting forward to keep the airway clear. Then he or she should feel in the mouth for the presence of a foreign object. After these steps, if there is still an obstruction, the rescuer should turn the victim on the side and clap the victim on the back vigorously with the flat of the hand. If this does not remove the obstruction, the rescuer should perform the manual thrust, or Heimlich maneuver, discussed later in this appendix.

When the rescuer is sure no obstruction exists, he or she should continue artificial ventilation. In the adult, breathing is done 12 times a minute or once every 5 seconds. In a child 1 to 8 years old, breathing is done 15 times a minute, and, in the infant, it is done 20 times a minute (see Figure D.3).

Similar to the change in number of breaths per minute, the volume of breath depends on the age of the victim. For an adult, the rescuer should exhale one full breath. This provides about one pint of air that contains 18% oxygen, slightly less than the 21% oxygen in the air we normally breathe. This oxygen content easily meets the needs of the brain and the body. For an infant, a cheekful of air is sufficient. A child needs half a breath.

Artificial Circulation: Closed-Chest Compression

In the same way that artificial ventilation simulates normal breathing, cardiac massage, or closed-chest compression, imitates the normal heartbeat. As already mentioned, artificial ventilation *must* be done in conjunction with closed-chest compression. Also, it is best if two people are involved in the resuscitation—one to do the ventilation and one to do the caridac massage.

In closed-chest compression, the lower half of the **sternum**, or breast bone, is rhythmically compressed at a rate of 60 times a minute in the adult. This increases the average systolic blood pressure to about half the normal level (40 instead of 80–100), and the rate of flow of blood to about one-third of normal (Mackenzie, Taylor, McDonald, et al., 1964). While this does not completely substitute for the heart's actions, this amount of increase is adequate to keep the brain and body functioning until the victim can receive more sophisticated care.

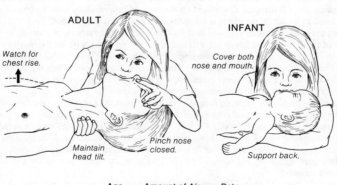

Age	Amount of Air	Rate
Adult	full breath	12/min
Child	½ breath	15/min
Infant	cheekful	20/min

Figure D.3.   Artificial ventilation.

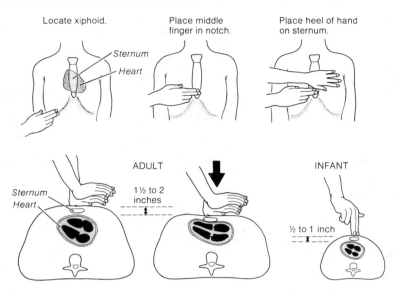

Figure D.4.   Closed-chest, or cardiac, compression. Note the different placement of the hands and the depth of compression in adults and infants.

To perform closed-chest compression, the first step is to locate the heart, which lies slightly to the left of the mid-chest region, between the sternum and the spine (Figure D.4). The rescuer's hands are first placed on the abdomen and then moved up in the midline until they reach the notch at the bottom of the rib cage. Located here is a flexible piece of cartilage called the *xiphoid process*. Two finger breadths above this notch is where the bottom of one hand should touch, placed heel down on the sternum. The second hand rests on top of the first with the fingers interlocked or near each other (see Figure D.4). It is important that only the heel of the hand touch the chest, not the fingers. Otherwise, one or more ribs might be fractured.

Once the hands are in place, the rescuer is ready to perform the compression. To do this, the rescuer should kneel alongside the victim and lean over the victim with his or her arms extended so that the elbows lock and the entire force is directed downward on the heart. Compressions must be smooth, rhythmical, regular, and deep. In an adult, the chest is compressed 1½ to 2 inches (Taylor, Tucker, Greene, et al., 1977), 60 times a minute. Each compression lasts half a second, and the release of pressure continues for an equal amount of time. When the hands are relaxed, they should remain on the sternum to maintain the correct position. To keep count, the rescuer doing the cardiac compressions should count, "One and two and three and four and five." On the count of five, the second rescuer breathes into the victim's mouth just as the first rescuer is releasing the chest compression (Figure D.5). The rhythm of the two procedures is maintained without stopping until the victim is either resuscitated or declared dead.

For an infant or child, the procedure is modified. Since the child's heart is smaller and situated higher in the body, the placement of the hand is different. For an infant, only two fingers are used to compress the chest rather than two hands (see Figure D.4). With the fingers placed on the sternum at the level of the nipples, compressions are ½ to 1 inch in depth, and the rate of compression is 100 times per minute. The count also changes and is one-two-three-four-five-breathe. For a child 1 to 8 years old, the heel of one hand is used and placement is midway between the nipples and xiphoid. Compressions are 1 to 1½ inches and the rate is 80 per minute.

On infants and young children, CPR can be performed by a single rescuer. However, this procedure is quite difficult for one person to do alone on an adult for a prolonged period of time. If only one rescuer is available, a series of 15 chest compressions is done followed by 2 quick breaths, and the rate of compression increases to 80 a minute.

With 2 rescuers available, the ratio of chest compressions to breaths is 5 to 1. Also, when two rescuers are available, it is advisable to take turns doing the ventilation and the compression. The chest compressions are especially exhausting work and may be needed for some time before help arrives. When

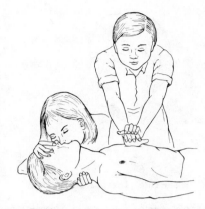

	Position of Hand	Compression	Rate	Ratio
Adult	heel	1½ to 2"	60/min	5:1
Child	heel	1 to 1½"	80/min	5:1
Infant	tips of index and middle fingers	½ to 1"	100/min	5:1

Figure D.5.   Cardiopulmonary resuscitation with two rescuers. For purposes of illustration, both rescuers are placed on the same side. In practice, the rescuers would be on opposite sides.

changing positions, the following procedure is used: The rescuers kneel on opposite sides of the victim so as not to interfere with each other's movements. The leader is always the one doing the cardiac massage. The count remains, "One and two and three and four and five." After the count of five, the rescuer doing the ventilations breathes into the victim's mouth. When it is time to switch, they change positions on the count of three. The person previously doing the artificial ventilation completes the last two chest compressions, and the rescuer formerly doing the compressions breathes into the victim's mouth after the count of five.

When Is CPR Stopped?

Ideally, CPR is continued until the victim starts breathing on his or her own and has a strong pulse. This may happen within minutes, or it may take hours. So long as the person continues to have adequate ventilation and circulation from CPR, he or she should not suffer further brain damage.

COMPLICATIONS OF CPR

Performing CPR is not without risks. If the rescuer's fingers are pressed against the chest wall, especially on a child, they might fracture some ribs. Also, if the hands are placed too low on the chest, they may injure the abdominal organs. With artificial ventilation, the extension of the neck of a victim of a car accident may worsen a spinal injury. Finally, trying to flatten a swollen stomach manually may induce vomiting and lead to aspiration pneumonia.

Thus, while CPR is a lifesaving technique, it must only be undertaken by a person who is adequately trained. Many schools and hospitals offer free minicourses in CPR. If someone who is attempting CPR does somehow injure the victim, he or she is protected in a number of states by what are called Good Samaritan laws. These laws prevent a victim (or his or her family) from suing someone who tried to administer lifesaving techniques.

THE MANUAL THRUST, OR HEIMLICH MANEUVER

Obstructed breathing may occur as part of a cardiac arrest. However, more often it happens to a person who has choked on a foreign object. The rapid use of the manual thrust, or Heimlich maneuver, to remove the obstacle has proved lifesaving in many of these instances.

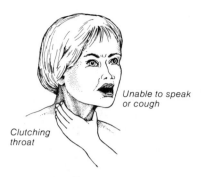

Unable to speak or cough

Clutching throat

Figure D.6. Universal choking sign.

The classic example of this situation is the "café coronary." In these cases, while eating meat or other bulky foods at a restaurant, an adult suddenly stands up, holds his or her fingers against the voice box, and gasps for breath (Figure D.6). The victim is often unable to make any sound. Respiratory difficulty increases and the lips turn blue. If the victim is not helped immediately, he or she will soon lose consciousness and stop breathing. Cardiac arrest will follow moments later, and the victim will die. Children, too, may experience life-threatening choking. While the objects swallowed by children are often different from the items on which adults usually choke, the symptoms remain the same. The procedure for helping them, the manual thrust, is also the same.

The only instance in which the manual thrust should not be used is when an obstruction is caused by an infection. For example, a child with severe croup may gradually develop an obstructed airway. Since the obstruction is due to swelling, not a lodging of a foreign object, manual thrusts will not help. However, because the obstruction develops more slowly with infection, a parent usually has time to get the child to a hospital where he or she can receive medical attention.

To clear a foreign object from a person's airway, a series of four back blows are first given. If this is not successful, the manual thrust is used. This procedure abruptly increases the pressure within the abdomen or chest and forces the foreign body to pop out like a cork from a champagne bottle. Four thrusts normally suffice.

The manual thrust is done either in a standing or in a lying position (Ruben & MacNaughton, 1978). In the standing position, the rescuer places him- or herself behind the victim. The rescuer wraps his or her arms around the victim's abdomen, midway between the bottom of the rib cage and the hips (Figure D.7). The other hand covers the fist. With a sudden thrust, the fist is brought inward and up, pressing against the victim's abdomen. This is repeated until the object is expelled.

For an unconscious victim, the lying-down position is used. The victim rests supine, and the rescuer straddles the victim's hips. The heel of one hand is placed against the victim's abdomen midway between the hips and the rib cage. The second hand rests on top of the first, and thrusting motions identical to those used in the standing position are administered until the obstruction is dislodged. A similar method may be used on the chest by placing the hands just above the notch of the sternum and pushing inward and up. This method is preferable for children, in whom a sudden change in abdominal pressure may injure internal body organs.

When a person is alone and begins choking, he or she may perform this maneuver by suddenly pushing his or her abdomen against the back of a chair. This will often increase the pressure within the abdomen sufficiently to dislodge the object.

CONCLUSION

CPR, when done appropriately, is a safe and effective procedure for treating respiratory and cardiac arrest. Manual thrust is equally useful for treating choking victims. Remember, however, that training is required to perform cardiopulmonary resuscitation correctly. With increased public training and awareness, more people can effectively use these methods.

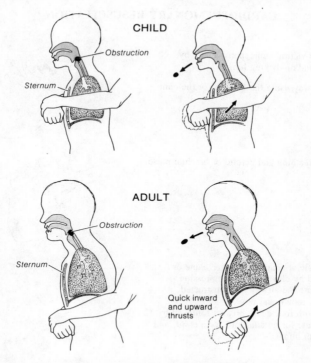

Figure D.7. Manual thrust, or Heimlich maneuver.

REFERENCES

American Heart Association (1980). Standards and guidelines for cardiopulmonary resuscitation and emergency cardiac care. *Journal of the American Medical Association, 244,* 453–494.

Black, P.M. (1978). Brain death. *New England Journal of Medicine, 299,* 338–344.

Copley, D.P., Mantle, J.A., Rogers, W.J., et al. (1977). Improved outcome for prehospital cardiopulmonary collapse with resuscitation by bystanders. *Circulation, 56,* 901–905.

Heimlich, H.J. (1975). A lifesaving maneuver to prevent food choking. *Journal of the American Medical Association, 234,* 398–401.

Lund, I., & Skulberg, A. (1976). Cardiopulmonary resuscitation by lay people. *Lancet, 2,* 702–704.

Mackenzie, G.J., Taylor, S.H., McDonald, A.H., et al. (1964). Hemodynamic effects of external cardiac compression. *Lancet, 1,* 1342–1349.

Morikawa, S., Safer, P., & De Carlo, J. (1961). Influence of the head-jaw position upon upper airway patency. *Anesthesiology, 22,* 265–270.

Ruben, H., & MacNaughton, F.I. (1978). The treatment of food choking. *Practitioner, 221,* 725–729.

Taylor, G.J., Tucker, W.M., Greene, H.L., et al. (1977). Importance of prolonged compression during cardiopulmonary resuscitation in man. *New England Journal of Medicine, 296,* 1515–1517.

CARDIOPULMONARY RESUSCITATION

1. Establish the victim's unresponsiveness by shouting at and/or shaking him.

2. Open the airway using the head tilt or the chin pull.

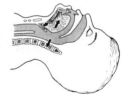

3. Check for breathing and carotid or brachial pulse.

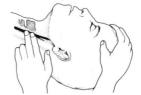

4. Perform artificial ventilation either alone or accompanied by closed-chest compression.
   a. Make sure the airway is unobstructed.
   b. Seal the mouth and nose.
   c. Begin with four quick breaths followed by 12 per minute for an adult, 15 for a child, and 20 for an infant.

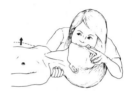

5. When performing closed-chest compression, always also administer artificial ventilation.
   a. Correctly place hands.
   b. Press down 1½ to 2 inches in an adult, 1 to 1½ inches in a child, and ½ to 1 inch in an infant.
   c. Maintain smooth, deep, rhythmical compressions.
   d. Repeat 60 times a minute in an adult (80 if there is only one rescuer), 80 times a minute in a child, and 100 times a minute in an infant.
   e. Maintain the ratio of 5 compressions to 1 breath except when only one rescuer is available. Then, the ratio is 15 to 2.

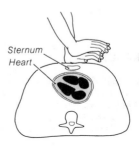

Sternum
Heart

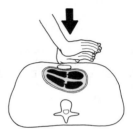

THE MANUAL THRUST, OR HEIMLICH MANEUVER

1. Try a series of four back blows.

2. If these are unsuccessful in removing the obstruction, either have the victim lie down or stand behind him.

3. Place a fisted hand between the rib cage and hips.

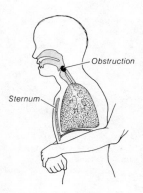

4. Do four thrusts pressing inward and up.

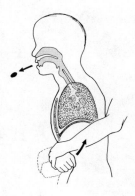

Index

187, 239–240
social-adaptive skills development, 186
visual skills development, 208–209
growth during
of brain, 110, 154–155
height, 110, 126, 167
weight, 110, 127
hyperactivity during, see Hyperactivity
and nutrition, 109–128
effects of malnutrition, 110–111
seizures during, 328–330
Chisholm, Julian, 120
Chloralhydrate, 146
Chloride, in body, 119
effects of imbalance in, 119
Chlorpromazine, see Thorazine
Choking, lifesaving technique for, 437–438
Choreoathetoid cerebral palsy, see Choreoathetosis
Choreoathetosis, 160, 302, 309, 312, 316, 319,
399
Chorionic gonadotrophin, 39, 399
Chorionic villus biopsy, 29–30
benefits of, 29
description of procedure, 29
risks associated with, 30
Chorioretinitis, 200, 399
Choroid, 200, 201, 205, 206, 213, 399
Choroid plexus, 162, 163, 399
Chromatid, 3, 399
Chromosomal abnormalities and malformations,
18, 20, 42, 81, 300
causes of, 18, 42
general characteristics of, 42
incidence of, 42
number of stillbirths, 60
prenatal diagnosis of, 25–27, 29–32, 50,
365–368
see also Deletion; Nondisjunction; Translocation
Chromosomes, 1–2
karyotyping of, 4, 8
see also Genes
Chronic alcoholics, incidence of malformed children among, 47–48
Chronic illness
learning problems associated with, 285
maternal, effect on labor and delivery, 57
Chronic sorrow, 353
Cilia, 39, 399
Cimetidine, see Tagamet
Circulatory system, changes in, at birth, 71–73,
90–91
Clancy Scale of Autistic Features, 254
Classrooms, see Educational methods and settings
Cleft lip and palate
causes of, 11, 21, 43, 139

dental problems associated with, 139
exact time of occurrence, 41
hearing loss associated with, 139, 227
in infants of epileptic mothers taking Dilantin,
46
and nutrition in infants, 139
and problems of voice production, 139, 244
Clinical Linguistic and Auditory Milestones
Scale (CLAMS), 245
Clonazepam, see Clonopin
Clonopin, in treatment of epilepsy, 333, 339,
340, 341
side effects of, 341
Clonus, 160, 237, 304, 399
Closed-chest compression, 435–437
see also Cardiopulmonary resuscitation
Club foot, 50, 51, 169, 180
CMV infection, see Cytomegalovirus
Cobalt treatment, of pregnant women with can-
cer, 399
associated with birth defects, 44
Cochlea, 224, 225, 226, 399
Code of Federal Regulations, 384, 385
Cognitive skills development, see Intellectual
development
Cognitive tests, for children, 286–287
Colase, 135
Collagen, formation of, 115
Coloboma, 200
Colon, 130, 131
Color blindness, 17, 205
Color-coding method, in treatment of learning
disabilities, 292
Communication
alternative methods of, 234, 239–240, 255
oral-only versus manual-only, 234
role of temporal lobe in, 156, 241–242
skill development, 183–184, 185–186,
239–240
see also Language
Communication boards, 247, 255
Communication disorders, 243, 244–245
see also Language disorders
Complement system, 74, 75
Computer programs, for use with learning dis-
abilities
Bank Street Writer, 294
BASIC, 294
Logo, 294
Mastertype, 294
Superpilot, 294
Computerized brain scan
to diagnose epilepsy, 336, 337
to diagnose intraventricular hemorrhage, 77
Computers, for handicapped children, 216, 247,
294, 317–319
Concrete operations, Piagetian stage of intellec-
tual development, 187–188

Movement—*continued*
177–179, 301–303, 304–308
and the neuromuscular junction, 175–177
role of brain in, 155, 157, 158, 179, 301, 302, 303
role of peripheral nervous system in, 175, 177
types of, 174–175, 176
see also Muscles; Primitive reflexes
Mucopolysaccharide disorders, 139, 402
Mucous secretions, as defense mechanism against infections, 75
Multiple sclerosis, 402
and hearing loss, 233
Muscle fiber, 174, 175, 176
effect of Valium on, 314
Muscles, 39, 41, 172, 174, 175
agonists and antagonists, 177
and movement
diseases and disorders affecting, 155, 160, 177–179, 180, 301–303, 304–308
maintenance of normal tone, 160
and the neuromuscular junction, 175–177
and primitive reflexes, 88, 304–307
role of brain in, 155, 158, 179, 301
role of peripheral nervous system in, 160
Muscular dystrophy, 17, 178–179
see also Duchenne muscular dystrophy
Musculoskeletal system, 167–180
bones, 167–172
diseases and disorders of, 60, 105, 155, 160, 170, 171, 177–179, 180, 301–303, 304–308
joints, 172–174
ligaments and tendons, 174
muscles, 175–177
Mutations, 13, 402
causes of, 13
heritability of, 13
single-gene, 13–18
see also Inborn errors of metabolism; Malformations
Myasthenia gravis, 178
characteristics of, 178
treatment for, 178
Myelin, 152, 159
Myelination, 152, 182, 402
Myoclonic seizures, 333, 402
control of, 341
Myopia, 201, 202, 203
Myosin, 175, 402
Myringotomy, 227, 232, 402
Mysoline, in treatment of epilepsy, 46–47, 339, 340, 341, 342
side effects of, 341

Naloxone, 194
Naltrexone, 194
Narcolepsy, 270

Nasogastric tube feeding, 135, 402
National Commission for the Protection of Human Subjects, 373
National organizations, serving handicapped children and their families, 415–425
Nearsightedness, *see* Myopia
Negative reinforcement, 268
Neonatal period, 69–81
causes of illness and death during, 73–81
congenital defects, 81
hypoglycemia, 80
infections, 58, 74–76, 30
intracranial hemorrhage, 76–78
jaundice, 78–80
incidence of serious illness during, 73
mortality rate during, 73, 74
physiological changes at birth, 71–73, 89
primitive reflexes during, 304–307
seizures during, 327–330
survival rate during, 81, 94
and weight gain, 110
Neostigmine, 178
Nerve cells, *see* Neurons
Nervous system, *see* Autonomic nervous system; Central nervous system; Peripheral nervous system
Nervous system disorders, 13, 206, 254
see also Tay-Sachs disease
Neural fold, 150
Neural plate, 150
Neural tube, 40, 150, 402
improper closure of, 43
Neuroectoderm, 200, 202, 402
Neurofibromatosis
characteristics of, 411
incidence of, 411
Neuromuscular diseases, 177–179
see also Cerebral palsy
Neuromuscular junction, 175
diseases of, 178
Neurons
arrangement of, in brain and spinal cord, 151–153
depolarization of, 327, 338
description of, 2, 150–151
effect of seizures on, 325–326, 328
limited recovery of, after injury, 2
and message transmission, 153
Neuropsychological approach, in treatment of learning disabilities, 292
Neurosurgery
in treatment of cerebral palsy, 316–317
in treatment of dystonia musculorum deformans, 179
in treatment of epilepsy, 342
Neurotransmitters, 153, 178, 402
Newborn screening programs
to detect inborn errors of metabolism, 100
hypothyroidism, 103

Parents—*continued*
  as advocates, 392
  counseling and support for, 256, 273, 311, 359–360, 415–432
  effects of disability on, 352–355
  identifying developmental delay in child, 191–192
  role of, in care, 215–216, 264, 271, 285–286, 310, 311, 359, 360
  see also Families, of handicapped children
  mentally retarded persons as, 374
Parietal lobe, 154, 282
  description of, 155, 156
  function of, 156, 295
Parkinson's disease, 403
  effects of, 157, 403
  treatment of, 179
Partial seizures, 333–336
  complex, 331–336
    control of, with anticonvulsants, 340, 341
    control of, with surgery, 342
  simple, 333
Patent ductus arteriosus, in premature infants, 90–91, 319
Pathological fractures, 171
Patterning
  in treatment of cerebral palsy, 311
  in treatment of visual-perceptual deficits, 290
Pauling, Linus, 117
Pavlik harness, 169, 403
Peabody Picture Vocabulary Test (PPVT), 246
Pemoline, in treatment of ADD-H, 269, 272–273
Penicillamine, 120, 403
PEP, *see* Positive end expiratory pressure
Perceptual deficits, *see* Visual-perceptual deficits
Periactin, as appetite stimulant, 134
Perilymph, 224, 225
Perinatal deaths, causes of, 56, 60–61, 103, 105, 110, 123
Periodontal disease, 140, 142–143, 403
  causes of, 142
  in children with handicaps, 142, 143, 145
  and use of Dilantin, 143
  treatment of, 142, 143
Periosteum, 168, 403
Peripheral nervous system, 149, 158, 160, 164, 175, 403
  description of, 160
  diseases of, 177–178, 180
  effects of damage to, 160, 177
  function of, 160
Petit mal seizures, 327, 330, 332
  control of, 341, 343
  EEG pattern in, 332
Phagocytes, 74, 403
Phalanges, 167, 403
Pharyngeal arches, 40, 139

see also Cleft lip and palate
Pharynx, 129, 130, 403
Phenobarbital
  side effects of, 117, 329, 341
    hyperactivity, 265
    teratogenic effects in mother on fetus, 46
  in treatment of epilepsy, 338, 339, 340–341
    as prophylactic, 329
  in treatment of febrile convulsions, 329, 345
Phenothiazines, 194, 403
  side effects of, 273
  in treatment of ADD-H, 269, 273
  in treatment of hyperactive children with mental retardation, 273
Phenylalanine, 42, 100, 101
Phenylalanine hydroxylase, 100
Phenylketonuria (PKU), 99, 100, 253, 403
  cause of, 11, 42, 100, 411
  characteristics of, 100, 411
  diagnosis of, 30
    newborn screening, 100, 362, 411
  incidence of, 100, 411
  infantile spasms in, 333
  treatment of, 42, 101–102, 411
Phenytoin, *see* Dilantin
Phocomelia, 45, 403
  cause of, 11, 45
Phoneme, 240, 403
Phosphorus, in body, 119
  effects of deficiencies in, 119
  sources of, 119
Physical activity, in treatment of cerebral palsy, 311–312
Physical therapy, in treatment of cerebral palsy, 311
Pia mater, 76, 159
Piagetian theory of intellectual development, 186–188
  stages of
    concrete operations, 186, 187–188
    formal operations, 186, 188
    preoperational, 186, 187
    sensorimotor, 186, 187
Pica, 120, 403
  behavior modification to decrease, 120
Pincer grasp, development of, 185
Pivot joint, 173, 174
PKU, *see* Phenylketonuria
Placenta, 403
  fetal contraction of infection through, 75
  formation of, 40
  function of, 41, 48, 71, 72
  position of
    abruptio, 59, 63, 300, 397
    identifying by ultrasound, 62–63
    previa, 57, 58, 63, 65, 403
Placenta previa, 56, 57, 58–59, 63, 65, 403
  cause of, 58–59

Visual impairment—*continued*
color blindness, 17, 205
hypermetropia, 201, 202
myopia, 201, 202
night blindness, 115, 205–206
presbyopia, 203, 403
refractive errors, 210–211
retinitis pigmentosa, 206, 411
retinoblastoma, 214, 404
retrolental fibroplasia (retinopathy of prematurity), 201, 89–90, 212, 213, 217,
218
strabismus, 158, 206, 207, 208, 309, 404
upward gaze paralysis, 79, 309
see also Blindness
Visual pathway, 206, 207
Visual-perceptual deficits
diagnosis, 283 284–285, 287
tests for, 288
disabilities with which associated
ADD, 263
cerebral palsy, 309
mental retardation, 254
treatment of, 290-291
Visual-perceptual tests, for children, 288
Visual sequential memory, 288, 405
Vitamins, 130
nutritional role of, 114–118
Vitamin A
effects of deficiencies in, 205–206
effects of megadoses of, 115, 123
nutritional role of, 115
recommended daily allowance, 116
sources of, 115
Vitamin B complex
nutritional role of, 115
recommended daily allowances, 116
sources of, 115
Vitamin B$_1$, *see* Thiamine
Vitamin B$_2$, *see* Riboflavin
Vitamin B$_6$, *see* Pyridoxine
Vitamin B$_{12}$, *see* Cyanocobalamin
Vitamin C
megadoses of, 117
nutritional role of, 115
recommended daily allowance, 116
sources of, 117
Vitamin D, 115, 171
effects of megadoses of, 123
nutritional role of, 117
potential deficiencies of, in vegetarianism,
122
recommended daily allowance, 116
sources of, 117
Vitamin E, 117
Vitamin K, 117–118
Vitreous humor, 200, 201, 202, 203, 213, 405
Vocational education and training, of individuals
with handicaps, 382–383

Vocational rehabilitation, of individuals with
handicaps, 383
Voice production, problems of, 243
incidence of, 243
Voluntary movement
diseases and disorders affecting, 155, 160,
177–179, 180, 301–303, 304–308
and integration of primitive reflexes, 304
see also Primitive reflexes
role of brain in, 155, 157, 158, 179, 301
role of peripheral nervous system in, 160
see also Movement; Muscles
Von Recklinghausen's disease, *see* Neurofibromatosis

Walking, 308
ataxic, 158
development of, 185
impairments of
from cerebral palsy, 308, 309
from club foot, 169
from dystonia musculorum deformans, 179
from muscular dystrophy, 178
Water, in body, 118–119
Wechsler Intelligence Scale for Children–
Revised (WISC-R), 190–191, 214,
286–287, 295
subtests of, 190–191, 286–287
test scores of children with ADD-H, 262, 264
testing age range, 190
type of score attained, 190–191
Wechsler Preschool and Primary Scale of Intelligence, (WPPSI), 246, 286
Weight, and growth during childhood, 110
charts of
for boys and girls, 127
for newborns, by gestational age, 86
Wepman Auditory Discrimination Test, 246,
288
Werdnig-Hoffmann Syndrome, 177, 405
characteristics of, 413
treatment of, 413
Wernicke's area, 156
and the control of receptive language, 241
effect of damage to, 245
Wheelchairs, *see* Chairs
White matter
in brain, 152, 155
in spinal cord, 159
Wide Range Achievement Tests (WRAT), 288
WISC-R, *see* Wechsler Intelligence Scale for
Children–Revised
Woodcock-Johnson Psychoeducational Battery,
288
Word Recognition Test, 289
WRAT battery, *see* Wide Range Achievement
Tests

About the Authors

Mark Levitt Batshaw, M.D., is Associate Professor of Pediatrics at The Johns Hopkins University School of Medicine, and Developmental Pediatrician at The Kennedy Institute for Handicapped Children. Associated with The Johns Hopkins Medical Institutions since 1973, Dr. Batshaw has had extensive experience in treating children with developmental disabilities, and has followed the development of more than 200 children with multiple handicaps over a 10-year period.

Dr. Batshaw is recognized as an authority on inborn errors of metabolism. In recent years, he has had more than 40 papers published in this field, including articles in such highly respected journals as *The New England Journal of Medicine, Pediatrics, Lancet, Clinical Genetics, Science,* and *Journal of Pediatrics.* The recipient of major grants from the National Foundation March of Dimes and the National Institutes of Health, Dr. Batshaw is currently conducting research involving neurochemicals and the metabolism of ammonia and genetic disorders that lead to a buildup of this toxic substance with subsequent development of mental retardation.

Among his varied professional activities, Dr. Batshaw has been an invited speaker on numerous occasions before professional societies. Dr. Batshaw is a Fellow of the American Academy of Pediatrics and the Royal College of Physicians and Surgeons, as well as a member of the Society for Pediatric Research, the Society for Inherited Metabolic Disorders, and the Society for Developmental Pediatrics.

Yvonne M. Perret, M.S.W., is an inpatient psychiatric social worker, Walter P. Carter Center, State Mental Health and Mental Retardation Center, Baltimore, Maryland. Previously, she was a developmental research associate at The Kennedy Institute for Handicapped Children, where she coordinated a research project on premature infants. She has been involved with social work and family studies since 1968.

Before joining The Kennedy Institute, she served as staff director for the Project on Women in Midlife Development at Cornell University. During this time, Ms. Perret also served as developmental editor for *Human Development,* by Karen Freiberg (Duxbury Press, 1979). Earlier casework and medical social work positions involved work in counseling and a variety of public welfare related issues such as child abuse and adoptions. She has counseled chronically ill persons and their families, as well as parents and adolescents. In addition, she has been involved in foster care and has worked with single parents.

Besides her social work experience, Ms. Perret has a master's degree in journalism from the Newhouse School at Syracuse University. She has several years' experience as a writer and editor, and has published articles on law, the environment, health care, and social work.